Interleukin Protocols

METHODS IN MOLECULAR MEDICINE™

John M. Walker, SERIES EDITOR

METHODS IN MOLECULAR MEDICINE™

Interleukin Protocols

Edited by

Luke A. J. O'Neill

*Department of Biochemistry and Biotechnology Institute,
Trinity College, Dublin, Ireland*

and

Andrew Bowie

*Department of Pharmacology, Conway Institute of Biomolecular
and Biomedical Research, University College Dublin, Dublin, Ireland*

Humana Press ✳ Totowa, New Jersey

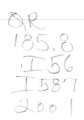

© 2001 Humana Press Inc.
999 Riverview Drive, Suite 208
Totowa, New Jersey 07512

The content and opinions expressed in this book are the sole work of the authors and editors, who have warranted due diligence in the creation and issuance of their work. The publisher, editors, and authors are not responsible for errors or omissions or for any consequences arising from the information or opinions presented in this book and make no warranty, express or implied, with respect to its contents.

This publication is printed on acid-free paper. ∞
ANSI Z39.48-1984 (American Standards Institute) Permanence of Paper for Printed Library Materials.

Production Editor: Jessica Jannicelli
Cover design by Patricia Cleary.

For additional copies, pricing for bulk purchases, and/or information about other Humana titles, contact Humana at the above address or at any of the following numbers: Tel.: 973-256-1699; Fax: 973-256-8341; E-mail: humana@humanapr.com; Website: http://humanapress.com

Photocopy Authorization Policy:

Printed in the United States of America. 10 9 8 7 6 5 4 3 2 1

Library of Congress Cataloging in Publication Data

Interleukin protocols / edited by Luke A. J. O'Neill and Andrew Bowie.
        p. cm. -- (Methods in molecular medicine ; 60)
     Includes bibliographical references and index.
     ISBN 0-89603-738-X (alk. paper)
     1. Interleukins--Laboratory manuals. I. O'Neill, Luke A. J. II. Bowie, Andrew. III.
Series.

     QR185.8.I56 I587 2001
     616.07'9--dc21

                                                                          2001016960

Preface

Interleukins are a family of proteins that regulate the maturation, differentiation, or activation of cells involved in immunity and inflammation, and belong to a broader family termed cytokines. Collectively these proteins are the key orchestrators of host defense and the response to tissue injury. There are currently 23 different interleukins (numbered from IL-1 to IL-23), although the full extent of the interleukin family will only become clear upon analysis of the human genome sequence. Most important, interleukins are central to the pathogenesis of a wide range of diseases that involve an immune component, including such conditions as rheumatoid arthritis, multiple sclerosis, ulcerative colitis, psoriasis, and asthma. Interleukins have also been implicated in other conditions, including cancer, migraine, myocardial infarction, and depression.

In essence, when cells are activated by interleukins, a program of gene expression is initiated in the target cell that alters the cell's phenotype, leading to enhanced immune reactivity, inflammation, and/or proliferation. Interleukins are therefore at the core of the cellular basis for many diseases. They are the subject of intense investigation by biomedical researchers and the targeting or use of interleukins in the clinic is proceeding apace. Approaches such as targeting IL-4 in asthma or IL-1 in joint disease are being pursued, and it is likely that in the next 5–10 years a number of new therapies based on either inhibiting or administering interleukins will be available. In addition, the assaying of interleukins has a role in the diagnosis and prognosis of disease, and polymorphisms in interleukin genes may well be found to predispose individuals to disease.

The basis for these many advances in interleukin research lies in the use of a range of methodologies for their study. In *Interleukin Protocols* we have brought together a critical mass of chapters covering the major techniques currently available to researchers in this area. The book is divided into five sections. Parts I and II concern a range of methods for assaying interleukin protein and mRNA. The ELISA is the mainstay of assaying interleukin protein production and the chapters here cover the basic methodologies, where to purchase reagents and also recent developments in the use of ELISA. The use of FACS as a method of assaying interleukins intracellularly has been an important advance and is also covered. The ability to measure interleukin mRNA is another important technique in interleukin research and several chapters describe quantitative methods that mainly rely on RT-PCR and RNAse protection. Part II gives examples of how to measure specific interleukins in order to illustrate the approaches that can be used for investigators interested in a particular interleukin.

Part III covers the assays of interleukins in specific pathologies, including breast cancer, depression, psoriasis, Grave's disease, migraine, and myocardial infarction. Part IV is related to Part III in that it also concerns pathologies, but has as its focus the assaying of interleukins in different biological fluids relevant to disease. These include peritoneal fluids, sputum from asthma patients, synovial fluid from arthritic joints, and cerebrospinal fluid from patients with meningitis. More important, this section covers the difficulties associated with the measuring of interleukins in such fluids. Finally, Part V concerns newer methods in the study of interleukin signal transduction, analysis of polymorphisms in interleukin genes, and the use of cDNA arrays, areas that will surely expand greatly in the next years as the feasibility of assaying the consequences of interleukin action in disease becomes more apparent.

Interleukin Protocols will therefore be of interest to a wide range of investigators, from molecular and cell biologists to immunologists to clinical investigators. The discovery of interleukins and the analysis of their role in disease represent major advances in molecular medicine. The methods described will help researchers continue to advance, ultimately leading to better diagnosis, prognosis, and treatment of many diseases where there remains an unmet medical need.

Luke A. J. O'Neill
Andrew Bowie

Contents

Contents   *ix*

Contributors

JEFFREY K. ACTOR • *Program in Molecular Pathology, University of Texas-Houston Medical School, Houston, TX*

FRANCO AMEGLIO • *Istituto San Gallicano, Polo Oncologico e Dermatologico, Istituti Fisioterapici Ospitalieri, IRCCS, Rome, Italy*

HYMIE ANISMAN • *Institute of Neuroscience, Carleton University; and Department of Psychiatry, Institute of Mental Health Research, Royal Ottawa Hospital, Ontario, Canada*

KHUSRU ASADULLAH • *Experimental Dermatology, Schering, AG, Berlin, Germany*

EMMANUELLE ASTOUL • *Lymphocyte Activation Laboratory, Imperial Cancer Research Fund, London, UK*

VERÓNICA ATHIÉ-MORALES • *Lymphocyte Activation Laboratory, Imperial Cancer Research Fund, London, UK*

MONA BAJAJ-ELLIOTT • *Digestive Diseases Research Centre, St. Bartholomew's and the Royal London School of Medicine and Dentistry, London, UK*

ANTONIA BASSI • *Headache-Unit Internal Medicine, DIMIMP, University of Bari, Bari, Italy*

DAVID BOUCHIER-HAYES • *Department of Surgery, Royal College of Surgeons in Ireland, Beaumont Hospital, Dublin, Ireland*

ANDREW BOWIE • *Department of Pharmacology, Conway Institute of Biomolecular and Biomedical Research, University College Dublin, Dublin, Ireland*

PER BRANDTZAEG • *Laboratory for Immunohistochemistry and Immunopathology, Institute of Pathology, University of Oslo, The National Hospital, Oslo, Norway*

PAUL BRENNAN • *Department of Medicine, University of Wales College of Medicine, Wales, UK*

VINCENZO CENTONZE • *Headache-Unit Internal Medicine, DMIMP, University of Bari, Bari, Italy*

LUCIANO D'AURIA • *Istituto San Gallicano, Polo Oncologico e Dermatologico, Istituti Fisioterapici Ospitalieri, IRCCS, Rome, Italy*

FABRIZIO DE BENEDETTI • *Dipartimento di Scienze Pediatriche, IRCSS Policlinico San Matteo, Universitá degli Studi di Pavia, Pavia, Italy*

xi

JOHN A. DI BATTISTA • *Osteoarthritis Research Unit, Hopital Notre-Dame, Centre Hospitalier de l'Université de Montréal, Montréal, Québec, Canada*

BENJAMIN F. DICKENS • *Immunochemistry Laboratory, George Washington University Medical Center, Washington, D.C.*

WOLF DIETRICH DOECKE • *Department of Medical Immunology, Medical School Charité, Humboldt University Berlin, Berlin, Germany*

AMOS DOUVDEVANI • *Soroka Medical Center and Ben-Gurion University, Beer Sheva, Israel*

ROMAN DZIARSKI • *Northwest Center for Medical Education, Indiana University School of Medicine, Gary, IN*

EMAD M. EL-OMAR • *Department of Medicine and Therapeutics, Aberdeen University, Aberdeen, Scotland, UK*

DIANE ERICKSON • *MJ Research, Waltham, MA*

DEIRDRE FOLEY • *Department of Surgery, Royal College of Surgeons in Ireland, Beaumont Hospital, Dublin, Ireland*

PETER G. GIBSON • *Department of Respiratory and Sleep Medicine, Airways Research Centre, John Hunter Hospital, Australia*

MAREK GLEZERMAN • *Department of Obstetrics and Gynecology, Wolfson Medical Center, Holon and Sackler School of Medicine, Tel Aviv University, Israel*

CATHERINE GREENE • *Respiratory Research Division, Department of Medicine, Royal College of Surgeons in Ireland, Education and Research Centre, Dublin, Ireland*

JENNA GRIFFITHS • *Department of Psychiatry, University of Ottawa, Institute of Mental Health Research, Royal Ottawa Hospital, Ontario, Canada*

ANTJE HAEUSSLER-QUADE • *Department of Dermatology, Medical School Charité, Humboldt University Berlin, Berlin, Germany*

JUDITH HARMEY • *Department of Surgery, Royal College of Surgeons in Ireland, Beaumont Hospital, Dublin, Ireland*

ALMUTH CHRISTINE HAUER • *Department of Pediatrics, University of Graz, Austria*

AMANDA HAVERTY • *Department of Surgery, Royal College of Surgeons in Ireland, Beaumont Hospital, Dublin, Ireland*

SHAWN HAYLEY • *Institute of Neuroscience, Carleton University, Ontario, Canada*

MAHMOUD HULEIHEL • *Department of Microbiology and Immunology, Department of Obstetrics and Gynecology, Soroka Medical Center of Kupat Holim, Faculty of Health Sciences, Ben-Gurion University of the Negev, Beer-Sheva, Israel*

FINN-EIRIK JOHANSEN • *Laboratory for Immunohistochemistry and Immunopathology, Institute of Pathology, University of Oslo, The National Hospital, Oslo, Norway*

JAN KOMOROWSKI • *Institute of Endocrinology, Medical University of Lodz, Lodz, Poland*

GIUSEPPE LACEDRA • *Department of Internal Medicine, Immunology and Infectious Diseases, University of Bari, Bari, Italy*

ELI LEWIS • *Soroka Medical Center and Ben-Gurion University, Beer Sheva, Israel*

MOSHE LIGUMSKY • *Gastroenterology Unit, Division of Medicine, Hadassah Medical Center and Hebrew University, Hadassah Medical School, Jerusalem, Israel*

EITAN LUNENFELD • *Department of Obstetrics and Gynecology and Soroka Medical Center of Kupat Holim, Beer-Sheva, Israel; and Faculty of Health Sciences, Ben-Gurion University of the Negev, Beer-Sheba, Israel*

MARIAROSARIA MARINARO • *Departments of Surgery and Pathology, University of Foggia, Italy*

JOHANNE MARTEL-PELLETIER • *Osteoarthritis Research Unit, Hopital Notre-Dame, Centre Hospitalier de l'Université de Montréal, Montréal, Québec, Canada*

ZUL MERALI • *Department of Psychiatry, Royal Ottawa Hospital, Institute of Mental Health Research; and Department of Cellular and Molecular Medicine, University of Ottawa and School of Psychology, Ontario, Canada*

MARK D. MOODY • *Pierce-Endogen, Inc., Woburn, MA*

PAUL N. MOYNAGH • *Department of Pharmacology, Conway Institute of Biomolecular and Biomedical Research, University College Dublin, Dublin, Ireland*

IRENE MUNNO • *Department of Internal Medicine, Immunology and Infectious Diseases, University of Bari, Bari, Italy*

KEVIN P. MURPHY • *Pierce-Endogen, Inc., Woburn, MA*

HOVAV NECHUSHTAN • *Department of Oncology, Hadassah Medical Center and Hebrew University, Hadassah Medical School, Jerusalem, Israel*

ELLEN M. NILSEN • *Laboratory for Immunohistochemistry and Immunopathology, Institute of Pathology, University of Oslo, The National Hospital, Oslo, Norway*

MIKIO NISHIDA • *Department of Clinical Pharmacy, Meijo University, Nagoya, Japan*

MAURICE O'DONOGHUE • *Department of Microbiology, University College Cork, Cork, Ireland*

YOSHIHIRO OKAMOTO • *Department of Clinical Pharmacy, Faculty of Pharmacy, Meijo University, Nagoya, Japan*

LIAM O'MAHONY • *Department of Microbiology and National Food Biotechnology Centre, University College Cork, Cork, Ireland*

LUKE O'NEILL • *Department of Biochemistry and Biotechnology Institute, Trinity College Dublin, Ireland*

CSABA PAZMANY • *Department of Biology and Biotechnology, Worcester Polytechnic Institute, Worcester, MA*

JEAN-PIERRE PELLETIER • *Osteoarthritis Research Unit, Hopital Notre-Dame, Centre Hospitalier de l'Université de Montréal, Montréal, Québec, Canada*

NIKOLAI PETROVSKY • *NHSC Autoimmunity Research Unit, Canberra Clinical School, University of Sydney, Canberra, Australia*

TERRY M. PHILLIPS • *Ultramicro Analytical Immunochemistry Resource, National Institutes of Health, Bethesda, MD*

RADEK PUDIL • *Department of Medicine, Charles University Faculty of Medicine, Czech Republic*

JUHA PUNNONEN • *Department of Medical Microbiology, University of Turku, Finland and Maxygen, Inc., Redwood City, CA*

REIJO PUNNONEN • *Medical School, Department of Obstetrics and Gynecology, University of Tampere; and Department of Obstetrics and Gynecology, University Hospital of Tampere, Tampere, Finland*

ARUN V. RAVINDRAN • *Department of Psychiatry, University of Ottawa, Institute of Mental Health Research, Royal Ottawa Hospital, Ontario, Canada*

EHUD RAZIN • *Department of Biochemistry, Hebrew University, Hadassah Medical School, Jerusalem, Israel*

JODIE L. SIMPSON • *Department of Respiratory and Sleep Medicine, Airways Research Centre, John Hunter Hospital, Australia*

WOLFRAM STERRY • *Department of Dermatology, Medical School Charité, Humboldt University Berlin, Berlin, Germany*

GINETTE TARDIF • *Osteoarthritis Research Unit, Hopital Notre-Dame, Centre Hospitalier de l'Université de Montréal, Montréal, Québec, Canada*

ARCHANA THAKUR • *Cooperative Research Centre for Eye Research and Technology, University of New South Wales, Sydney, Australia*

SCOTT W. VAN ARSDELL • *Pierce-Endogen, Inc., Woburn, MA*

HANS-DIETER VOLK • *Department of Medical Immunology, Medical School Charité, Humboldt University Berlin, Berlin, Germany*

ZHENG-MING WANG • *Northwest Center for Medical Education, Indiana University School of Medicine, Gary, IN*

STEPHEN G. WARD • *Department of Pharmacy and Pharmacology, Bath University, Claverton Down, Bath, UK*

MICHAL WEILER • *Soroka Medical Center and Ben-Gurion University, Beer Sheva, Israel*

Lᴥᴀɴɴᴇ Wᴇsᴛᴏɴ • *Cellular Tissue Typing, Australian Red Cross Blood Service-New South Wales, Sydney, Australia*
Mᴀʀᴋ D. P. Wɪʟʟᴄᴏx • *Cooperative Research Centre for Eye Research and Technology, University of New South Wales, Sydney, Australia*
Tᴏsʜɪʏᴜᴋɪ Yᴏᴋᴏʏᴀᴍᴀ • *Department of Pediatrics, Okayama Municipal Hospital, Okayama, Japan*

I

General Methods for Assaying Interleukin Protein and mRNA

1

ELISAs and Interleukin Research

Catherine Greene

1. Introduction

1.1. Overview and Application of ELISAs

ELISA (enzyme-linked immunosorbent assay) is a powerful, versatile, precise, and reliable quantitative technique for the measurement of antigens or antibodies in biologic samples. The ELISA technique is a widely used tool in biologic and biomedical research; it has been modified and adapted for multiple applications since its development almost 30 years ago *(1)*. As the most commonly used immunoassay technique, ELISA provides the basis for numerous tests in the study of infectious diseases, epidemiology, endocrinology, and immunology. The development of specific ELISA antibodies and reagents has helped to revolutionize the field of immunology, in particular by providing a simple, rapid, and reproducible method of evaluating the role of immune mediators in disease processes.

ELISA was pioneered by Engall and Perlmann *(2)* and developed by Van Weemen and Schuurs *(3)* in the early 1970s. As the name suggests, ELISA exploits the use of an enzyme attached to one reagent in the test. Addition of a chromogenic, chemiluminescent, or fluorimetric enzyme substrate causes a reaction that can be quantified visually, photometrically, or by fluorimetry. ELISA is a particularly useful technique because of its high sensitivity and precision; it is also practical in that large numbers of samples can be rapidly analyzed. The most commonly used and versatile ELISA is the solid-phase heterogeneous ELISA which relies on the ability of proteins or carbohydrates to attach to a solid phase passively by adsorption. Subsequent reagents are added, and incubated, and the unreacted materials can be washed away. The

From: *Methods in Molecular Medicine, vol. 60: Interleukin Protocols*
Edited by: L. A. J. O'Neill and A. Bowie © Humana Press Inc., Totowa, NJ

resulting color reaction following addition of enzyme substrate can be read using specially designed 96-well-format spectrophotometers. Quantification of antigen or antibody is made with reference to a suitable standard curve on the same plate.

1.2. Solid-Phase Heterogenous ELISAs

A number of different ELISA schemes have been developed for a variety of purposes *(4)*; however, solid-phase heterogeneous ELISAs can be classified into four groups: direct, indirect, competition, and sandwich *(5)*.

1.2.1. Direct ELISA

In direct "antigen" ELISA **(Fig. 1A)**, an antigen is immobilized onto a solid phase and incubated with enzyme-labeled antiserum. This technique is used primarily in the estimation of the antibody titer of antispecies conjugates, in particular IgG monoclonal antibodies. In contrast, direct "antibody" ELISA involves the adsorption of IgG antibodies to a solid phase followed by incubation with enzyme-conjugated antigen. This method has little use diagnostically, as antigens are rarely labeled.

1.2.2. Indirect ELISA

The specificity of an indirect ELISA **(Fig. 1B)** is directed by antigen bound to a solid phase. This method is widely employed for the detection and/or titration of specific antibodies from serum samples. Bound antibody is detected with an antispecies antibody conjugated to an enzyme.

1.2.3. Competition ELISA

Competition ELISA is used for the detection and measurement of antibody or antigen concentrations and can be direct or indirect. In competition assays, two reactants compete for binding to a third. This technique is similar to inhibition or blocking assays; however, competition ELISA involves the simultaneous rather than stepwise addition of the two competitors. Readers are directed elsewhere for a comprehensive description of different competition ELISAs *(5)*.

1.2.4. Sandwich ELISA

An antigen-specific IgG monoclonal "capture" antibody is coated onto a solid phase in the direct sandwich ELISA technique **(Fig. 1C)**. Following incubation of the test sample, containing antigen, enzyme-labeled antibody (which can be the same as or different from the capture antibody) is used to detect the trapped antigen. A modification of this ELISA method is the indirect sandwich ELISA technique **(Fig. 1Di)**. Here the secondary antibody used to detect bound antigen is not enzyme-labeled and is produced in a different species from the

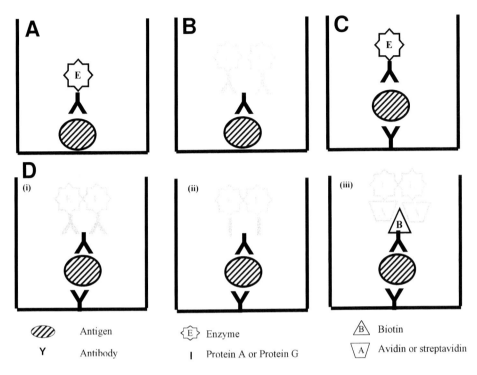

Fig. 1. Basic ELISA techniques.

capture antibody. Addition of a species-specific antiserum enzyme-conjugate that does not react with the adsorbed primary capture antibody, as well as subsequent substrate incubation, enables colorimetric detection. Often digoxigenin-conjugated antibodies are used as secondary antibodies, and detection is achieved using antidigoxigenin enzyme-conjugates. Further modifications of this method rely on the binding affinities of protein A (or protein G) for mammalian IgGs or biotin-avidin/streptavidin interactions (**Fig. 1Dii** and **iii**). The indirect sandwich ELISA is the method of choice for quantifying interleukins in test samples and is dealt with in more detail below.

2. Materials

A wide range of sandwich ELISA reagents for the detection and quantification of interleukins from different species have been developed. Polyclonal, monoclonal, and matched capture and secondary antibody pairs are available commercially (*see* **Note 1**). These can be used in combination with recombinant and purified interleukin proteins for use as standards, enzyme-conjugated IgGs, and detection reagents. ELISA immunoassay kits for the quantification of interleukins in cell culture supernatants and biologic fluids have been developed by a number of manufacturers. Kits, although expensive, provide all the reagents required to complete an ELISA, and because all steps have been optimized, these are highly sensitive and accurate (*see* **Note 2**).

3. Methods
3.1. Outline of Sandwich ELISA Protocol

The sandwich ELISA technique has been widely used in interleukin research. Similar to other ELISA methods, the sandwich technique involves the stepwise addition of reactants in order to reach a defined endpoint. Stages include (a) adsorption of antibody to a solid phase, (b) separation of unbound and free reactants by washing, (c) blocking of additional unbound sites on the solid phase, (d) addition and incubation of test samples, (e) addition of enzyme-labeled reagent, (f) addition of detection system and termination of reaction, and (g) visual, photometric, or fluorimetric reading of the assay. Interleukin sandwich ELISAs are highly specific because the antibodies used are directed against two specific epitopes of the interleukin being assayed. **Figure 2** shows a schematic of the general procedure. Each of these steps can be affected by a number of variables.

3.1.1. Immobilization of Primary Capture Antibody on Solid Phase

This initial step is often referred to as "coating" and involves the passive adsorption of antibody to a solid phase. The most widely used solid phase is the plastic matrix of flat-bottomed polyvinyl chloride or polystyrene 96-well microtiter plates. Either rigid or flexible plates may be used. Plates with removable wells and strips are also available, but these are a more expensive option. Tissue culture grade plates should not be used as they give much more variability than those specifically made for ELISA *(4)*.

Adsorption occurs due to hydrophobic interactions between nonpolar regions of the antibody and the plastic. These interactions are independent of the net charge of the antibody. Concentration, time, temperature, and pH are important factors in the rate and extent of coating. In general, a concentration range of $1–10$ µg/mL in a 50-µl, vol is a good guide to the level of antibody needed to saturate available sites. Rotation of the plates can significantly decrease the time required for optimal coating, by effectively increasing the diffusion coefficient of the attaching molecule. Intuitively, higher temperatures lead to concomitant increases in the rate of binding. A number of different coating regimens and coating buffers are used (*see* **Note 3**). This step must be optimized for each ELISA. Theoretically, saturation of the finite capacity of the plastic surface or desorption due to leaching may mitigate against successful coating. However, they do not have a significant effect in practice.

Dilute anti-interleukin capture antibody in coating buffer
Add 100 μl per well, seal plate.

⬇ **4 °C overnight**

Aspirate and wash x3 with 300 μl per well PBS/Tween
Add 200 μl blocking buffer per well, seal plate.

⬇ **RT 1-2 h**

Wash x3.
Add standards and samples, 100 μl per well, seal plate

⬇ **RT 2 h or 4 °C overnight**

Wash x3.
Dilute biotinylated anti-interleukin detection antibody in blocking buffer/Tween
Add 100 μl per well, seal plate.

⬇ **RT 1-2 h**

Wash x3.
Dilute avidin- or streptavidin-enzyme conjugate in blocking buffer/Tween.
Add 100 μl per well, seal plate.

⬇ **RT 30-60 min**

Wash x3.
Prepare substrate solution. Add 100 μl per well.
Allow color reaction to develop in dark

⬇ **RT 10-80 min**

(OPTIONAL) - Add 50 μl stop solution per well.

Read optical density for each well at correct wavelength.

Fig. 2. General procedure for indirect sandwich ELISA.

3.1.2. Washing

The purpose of washing is to separate bound and free (unbound) reagents. Washing is usually performed at least three times for each well using 0.1 M Tris-HCl or phosphate-buffered saline (PBS), pH 7.4, to maintain isotonicity. Generally flooding of the wells is sufficient to remove unbound reagents with optional soak times of 1–5 min after each addition. The incorporation of detergent in the wash buffer (0.05 % [v/v] Tween-20) adds stringency but does not appear to contribute significantly to the wash procedure and does require that extra care be taken to avoid excessive foaming. A number of different washing methods can be used including immersion or specialist plate washers. The most efficient and cost-effective methods employ wash bottles or multichannel pipets, followed by blotting of the plates onto absorbent paper with gentle tapping to remove residual wash buffer from the wells. After washing, coated plates may be used immediately or washed with distilled water, dried thoroughly, sealed in an airtight container, and stored at 4°C for 6–12 mo.

3.1.3. Blocking

Nonspecific adsorption of protein to available plastic sites not occupied by the primary capture antibody can lead to high background color at the completion of an ELISA. Prevention of these nonspecific adsorption events is achieved by incorporating a blocking step in the ELISA procedure. The most commonly used ELISA blocking agents are detergents and proteins. Both nonionic and anionic detergents can be used at low concentrations to prevent nonspecific adsorption, with Tween-20, Tween-80, Triton X-100, and sodium dodecyl sulfate (SDS) proving very effective. Bovine serum albumin (BSA), human serum albumin, fetal calf serum (FCS), casein, casein hydrolysate, and gelatin are also widely used (*see* **Note 4**). Common blocking buffers are PBS containing 1% BSA and 0.05% Tween-20 or PBS/10% FCS. These solutions are made up in small volumes as required as they are prone to contamination. However, short-term storage (1–2 d) at 4°C is possible.

3.1.4. Addition and Incubation of Test Samples

Samples tested in ELISA are most commonly cell culture supernatants, serum, or plasma. However, any biologic fluid can be assayed for interleukin levels using this technique, e.g., saliva, lavage fluids, exudates, urine, etc. Sample addition requires accurate dispensing of small volumes (50–100 μL) into each well and should be carried out in duplicate or triplicate. To eliminate nonspecific binding events further, especially when measuring antigen concentrations in complex fluids such as serum or cerebrospinal fluid, dilution in PBS with a wetting agent (e.g., 0.05% Tween-20) is recommended. It is also suggested that diluents that include irrelevant Igs be used when measuring antigen levels in these fluids (*6*). In addition, complete thawing of sample materials prior to addition must be ensured so that proteins are homogenously dispersed in the sample.

By including serial dilutions of a standard antigen solution, a standard or calibration curve can be generated (**Fig. 3**). The linear region of standard curves for most commercially available interleukin ELISAs can usually be obtained in a series of seven twofold dilutions. In general, it is recommended that doubling dilutions ranging from 1000 pg/mL to 15 pg/mL be used for recombinant interleukin standards. It is important to remember to include

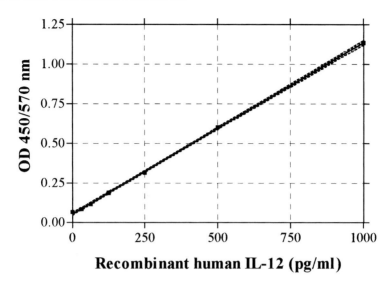

Fig. 3. Standard curve from an R & D Systems Quantikine sandwich ELISA that measures IL-12 protein levels.

"blank" wells to which no standard or sample has been added. High background readings in blank wells may indicate that more stringent washing procedures are required. Reactions between antibodies and antigens depend on distribution, time, temperature, and buffer conditions. Similar to the coating step, it is advisable to test a variety of conditions. Some manufacturers recommend overnight incubation of standards and samples for optimal sensitivity (*see* **Note 5**).

3.1.5. Addition of Secondary Antibody and Enzyme-Labeled Reagent

After removal of unbound standard and sample, captured antigens are detected by incubation with secondary antibodies. To determine the lowest background and optimal signal for an ELISA, titration of capture and secondary antibodies is recommended. If possible, the secondary antibody should be raised in a different species from the capture antibody and should recognize a different epitope on the bound antigen. Unmodified secondary antibody can be detected with species-specific enzyme-conjugated antiserum. Alternative methods involve the conjugation of enzymes to pseudo-immune reactors such as protein A or protein G, which bind mammalian IgGs, or indirect biotin-avidin/streptavidin systems **(Fig. 1D)**. Digoxigenin-conjugated secondary antibodies are also routinely used.

A wide variety of enzymes have been used as conjugates including acetyl cholinesterase, cytochrome C, glucoamylase, glucose oxidase, β-D-glucouronidase, lactate dehydrogenase, lactoperoxidase, ribonuclease, and tyrosinase *(7)*. Horseradish peroxidase (HRP), alkaline phosphatase (AP), β-galactosidase, and urease are the four most commonly used enzymes in ELISA. These enzymes are stable and highly reactive, available in pure form, yield stable conjugates, and are cheap and safe to use. HRP has emerged as the clear favorite due to its low cost, easy conjugation, and wide variety of substrates.

Many enzyme conjugates are available commercially, but, if required, individuals can generate their own relatively easily *(8)* (*see* **Note 6**).

3.1.6. Detection of Signal and Termination of Reaction

The kinetics of color development depend on a variety of physiochemical parameters including buffer composition and pH, reaction temperature, substrate, enzyme and product stability, and/or cofactor concentration and stability. Reaction conditions for colorimetric ELISA enzyme/substrate systems are summarized in **Table 1**. Enzyme substrates should be chosen that provide a sensitive detection method for the enzyme-conjugate and should ideally yield a soluble stable colored product with a high extinction coefficient, i.e., dense color per unit degraded. Substrates should also be cheap, safe and easy to use.

HRP is a widely used enzyme for which a variety of substrates, oxidizable by H_2O_2, are available. This enzyme is active over a broad pH range with respect to H_2O_2, but the optimum pH is dependent on the chromogen used. HRP is more stable in 0.1 M citrate than 0.1 M phosphate buffers, and its activity is potently inhibited by sodium azide. A number of HRP substrates are commonly used; however, *o*-phenylenediamine (OPD) is probably the most widely used. It is completely soluble as a 1% solution in methanol and yields an orange color with a high extinction coefficient at 492 nm after addition of 1/4 vol of 2 M H_2SO_4; however, OPD is photosensitive, and care must be taken to protect substrate-solutions from light. Other HRP substrates that are commonly used are 2,2'-azino diethylbenzothiazoline-sulfonic acid (ABTS), 5-aminosalicylic acid (5AS) and tetramethylbenzidine (TMB). Certain of these substrate solutions (OPD and ABTS) can be made up in batches and stored frozen, without the addition of H_2O_2. This can reduce interassay variation.

The activity of AP is dependent on inorganic Mg^{2+} and is optimal above pH 8.0. Two different AP enzymes can be used—bacterial AP, which has a pH optimum of 8.1 in 0.1 M Tris-HCl buffer, and intestinal mucosal AP, which hydrolyzes its substrate most effectively in a 10% diethanolamine buffer, pH 9.8. The AP substrate paranitrophenyl phosphate (pnpp) is easy to use and produces linear color development over time. Inorganic phosphate and EDTA have strong inhibitory effects on AP; therefore wash buffers should be Tris- rather than phosphate-based. Nonionic detergents do not appear to affect this enzyme's activity.

Urea is hydrolyzed into ammonia and bicarbonate by urease. The recommended substrate solution for ELISA contains urea and a pH indicator,

Table 1
Common Colorimetric Enzyme/Substrate Systems for ELISA[a]

Enzyme	Substrate	Dye	Buffer	Color change/wavelength (nm)		Stop solution
				Nonstopped	Stopped	
HRP	H_2O_2 (0.004%)	OPD (0.04%)	Sodium citrate (0.1 M), pH 5.0	Green/orange (450)	Orange/brown (492)	2 M H_2SO_4
	H_2O_2 (0.002%)	ABTS (0.04%)	Phosphate/citrate (0.1 M), pH 4.2	Green (414)	Green (414)	20% SDS/ 50% DMF
	H_2O_2 (0.004%)	TMB	Acetate buffer (0.1 M), pH 5.6	Blue (650)	Yellow (450)	1% SDS
	H_2O_2 (0.006%)	5AS (0.04%)	Phosphate (0.2 M), pH 6.8	Brown (450)	Brown (450)	No stop
AP	pnpp (2.5 mM)	pnpp (0.01%)	Diethanolamine (10 mM) and $MgCL_2$ (0.5 mM), pH 9.5	Yellow/green (405)	Yellow/green (405)	2 M sodium carbonate
β-gal	ONPG (3 mM)	ONPG (0.07%)	Potassium phosphate buffer with $MgCL_2$, 2ME (0.01 M), pH 7.5	Yellow (420)	Yellow (420)	2 M sodium carbonate
Urease	Urea	BC	pH 4.8	Purple (588)	Purple (588)	1% merthiolate

[a]Abbreviations: HRP, horseradish peroxidase; AP, alkaline phosphatase; β-gal, β-galactosidase; H_2O_2, hydrogen peroxide; pnpp, paranitrophenyl phosphate; ONPG, O-nitrophenyl β-D-galactopyranoside; OPD, ortho-phenylene diamine; TMB, tetra-methylbenzidine; ABTS, 2,2'-azino di-ethylbenzothiazoline-sulfonic acid; 5AS, 5-aminosalicylic acid; BC, bromocresol; $MgCl_2$, magnesium chloride; 2ME, 2-mercaptoethanol; H_2SO_4, sulphuric acid; SDS, sodium dodecyl sulphate; DMF, dimethyl formamide. Adapted from **ref. 5**.

bromocresol purple. The released ammonia increases the pH and changes the color of the indicator from yellow to purple. Since the reaction is dependent on pH, it is important to remove all traces of alkaline buffers (e.g., PBS, pH 7.4) prior to substrate addition. This can be ensured by washing finally in distilled water.

β-Galactosidase activity is determined by the development of a yellow color after addition of O-nitrophenyl β-D-galactopyranoside (ONPG) in potassium phosphate buffer containing 1 mM $MgCl_2$ and 10 mM 2-mercaptoethanol. The amount of bound enzyme can be determined by measuring the optical density of each sample at 420 nm. An alternative to ONPG is chlorophenolred-β-D-galactopyranoside (CRPG). This substrate produces a dark red color that can be read at 474 or 578 nm.

Chemiluminescent ELISA substrates are available for a number of these enzyme systems. These can provide greater sensitivity than colorimetric substrates. However, microplate chemiluminescence readers or tube-format luminometers are required to interpret results. For researchers who have access to a fluorimeter, the use of fluorimetric ELISA substrates is possible.

3.1.7. Termination of Reaction

The addition of denaturants or strong acids or bases can stop enzymic activity by quickly denaturing enzymes. Reagents such as 2 M H_2SO_4 or 1% SDS inhibit HRP. These and other agents (**Table 1**) are used to terminate color development in ELISA and are referred to as *stop solutions*. Termination can increase the sensitivity of an ELISA; however, the volume of a stop reagent must remain constant per well since photometric readings are affected if the total volume of reactant varies between wells.

3.1.8. Reading of the Assay

At the completion of a chromogenic ELISA, the optical density of each well is measured using a microtiter plate reader set at the appropriate wavelength for the enzyme/substrate system used. Alternative methods that employ chemiluminescent or fluorimetric substrates require the use of specialist light detectors or fluorimeters. Raw data generated are generally expressed as absorbance, light, or fluorescence units. To calculate assays results, mean values for duplicate or triplicate standards are calculated, and a standard curve is plotted of optical density, light units, or fluorescence light units vs concentration. The best curve is fitted using suitable regression analysis *(9)*. The concentration of antigen in an unknown sample is read by taking, for example, the mean of optical density of the sample on the y-axis and extending a horizontal line to the standard curve. At the point of intersection, a vertical line is extended to the x-axis, and the corresponding antigen concentration is read. If samples have been diluted, the concentration read from the standard curve must be multiplied by the dilution factor. Alternatively, results can be calculated from the slope of the curve either arithmetically or using computer software such as Excel or Prism.

"By eye" assessment of colorimetric ELISAs may be acceptable where a "yes or no" answer is required. Subjective visual assessment can also be used to determine titers by comparison with known positive and negative samples, although it is not a generally accepted method for quantitative evaluation.

3.2. Interleukin mRNA ELISAs

Recently a number of new products based on the ELISA method have been developed for the detection and quantification of interleukin (IL) mRNAs. In the Quantikine mRNA system from R&D Systems, interleukin mRNA transcripts are double-labeled with biotin- and digoxigenin-conjugated interleukin-specific oligonucleotides. Streptavidin-coated wells are used to capture the transcripts via interaction with biotin. These captured transcripts can subsequently be detected using an enzyme-conjugated antidigoxigenin antibody and substrate. Kits currently available detect IL-1β, IL-2, and IL-6 mRNAs (www.rndsystems.co.uk). An alternative method developed by BioSource International is the CytoXpress Quantitative PCR Detection Kit. Competitive reverse transcription polymerase chain reaction (RT-PCR) using biotinylated interleukin-specific oligonucelotides amplifies biotin-labeled interleukin products. These biotinylated amplicons are hybridized to interleukin-specific capture oligonucleotides, and addition of an enzyme-streptavidin conjugate enables mRNA quantitation following addition of chromogen (www.biosource.com). Both methods are quantitative, reproducible, and user friendly.

4. Notes

1. Numerous antibodies and reagents are commercially available for interleukin ELISA. The names of some major suppliers are shown below:
   Biodesign International
   Biotrend Chemikalien
   Calbiochem
   Chemicon
   Fitzgerald Industries International
   ICN Pharmaceuticals
   Pharmingen
   R & D Systems
   Research Diagnostics
   US Biologicals
   More detailed lists can be found on Anderson's webalog (www.atcg.com) and "The online ordering site for biologists and biochemists" (condor.bcm.tmc.edu/buying.html).

2. The quality of water can be a major problem in standardization of assays. Thus, kits that supply water, at least for initial dilutions of stock regents, are recommended. Otherwise the use of triple-distilled water is advisable for dilution of reagents and buffers.

3. For example, 37°C for 1–3 h, room temperature for 1–3 h, or 4°C overnight. Frequently used coating buffers include 20 mM Tris-HCl, pH 8.5, or 10 mM PBS, pH 7.2. However, the most effective is 50 mM carbonate, pH 9.6 (Voller's buffer). This buffer should be stored at room temperature for no more than 2 wk.

4. Other agents such as dextran sulphate and nonfat dried milk may have applications for some assays; however, it is important to note that certain blocking agents may be unsuitable for use with some enzyme systems, e.g., skim milk cannot be used in assays based on biotin-avidin interactions or urease.

5. In general a 2-h incubation is sufficient, although incubation times should be increased for viscous samples, e.g., 1/20 serum, or samples with low amounts of antigen. Increasing the rate of contact between the coating material and the plastic by rotation of the plates can decrease the incubation times required.

6. Enzymes are conjugated to reagents either directly via reactive groups on each or indirectly via bifunctional crosslinking agents. Glutaraldehyde and sodium periodate are two good crosslinkers. Other coupling agents such as *N-N'-O'*-phenylenedimaleimide or *p*-benzoquinone can also be used *(4)*. Following conjugation, residual unlabeled antibody and free enzyme must be removed by salt precipitation or gel filtration. Chemical modification of the enzyme or the antibody/immunoreactant can affect catalytic activity and reactive sites, respectively. Therefore it is important to choose a method that does not affect these parameters. Optimal conjugation should be simple, rapid, and reproducible and should generate a high yield of active reagent with long-term stability.

References

1. Avrameas, S., Nakane, P. K., Papamichail, M., and Pesce, A. J., eds. *Special Edition of the Journal of Immunological Methods, 25 Years of Immuoenzymatic Techniques*. International Congress, Athens, Greece, September, 1991.

2. Engvall, E. and Pearlmann, P. (1971) Enzyme-linked immunosorbent assay (ELISA). Quantitative assay of immunoglobulin G. *Immunochemistry* **8,** 871–879.

3. Van Weeman, B. K. and Schuurs, A. H. W. M. (1971) Immunoassay using antigen-enzyme conjugates. *FEBS Lett.* **15,** 232–236.

4. Kemeny, D. M. (1991) *A Practical Guide to ELISA*. Pergamon, NY, pp. 1–130.

5. Crowther, J. R. (1995) ELISA, theory and practice, in *Methods in Molecular Biology, vol. 42* (Crowther, J. R., ed.), Humana, Totowa, NJ, pp. 1–223.

6. Abrams, J. S. (1995) Immunoenzymatic assay of mouse and human cytokines using NIP-labelled anti-cytokine antibodies, in *Current Protocols in Immunology* (Coligan, J., Kruisbeek, A., Marguiles, D., Shevach, E., and Strober, W., eds.), John Wiley & Sons, NY, CD-ROM section 6.20.

7. Voller, A., Bidwell, D. E., and Bartlett, A., eds. (1979) *The Enzyme-Linked Immuosorbent Assay (ELISA)—A Guide with Abstracts of Microplate Applications.* Nuffield Laboratories of Comparative Medicine, The Zoological Society of London, London, pp. 1–125.
8. Ishikawa, E., Imagawa, M., Hashide, S., Yoshatake, S., Hagushi, Y., and Ueno, T. (1983) Enzyme labelling of antibodies and their fragments for enzyme immunoassays and immunological staining. *J. Immunoassay* **4,** 209–213.
9. Daly, L. E., Bourke, G. J., and McGilvray, J. (1995) Regression and correlation, in *Interpretation and Uses of Medical Statistics* (Daly, L. E., Bourke, G. J., and McGilvray, J., eds.), Blackwell Science, Oxford, pp. 157–163.

2

ELISPOT Technique for Assaying Interleukins

Almuth Christine Hauer and Mona Bajaj-Elliott

1. Introduction

The enzyme-linked immunosorbent assay (ELISA) spot (ELISPOT) procedure is basically a modification of the plaque techniques, hence its initial synonym ELISA plaque assay. Plaque assays allow the enumeration of antibody-secreting cells by diluting them in an environment in which the antibody formed by each individual cell produces a readily observable effect. Based on this principle, Czerkinsky and coworkers (1) first described a modification of this technique which could be used for the detection and enumeration of antibody-producing cells in vitro. In this modified assay, a suspension of single antibody-forming cells was incubated on a precoated solid phase, i.e., on a dish of immobilized antigen, to which specific antibody secreted during the incubation period would bind. This locally captured antibody was visualized after removal of the cells by treatment with an enzyme-conjugated anti-immunoglobulin and development of a color reaction by incorporating the substrate in a gel that was poured over the ground of the dish. Limited diffusion of the colored reaction product in the gel provided a series of macroscopic spots that were readily enumerated.

Since then the ELISPOT assay has been employed not only to enumerate specific as well as total immunoglobulin-secreting cells but also to detect a variety of cells secreting antigenic substances (2). Although Versteegen et al. (3) were the first to use this assay to detect human cells secreting interferon-γ (IFN-γ), an important modification of the ELISPOT assay employing nitro-cellulose membranes and epitope-specific monoclonal antibodies has made it more reproducible and sensitive in detecting cytokine-secreting cells at a single cell level (4). The advantage of this modification is the use of nitrocellulose plates as solid support instead of the former polystyrene surfaces. As they have a

From: *Methods in Molecular Medicine, vol. 60: Interleukin Protocols*
Edited by: L. A. J. O'Neill and A. Bowie © Humana Press Inc., Totowa, NJ

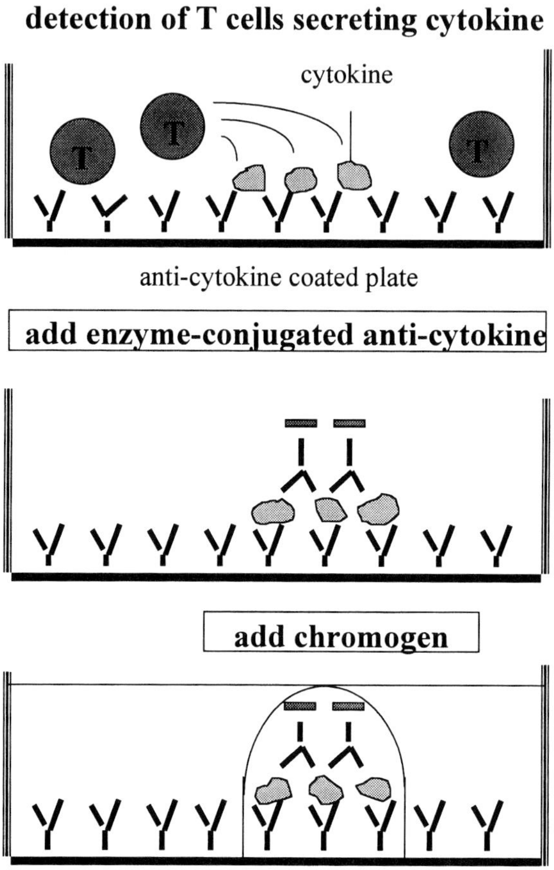

detection of T cells secreting cytokine

Fig. 1. Plates are coated with anti-cytokine and the captured cytokine is detected with enzyme-coupled antibody and visualized by addition of a chromogen.

higher protein binding capacity, requirements for relatively large amounts of expensive coating reagents can be minimized, and nitrocellulose plates are now routinely used for cytokine analysis by the ELISPOT method (*see* **Fig. 1**). Furthermore, this method became a well established technique for measuring cytokine synthesis, as it also has the benefit allowing cells secreting different cytokines to be compared with a common denominator, namely, the cell number. However, there remains the disadvantage that one has very little idea of how much cytokine each cell is secreting. This is the reverse problem of assays measuring cytokines in supernatants: Here one knows the exact concentration of cytokine but not how many cells are secreting the molecule.

In principle, the ELISPOT method can be used in a whole variety of settings: Cytokine secretion by peripheral as well as mucosal lymphocytes can be measured, both the spontaneous secretion and that after in vitro stimulation with various agents, but also after having positively or negatively selected for a number of cell subtypes, i.e., T-helper cells *(5,6)*. ELISPOT is equally used in settings involving animal experiments *(7)*. However, the technical details described in this chapter refer to work with human mononuclear cells only. The essential and overall determinant for the quality of the assay remains the initial preparation of the single cell suspension, i.e., the separation of peripheral lymphocytes or mucosal lymphocytes, and treatment of the cells before commencement of the assay.

2. Materials
2.1. Experimental Reagents and Buffers

This method requires sterile working conditions, and all steps should be performed in a laminar air flow hood. However, the final stage, including color development of the ELISPOTs, is performed at the bench.

The experimental reagents and buffers listed should be prepared as fresh as possible, but in convenient amounts; buffers such as phosphate-buffered saline (PBS), Tris-buffered saline (TBS), and the alkaline phosphate color substrate buffer can be prepared in advance (1-L aliquots) to the appropriate pH, filter-sterilized (0.2 μm), and stored until required. Reagent preparation, such as the dilution of antibodies and the preparation of the color substrate, should be done immediately before use. In case of the detecting secondary antibody, 1% fetal calf serum (FCS) has always to be added directly to the freshly prepared antibody.

If not otherwise stated, the general storage conditions are at 4°C for up to 2 mo.

1. RPMI-1640/10% FCS: RPMI-1640 serves as the principle cell medium for both peripheral and mucosal lymphocytes in this assay. It is also used for the individual cell dilutions. Supplementation with FCS is essential for cell viability: 10.3 g of RPMI-1640 powder (Sigma, Poole, Dorset, UK) and 2.0 g NaHCO$_3$ (20 mM; GIBCO, Paisley, Scotland) are dissolved in 900 mL MQ water and supplemented with 10% heat-inactivated FCS, 50 μL β$_2$-mercaptoethanol (Merck-BDH), 50 U/mL penicillin, 50 μg/mL streptomycin (ICN Flow), and 50 μg/mL Gentamicin (Roussel, Uxbridge, Middlesex, UK) and the pH adjusted to 7.4. The final volume is then made up to 1 L.
2. PBS: For 1 L of PBS, mix 7.02 g NaCl, 3.44 g Na$_2$HPO$_4$, and 0.79 g KH$_2$PO$_4$ and adjust to pH 7.4.
3. PBS/Tween-20: Tween-20 is a detergent, and its addition to the buffer reduces nonspecific binding of the antibodies, leading to low background. Tween-20 is stored at room temperature and should be added at a concentration of 0.05% (v/v) to the freshly prepared PBS.
4. TBS: 1 L TBS requires 8.0 g NaCl (Merck-BDH), 0.605g Tris(hydroxymethyl) methylamine (Merck-BDH), and 4.4 mL 1 N hydrochloric acid (Merck-BDH), adjusted to pH 7.6.
5. 5-Bromo-4-chloro-3-indoyl phosphate/nitro blue tetrazolium (BCIP/NBT) substrate solution (Bio-Rad, Hercules, CA): The reagents for the final step of the color development are obtained in a kit form consisting of:

    a. Two substrates (substrate A and substrate B) that are stored at –20°C in the dark and are stable up to 12 mo. Both substrates should only be taken out of the deep freeze for as short a period as possible, ideally placed on ice.

    b. An alkaline phosphatase substrate buffer that has to be prepared initially under sterile conditions following the manufacturer's instructions exactly, adjusted to pH 7.6 and filtered. It can be then stored at 4°C for up to 12 mo.

6. Ficoll-hypaque (Amersham-Pharmacia, UK): Ficoll is used in the isolation of peripheral mononuclear cells by density gradient centrifugation. It is in liquid form, ready to use, and can be stored at 4°C for up to 2–4 mo.

7. Hanks' balanced salt solution (HBSS-CMF, free of calcium and magnesium; Flow Laboratories, McLean, VA): HBSS helps to dissociate the epithelia from the underlying mesenchyme by complexing with Ca^{2+} ions. It can be stored at 4°C for up to 6 mo.

8. Collagenase (Type 1, Sigma): Collagenase is needed for the enzymatic digestion of mucosal specimens. It comes as a powder and is stored at –20°C.

9. Cycloheximide (Sigma): Cycloheximide is a protein synthesis inhibitor and thus affects the cell function directly. It can therefore be used in control experiments to ensure that one does not measure cytokines released from the cytoplasm of dead cells or membrane-bound cytokines being released into the medium.

10. Trypan blue (0.1%, Bioconcept, Switzerland): Small amounts of freshly prepared single cell suspensions are mixed with trypan blue in order to count the mononuclear cells and to determine the viability of cells. Trypan blue should always be freshly filtered immediately before use using a microfilter. It is stored at room temperature (RT), in the dark, for up to 6 mo.

2.2. Monoclonal Antibodies

We routinely use this assay to detect the secretion of cytokines such as IFN-γ, interleukin (IL)-4, IL-5, IL-10, and transforming growth factor-β (TGF-β) by peripheral blood and mucosal lymphocytes. The concentrations of the primary and secondary antibodies listed below have been optimized for our system (*5,6,8,9*). Although the reader may have to test and modify these conditions for his/her experiment, the range of concentrations and dilutions suggested may be a good starting point.

The set of monoclonal antibodies (MAbs) for each cytokine includes a primary ("capture") and a secondary ("detecting") antibody. The nitrocellulose plates are initially coated with the primary MAb; the cells secreting the particular cytokine will affinity bind to it, hence "capture." The secondary MAb is biotin labeled and recognizes a different epitope on the cytokine, thus leading to binding and sandwich formation with the antibody-cytokine complex. A further MAb, namely, streptavidin alkaline phosphatase, that binds to the biotinylated secondary MAb is always added, thus acting as the "universal" tertiary antibody of the assay.

All MAbs listed are stored in the dark at 4°C. They are diluted as indicated in their respective buffers immediately before use, resulting in a final concentration of MAb per culture well that equals 0.5–0.7 µg/100 µL (0.5–0.7 µg/culture well) for all the primary antibodies and 0.15–0.3 µg/100 µL (0.15–0.3 µg/culture well) for all the secondary antibodies.

1. IFN-γ antibodies (Chromogenix AB, Mölndal, Sweden): Stock concentrations are 100 µg/mL (capture) and 30 µg/500 µL (detecting).
2. IL-4 antibodies (Mabtech, Stockholm, Sweden): Stock concentrations are 100 µg/100 µL (capture and detecting).
3. IL-5 antibodies (Pharmingen, San Diego, CA): Stock concentrations are 500 µg/mL (capture and detecting).
4. IL-10 antibodies (Pharmingen): Stock concentrations are 500 µg/mL (capture and detecting).
5. TGF-β antibodies (R & D Systems, Minneapolis, MN): Stock concentrations are 500 µg/mL (capture) and 50 µg/mL (detecting).
6. Streptavidin alkaline phophatase (Mabtech): 1 mL.

3. Methods

ELISPOT is essentially an assay that analyzes the cytokine-secreting capacity of viable cells only! One should therefore proceed with the experiment as quickly as possible to keep the yield of viable cells high, i.e., within a maximum of 2–4 h after having obtained either blood sample or mucosal specimen. Cells have to be carefully worked with, and, after single cell separations have been prepared, cells should be always kept cold, on ice.

3.1. Separation of Peripheral Blood Mononuclear Cells

Peripheral blood mononuclear cells (PBMCs) are obtained from venous heparinized blood layered over a Ficoll-Hypaque density gradient using standard procedures (8):

1. A minimum of 2 mL of whole blood is mixed 1:1 with sterile RPMI-1640/10% FCS (i.e., 2 mL of RPMI-1640/10% FCS) and carefully layered over the same amount of Ficoll (i.e., 4 mL of Ficoll; see **Note 1**).
2. The blood layered over Ficoll is spun down in the centrifuge at 1500 rpm, *20°C, without brake* for 20–25 min (see **Note 2**).
3. Cells of the buffy coat (i.e., the interphase mononuclear cells) are carefully collected (**Fig. 2**) using a Pasteur pipet with a small rubber bulb adjusted (see **Note 3**), resuspended in 10–15 mL of RPMI-1640/10%FCS and washed three times at 1500 rpm, *4°C, with maximal brake*, for 10 min.
4. After resuspension in 1 mL of medium, the cell number is determined (**Fig. 3**) using a hemocytometer (see **Note 4**).
5. Viable cells are identified by trypan blue exclusion and should comprise more than 95% before use (see **Note 5**).
6. To specify the subtypes of the PBMCs further, small samples can be prepared at this stage either for immunostaining or for fluorescence-activated cell sorting (FACS) analysis (5).

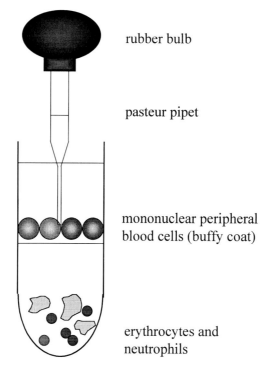

rubber bulb

pasteur pipet

mononuclear peripheral
blood cells (buffy coat)

erythrocytes and
neutrophils

Fig. 2. Suctioning of the buffy coat by a Pasteur pipet.

3.2. Isolation of Mucosal Mononuclear Cells

Mononuclear cells are isolated from biopsies by an enzymatic digestion process.

1. Specimens should be placed in cold RPMI-1640/10% FCS (i.e., 2 pinch biopsies in 10–15 mL medium) directly after the biopsy has been performed and should be processed within 2–4 h.
2. Then specimens are put into 20 mL of HBSS for 45–75 min at RT and washed (10 min, 1500 rpm, 4°C, maximal brake). This process allows the separation of the epithelia.
3. The remaining samples are then placed into RPMI-1640/10%FCS using a Pasteur pipet, and 1.5–5 mg collagenase/mL medium is added (*see* **Note 6**).
4. Tubes are incubated at 37°C in a 5% CO_2/95% air/water-saturated atmosphere with vigorous pipetting every 10–15 min, using a pasteur pipet with a small rubber bulb attached.
5. The enzyme treatment is finished when tissue pieces are dissolved to an almost homogenous cell suspension. This takes usually 3–5 h.
6. Cells are washed twice in RPMI-1640/10% FCS and resuspended in 10 mL of medium. Facultatively, they can then be filtered through a glass wool column (*see* **Note 7**).

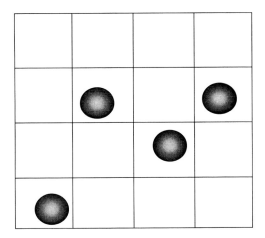

4 MNC*/16 hemocytometer squares =
0.4 x 10^6 MNC/ml
(10 µl cell suspension + 90 µl trypan blue)

* MNC: mononuclear cells

Fig. 3. Example for the determination of the cell number per volume using a hemocytometer.

7. After a final wash, cells are resuspended in 500 µL of RPMI-1640/10% FCS, counted, and left on ice while checking for viability (>95%) and purity (<5% epithelial cells) (*see* **Note 8**).
8. Cytocentrifuge preparations can be performed at this stage (a minimum of two per sample, with 5–10,000 cells/slide) and stored until immunostaining.

3.3. Enumeration of IFN-, IL-4-, IL-5-, and IL-10-Secreting Cells

Both diluted antibodies and single cell suspensions are always added in 100-µL vol to each well, using individual pipets. All washing steps are performed with 200-µL vol of the respective buffers, using a multichannel pipet. One should always perform assays involving peripheral blood mononuclear cells (MNCs) at least in triplicate or quadruplicate, adding 100,000–150,000 MNC/culture well, and assays with mucosal MNCs at least in duplicate, adding 5000–50,000 MNC/well.

1. Nitrocellulose-bottomed microtiter wells (Millipore Bedford, MA) are coated for 3 h at RT with the cytokine-specific monoclonal capture antibody, diluted in 100 µL sterile PBS per well (*see* **Note 9**). Plates should be agitated for 1–2 min directly after adding the antibody to ensure homogenous suspension.
2. After 3 h, unadsorbed antibody is removed by three washes with PBS (*see* **Note 10**).
3. Single cell suspensions in 100-µL vol are added to each well (*see* **Note 11**).

4. Cells are incubated for 20 h (or overnight) at 37°C in a humidified atmosphere of 5% CO_2 in air.
5. The cells are removed by washing the wells eight times with PBS/0.05% Tween.
6. A biotin-labeled cytokine-specific MAb is then used as a detecting antibody and added in 100-µL vol/well.
7. The plate is again agitated for 1–2 min and then left for an incubation period of 3 h at RT (*see* **Note 12**).
8. Wells are washed 6× with PBS/0.05% Tween.
9. Streptavidin alkaline phophatase is diluted 1:1000 in TBS and added at 100 µL/well; after agitation, the plate is incubated for 1 h at 37°C in the CO_2 incubator (*see* **Note 13**).
10. Wells are washed five times with TBS and finally once with the alkaline phosphatase substrate buffer.
11. Color substrate is freshly prepared (10 µL of substrate A and 10 µL of substrate B/1 mL of substrate buffer) and added in 100-µL aliquots to each culture well.
12. The plates are left at RT until dark blue spots appear (20–40 min).
13. The enzyme reaction is stopped by washing three times with distilled water. The wells are allowed to dry and the number of spots per well enumerated using a dissecting microscope (×25 magnification; *see* **Note 14**).
14. ELISPOT sizes can be determined by measuring the spot diameters on the basis of their optical density by computer-assisted image analysis (SeeScan, Cambridge, UK). With this equipment spots are visualized on a monitor and their diameter measured using a mouse-controlled cursor (*see* **Note 15**).

3.4. Control Experiments

To assess true spot formation, inhibition assays with cycloheximide can be performed. Cycloheximide inhibits protein synthesis, leading to subsequent downregulation of cytokine synthesis and secretion, and thus spot formation. This time-course experiment includes the following steps:

1. The single cell suspension of blood or mucosal lymphocytes, respectively, is assessed for its cell number, resuspended in 20–40 mL RPMI-1640/10% FCS, and aliquoted into four culture flasks (50-mL vol).
2. Two flasks are incubated for 3 h, and the other two for 5 h, with one at each time containing cycloheximide at a final concentration of 50 ng/mL.
3. After two subsequent washes, cell suspensions are added at 100-µL vol to the previously coated culture wells and the ELISPOT assay continued as usual.
4. Inhibition of spot formation by cycloheximide within a time-course of 3 and 5 h, respectively, can finally be calculated by comparing the spot numbers of wells containing cell suspensions with and without cycloheximide added.

3.5. Stimulation of Mononuclear Cells for the ELISPOT Assay

Both peripheral blood and mucosal MNCs can be stimulated before using them in the ELISPOT assay as usual. However, stimulation assays involving mucosal

MNCs will always depend on a sufficiently high cell yield at the beginning. Stimulants can either serve as positive controls (i.e., T-cell mitogens such as phytohemagglutinin) or in assays analyzing cytokine secretion upon stimulation with specific antigens (i.e., dietary antigens such as various cow's milk proteins).

1. A single cell suspension is prepared as usual, counted, tested for viability, and resuspended in 20 mL RPMI-1640/10% FCS.
2. This cell suspension is then aliquoted (i.e., 100,000 peripheral MNCs and 10–50,000 mucosal MNCs/aliquot). One aliquot serves as the unstimulated control and the remaining aliquots for adding the respective stimulating agents. All are incubated in culture flasks or 24-well plates in the CO_2 incubator overnight.
3. Cells are then washed, checked for viability, counted, and added to the previously coated wells in 100-µL vol, before the ELISPOT assay is continued as usual.

3.6. Using Selected Cell Subtypes

Single cell suspensions that have either been depleted of or enriched for a given cell population by magnetic separation techniques can equally be used for the ELISPOT assay.

1. A minimum of three wells per cytokine (ideally six wells for duplicate experiments) has to be coated in advance to ensure that the unselected cell fraction along with both the negative and the positive cell fraction can be set up.
2. After the separating procedures, cells have again to be counted, tested for viability, resuspended in cell medium, and added at 100-µL vol to the wells in order to continue with the assay as usual (**Figs. 4** and **5**).

4. Notes

1. This layering can be easily performed using a broad-end Pasteur pipet with a small rubber bulb in order to suck up the milliliter amounts of the suspended blood gently and repetitively and place them onto the Ficoll.
2. Because too much mixing of the layers will dramatically reduce the yield of lymphocytes, care is required when transferring the tube to the centrifuge. No brake on this centrifugation is recommended, as this helps to maintain the gradient established.
3. One should proceed with the Pasteur pipet directly to the buffy coat (the mononuclear cell layer) that appears at the interphase between the top (aqueous) and the bottom (Ficoll) layer and suck it up as complete as possible trying not to disturb the respective layers in the least (**Fig. 2**).
4. Cell suspension (10 µL) is diluted in 90 µL of trypan blue (0.1%) and quickly vortexed; a small amount of the mixture is then added to a hemocytometer. If there are enough cells, a minimum of 16 squares is counted; otherwise one should count 64 squares (example: 25 MNC/16 squares = 2.5×10^6/mL MNC; 136 MNC/16 squares: 13.6×10^6/mL MNC; **Fig. 3**).
5. This step has to be performed very fast, since trypan blue affects the viability of cells.
6. The amount of collagenase added can be adjusted individually according to one's experience through the experimental series. We found an amount of 2–2.5 mg/mL

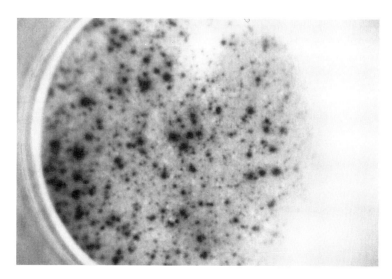

Fig. 4. Interleukin-4 ELISPOTS upon stimulation with β-lactoglobulin, by peripheral blood mononuclear cells (original magnification ×25).

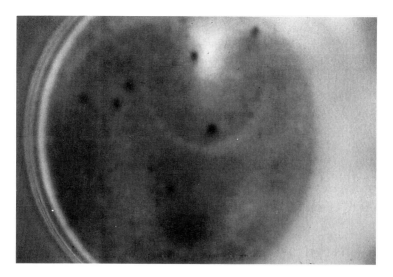

Fig. 5. Transforming growth factor-β ELISPOTS by peripheral blood mononuclear cells (original magnification ×25).

collagenase appropriate when dealing with Peyer's patches, whereas specimens from the ileal mucosa needed up to 5 mg collagenase/mL to digest well. However, prolonged exposure to collagenase will affect the viability of cells. Once single cell suspension is obtained, proceed rapidly to the next step.

7. This filtering procedure might be useful in getting rid of remaining mucus and cell debris. However, loss of viable cells is also likely. Therefore a balance needs to be achieved between the requested cell number and the purity of the cell suspension.

8. Of 2 mL blood one can expect between 1.0 and 10.0×10^6 MNC/mL, depending on the patient's age (i.e., newborns have much higher MNC numbers than adults), and of one pinch biopsy between 0.2 and 1.5×10^6 MNC/mL. In case of small mucosal specimens, there are often only few remaining cells. To count these, it is therefore easier to resuspend them in 200 μL of medium only and to have thus a higher concentration of cells per volume. One has then to adjust the final cell count with respect to the diluting volume chosen (i.e., a count of 1.0×10^6 MNC diluted in 200 μL equals 0.2×10^6 MNC diluted in 1000 μL).

9. To match the antibody concentration required per well, the aforementioned antibodies have to be diluted as follows:

   a. Primary ("capture") antibodies:

   IFN-γ: 1:10   (80 μL MAb/800 μL PBS for 8 wells = 100 μL diluted MAb/well)

   IL-4, IL-5, IL-10: 1:50   (16 μL MAb/800 μL PBS for 8 wells = 100 μL diluted MAb/well)

   TGF-β: 1:167   (4.8 μL MAb/800 μL PBS for 8 wells = 100 μL diluted MAb/well)

   b. Secondary ("detecting") antibodies:

   IFN-γ: 1:10   (80 μL MAb/800 μL PBS/0.05% Tween, supplemented with 8 μL FCS for 8 wells = 100 μL diluted MAb/well)

   IL-4, IL-5, IL-10: 1:50

   TGF-β: 1:714

10. Antibody is removed by swiftly reversing the plates onto absorbing tissue covering some of the bench. From now on, all working steps should be performed as fast as possible in order not to allow the bottoms of the culture wells to dry, as dried nitrocellulose will reduce the binding of the subsequent reagents. Better leave buffers of the final washes in the wells while preparing the necessary antibodies!

11. Assays involving blood lymphocytes should be performed at least in triplicate for each cytokine (about $1–1.3 \times 10^5$ cells/100 μL). Assays with mucosal cells should be done in duplicate. In contrast to previous reports *(8)*, we found it worthwhile not only to reduce the input of mucosal cells per well, but also to modify the cell input depending on the respective cytokines tested. Since spontaneous secretion of IFN-γ proved to be very high in our studies *(5,6)*, one might add only 0.5–1.0 instead of 5.0–7.0 $\times 10^4$ MNCs/well. Due to this variation, the enumeration of spot-forming cells is more precise and easier to reproduce, since artifactual background staining is minimized. For measurement of IL-4-, IL-5-, and IL-10-secretion, the appropriate cell input ranges from 1.5 to 4.0×10^4/well.

12. It is very important not to put the plates into the CO_2 incubator by mistake, because this can destroy the experiment.

13. It is important that the duration of this incubation be not less than 45 min and not more than 75 min.

14. The frequency of spot-forming cells (SFC)/10^5 input MNCs is derived based on the number of cells placed into the wells. The mean of the duplicate or triplicate experiments, respectively, should be taken as a result. The reproducibility and accuracy of the counts should always be double-checked by a second observer, ideally blinded. If there are abundant spots, a precise count is impossible, but in order to have at least a semiquantitative result, one should only count a quarter of the well's ground and multiply it by four. In such cases, it is worthwhile to blind oneself and do repetitive counts. One should absolutely have an interobserver comparison in such situations.

15. This determination depends on whether such equipment is at hand. One can then follow the technical instructions and the menu for "measurement of optical density." In wells with many homogenously distributed spots, a minimum of 20 random spots should be measured, whereas in wells with fewer spots, each single spot should be analyzed.

References

1. Czerkinsky, C., Nilsson, L.-A., Nygren, H., Ouchterlony, Ö., and Tarkowski, A. (1983) A solid-phase enzyme-linked immunospot (ELISPOT) assay for enumeration of specific antibody-secreting cells. *J. Immunol. Methods* **65,** 109–116.
2. Sedgwick, J. D. and Holt, P. G (1988) ELISA-plaque assay for the detection of single antibody-secreting cells, in *Theoretical and Technical Aspects of ELISA and Other Solid Phase Immunoassays* (Kemeny, D. M. and Challacombe, S. J., eds.), John Wiley, Oxford, pp. 241–257.
3. Versteegen, J. M. T., Logtenberg, T., and Ballieux, R. E. (1988) Enumeration of IFN-γ producing human lymphocytes by spot-ELISA. A method to detect lymphokine-producing lymphocytes at the single cell level. *J. Immunol. Methods* **111,** 25–34.
4. Czerkinsky, C., Anderson, G., Ekre, H.-P., Nilsson, L. A., Klareskog, L., and Ouchterlony, Ö. (1988) Reverse ELISPOT assay for clonal analysis of cytokine production. 1. Enumeration of gamma-interferon-secreting cells. *J. Immunol. Methods* **110,** 29–36.
5. Hauer, A. C., Breese E., Walker-Smith, J. A., and MacDonald, T. T. (1997) The frequency of cells secreting interferon-γ, interleukin-4, interleukin-5 and interleukin-10 in the blood and duodenal mucosa of children with cow's milk hypersensitivity. *Pediatr. Res.* **42,** 629–638.
6. Hauer, A. C., Bajaj-Elliott, M., Williams, C. B., Walker-Smith, J. A., and MacDonald, T. T. (1998) An analysis of interferon-γ, IL-4, IL-5 and IL-10 production by ELISPOT and quantitative reverse transcriptase-PCR in human Peyer's patches. *Cytokine* **10,** 627–634.
7. Culshaw, R. J., Bancroft, G. J., and McDonald, V. (1997) Gut intraepithelial lymphocytes induce immunity against cryptosporidium infection through a mechanism involving gamma interferon production. *Infect. Immun.* **65,** 3074–3079.
8. Karttunen, R., Karttunen, T., Ekre H.-P. T., and MacDonald, T. T. (1994) Interferon-γ and interleukin-4 secreting cells in the gastric antrum in *Helicobacter pylori*-positive and negative gastritis. *Gut* **36,** 341–345.
9. Hauer, A. C., Griessl, A., Riederer, M., and MacDonald, T. T. (1998) T Helper 2 (TH2) cytokines in the response of newborn human infants to cow's milk proteins. *J. Pediatr. Gastroenterol. Nutr.* **26,** 548.

3

Measurement of Interleukins by ELISPOT Assay with Particular Application to Dual-Color Analysis (Stardust Assay)

Yoshihiro Okamoto and Mikio Nishida

1. Introduction

The ordinary method for quantitative analysis of cytokines consists of measuring cytokines produced and accumulated in the supernatants of short-term cultures, by means of enzyme immunoassay. However, this approach provides only cumulative amounts in a fixed time, thus limiting the sensitivity of the technique, particularly when relatively few cells are producing lymphokines of interest. In addition, this strategy does not permit an estimation of the frequency of corresponding secreting cells.

The method based on immunoenzyme technology was developed for enumerating specific antibody-secreting cells (1). Since its original description, this method, termed an enzyme-linked immunospot assay (ELISPOT assay) or an enzyme-linked immunosorbent (ELISA) plaque assay, has been employed not only to detect antibody-secreting cells but also to enumerate a variety of cytokine-secreting cells (2–8). This method is a useful tool for quantitative analysis of cytokines at the single cell level. In fact, many researchers have reported significant results in cytokine research by using ELISPOT assay (9–17).

The schematic features of the technique for the detection of cytokine-secreting cells are illustrated in **Fig. 1**. The method is normally performed in a nitrocellulose-backed multiwell plate. Putative cytokine-secreting cells are added to wells that have been precoated with a capture-antibody specific for the cytokine. After an appropriate incubation time, the cells are removed and the site of secretion is revealed by addition of enzyme-coupled reagents, followed by a substrate that yields an insoluble product. Spots reveal the cytokine-secretion by single cells.

From: *Methods in Molecular Medicine, vol. 60: Interleukin Protocols*
Edited by: L. A. J. O'Neill and A. Bowie © Humana Press Inc., Totowa, NJ

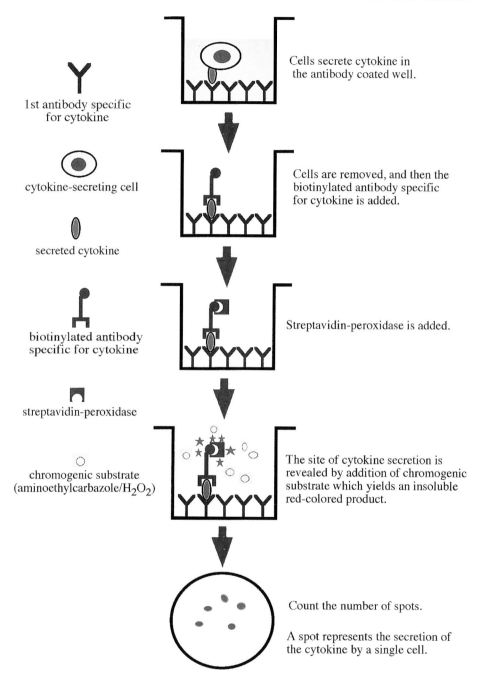

Fig. 1. Ordinal ELISPOT assay-procedure for detection and enumeration of cytokine-secreting cells.

In the present article, first a fundamental (ordinary) ELISPOT assay is described, and second a new device enabling simultaneous assay for plural numbers of cytokines is described.

2. Materials
2.1. Reagents and Buffers

1. Capture (first) antibody: Monoclonal antibody specific for the cytokine of interest. Many kinds of monoclonal antibodies specific for cytokines are commercially available.
2. Biotinylated anti-cytokine detecting antibody: Many kinds of biotinylated mono-clonal/polyclonal antibodies specific for cytokines are commercially available.
3. Streptavidin-horseradish peroxidase (HRP) (GIBCO BRL).
4. 30% Hydrogen peroxide (H_2O_2).
5. Bovine serum albumin (BSA).
6. Cell culture medium, e.g., RPMI-1640 containing 10% heat-inactivated fetal bovine serum (FBS).
7. Phosphate-buffered saline (PBS): Dissolve 80 g NaCl, 2.0 g KCl, 11.5 g Na_2HPO_4 and 2.0 g KH_2PO_4 in 900 mL distilled water (dH_2O). Check pH and adjust to 7.4 with 1 M NaOH if necessary. Make volume up to 1 L with dH_2O. Store at room temperature. Dilute 1 in 10 with dH_2O for use.
8. 0.05% Tween-20 in PBS (PBS-T): Add 0.5 mL Tween-20 to 1 L diluted PBS from above.
9. Blocking solution: 5% BSA in PBS.
10. 0.1 M sodium acetate buffer, pH 5.0: Add 148 mL 0.2 M acetic acid (=11.55 mL glacial acetic acid/L of dH_2O) to 352 mL of 0.2 M sodium acetate. Bring up to 1 L in dH_2O. Adjust pH to 5.0. Store at room temperature.
11. Substrate solution: Add 10 mg 3-amino-9-ethylcarbazole (AEC) to 1 mL of dimethylformamide (DMF) in a glass tube. Dissolve well. Add 30 mL 0.1 M sodium acetate buffer (pH 5.0). Pass through 0.45-µm filter to remove insoluble materials. Add 16 µL of 30% H_2O_2 immediately before use. The substrate solution should be prepared immediately before use and protected from light whenever possible. It is also possible to purchase commercial AEC substrate kit (e.g., from Vector).

2.2. Equipment

1. 37°C CO_2 incubator: It is important that the incubator be absolutely leveled to prevent cells from rolling to one side of the well.
2. Microscope (magnification; ×10–×40).
3. 96-well nitrocellulose-backed plate (Millipore Multiscreen HA plate).
4. Plate seal (Sumitomo Bakelite, Tokyo, Japan).

3. Methods
3.1. Basic ELISPOT Assay

1. Dilute first antibody to 2–10 µg/mL in PBS. Coat the wells of a 96-well nitrocel-lulose-backed plate with 100 µL diluted antibody per well (*see* **Notes 1** and **2**).

2. Seal the plate with Plate seal to prevent evaporation. Incubate overnight at 4°C.
3. Wash the plate three times with PBS-T (*see* **Note 3**).
4. Add 300 µL blocking solution.
5. Incubate for 2 h at room temperature.
6. Wash the plate three times with PBS.
7. Prepare cell suspension at different concentrations, e.g., 1×10^5 cells/mL, 2×10^4 cells/mL, and 4×10^3 cells/mL. Add 100 µL of each cell suspension per well, in triplicate (*see* **Notes 4** and **5**).
8. Incubate at 37°C in 5% CO_2 for 18 h (*see* **Note 5**).
9. Wash the plate five times with PBS-T.
10. Dilute biotinylated anti-cytokine detecting antibody to 2–5 µg/mL in PBS-T containing 1% BSA. Add 100 µL/well.
11. Seal the plate to prevent evaporation. Incubate overnight at 4°C.
12. Wash the plate five times with PBS-T.
13. Dilute streptavidin-peroxidase accurately to manufacturer's recommendation (e.g., GIBCO BRL, diluted 1:1000) in PBS-T containing 1% BSA. Add 100 µL per well (*see* **Note 6**).
14. Seal the plate to prevent evaporation. Incubate for 2 h at room temperature.
15. Wash the plate five times with PBS-T.
16. Add 100 µL of substrate solution to each well. Wait for maximal red spots to develop (this takes 5–30 min) at room temperature and under light protection.
17. Wash the plate with water. Remove the supporting manifold of the plate and air-dry plate for 30–60 min at room temperature. This helps reduce the background of each well.
18. Count the number of spots in each well under low magnification (approx ×40) with a microscope. A typical profile of an ELISPOT assay with AEC/H_2O_2 substrate is shown in **Fig. 2** (*see* **Notes 7–9**).

3.2. Useful Variation of ELISPOT Assay (Stardust Assay)

Variations of the ELISPOT assay have been developed by some investigators including us *(18–24)*. Recently we have developed a dual-color ELISPOT assay *(20)*, which was named the Stardust assay, by improving an ordinary ELISPOT assay described above. This new method enabled us to analyze two kinds of cytokine-secreting cells simultaneously. T-helper (Th) cells can be subdivided into at least two distinct functional subsets based on their cytokine secretion profiles *(25)*. The first type of clone (Th1) produces interleukin-2 (IL-2) and interferon-γ (IFN-γ), but not IL-4 or IL-5. The second type of clone (Th2) produces IL-4 and IL-5, but not IL-2 or IFN-γ. Furthermore, the presence of the third type (Th0) cell, which is a precursor of Th1 or Th2 cells, has been demonstrated to produce both Th1- and Th2-type cytokines *(26,27)*. The Stardust assay enabled us to differentiate these three subtypes of Th- cells in an identical well:

1. Coat a 96-well nitrocellulose-backed microtiter plate with 100 µL of the coating antibody mixture including an anti-mouse IL-2 monoclonal antibody (5 µg/mL;

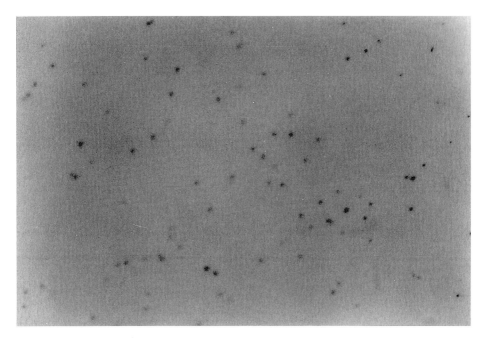

Fig. 2. Typical appearance obtained by ordinal ELISPOT assay. Spleen cells prepared from normal mice were added to anti-mouse IL-12 p35 monoclonal antibody (Genzyme) coated well. After an 18-h incubation at 37°C in a humidified atmosphere of 5% CO_2, spots were developed by sequential incubation with biotinylated anti-mouse IL-12 p70/p40 monoclonal antibody (Genzyme), streptavidin-HRP (GIBCO BRL) and chromogenic substrate (AEC/H_2O_2) (original magnification ×40).

Genzyme, Cambridge, MA) and an anti-mouse IL-4 monoclonal antibody (5 μg/mL, clone BVD4-1D11; Pharmingen, San Diego, CA) in PBS.

2. Seal the plate with Plate seal to prevent evaporation. Incubate overnight at 4°C.
3. Wash the plate three times with PBS-T (*see* **Note 3**).
4. Add 300 μL of blocking solution.
5. Incubate for 2 h at room temperature.
6. Wash the plate three times with PBS.
7. Prepare cell suspension at different concentrations, e.g., 1×10^5 cells/mL, 2×10^4 cells/mL, and 4×10^3 cells/mL. Add 100 μL of each cell suspension per well, in triplicate (*see* **Notes 4** and **5**).
8. Incubate at 37°C in 5% CO_2 for 18 h (*see* **Note 5**).
9. Wash the plate five times with PBS-T.
10. Add 100 μL of the detection antibody mixture including a rabbit polyclonal antibody for mouse IL-2 (2 μg/mL; Becton Dickinson, Bedford, MA) and a biotinylated monoclonal antibody for mouse IL-4 (2 μg/mL, clone BVD6-24G2; Pharmingen) in PBS-T containing 1% BSA/well.

11. Seal the plate to prevent evaporation. Incubate overnight at 4°C.
12. Wash the plate five times with PBS-T.
13. Add 100 µL of the mixture including a horseradish peroxidase-conjugated F(ab')$_2$ fragment donkey anti-rabbit IgG(H+L) (diluted 1: 5,000; Jackson ImmunoResearch, West Grove, PA) and a streptavidin-conjugated alkaline phosphatase (diluted 1:2,000, GIBCO BRL) per well.
14. Seal the plate to prevent evaporation. Incubate for 2 h at room temperature.
15. Wash the plate five times with PBS-T.
16. Expose wells to 100 µL of AEC/H$_2$O$_2$ substrate solution (Vector) and examine for red spots to identify IL-2. These reactions are developed for 5–7 min at room temperature.
17. Plates are then rinsed with PBS several times to eliminate excess reagents.
18. Next, 100 µL of the Vector blue substrate solution is added to each well, yielding light blue spots within 10–20 min to stain IL-4. The mixed-colored (indigo) spots correspond to both kinds of cytokine-secreting cells (*see* **Note 10**).
19. Count the number of spots in each well under low magnification (approx ×40) with a microscope.

In the system, the red spots corresponding to IL-2-secreting cells (Th1 cells) were developed with HRP and aminoethylcarbazole (AEC)/H$_2$O$_2$. The light blue spots corresponding to IL-4-secreting cells (Th2 cells) were developed with alkaline phosphatase and Vector blue (chromogenic substrate for alkaline phosphatase). The mixed colored (indigo) spots corresponding to both kinds of cytokine-secreting cells (Th0 cells) were developed with both chromogenic substrates **(Fig. 3)**. A photographic profile of different colored spots resembles "Stardust." Thus we call this technique the Stardust assay. With this system, we could detect the IL-2- and/or IL-4-secreting cells simultaneously in a murine spleen cell preparation **(Fig. 4A,B)**.

Recent studies revealed that the balance of cytokines secreted by different types of cells affected the state and progression of various diseases, including infectious, allergic, and autoimmune disorders *(28)*. This procedure provides a useful tool for quantitatively analyzing microlevels of dynamic immune responses. Practically we analyzed the changes in cytokine balance in collagen-induced arthritic (CIA) mice as an animal experimental model of human rheumatoid arthritis using the Stardust assay. We could obtain the valuable findings that at the prearthritic phase Th1 cells were dominant and after the onset of clinical arthritis there was a shift from a Th1-dominant to a Th2-dominant state (manuscript in preparation). We are now examining the clinical usefulness of the Stardust assay using human peripheral blood cells.

In summary, the ELISPOT assay is an efficient and sensitive technique for the enumeration of single cell-secreting cytokines. The ELISPOT assay and its variation are available to monitor the cytokine balance in diseases and should become one of the most powerful tools for cytokine research.

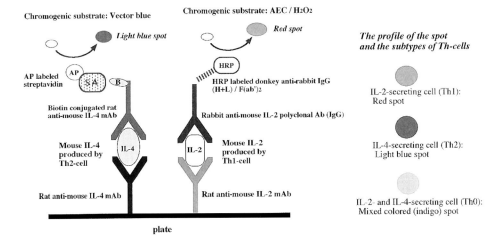

Fig. 3. Schematic representation of a dual-color detection (Stardust assay). Abbreviations: MAb, monoclonal antibody; AP, alkaline phosphatase; HRP, horseradish peroxidase; SA, streptavidin; B, biotin. Reprinted from *Immunopharmacology*, **39**, Okamoto, Y., et al., Development of a dual color enzyme-linked immunospot assay for simultaneous detection of murine T helper type-1- and T helper type 2-cells, pp. 107–116. Copyright 1998, with permission from Elsevier Science *(20)*.

4. Notes

1. Keep reagents and assay plate sterile at **steps 1–8**.
2. Higher concentration of coating antibody may give better results. However, an optimal concentration (usually 2–10 µg/mL) should be found by preliminary experiment.
3. For each wash, fill wells with approx 300 µL PBS(-T), soak for at least 1 min/wash, and invert plate to discard washing solution.
4. Various types of cell specimens are applied to this assay (e.g., spleen, lymph nodes, bone marrow for mice, mononuclear cells in peripheral blood for human, or a cell fraction purified from various sources). The cell suspension is prepared by washing cells extensively with incomplete medium, and then resuspending the cells in medium containing 10% heat-inactivated FBS. The cell specimen should be kept on ice until use. The viability of the cells should be assessed by trypan blue dye exclusion test before use to identify the number of living cells.
5. The optimal cell concentration and optimal time of incubation will differ in individual experiments. The cell specimen is sequentially diluted to detect the appropriate number of spots in a well, and the conditions to produce 10–200 spots/well should be used to count the total number of cytokine-secreting cells per sample. It is difficult to count the number of spots precisely when more than 200 spots per well were developed.
6. Streptavidin-alkaline phosphatase (AP) can be used alternatively for the enzyme-substrate system. As the chromogenic substrate for streptavidin-AP, the substrate

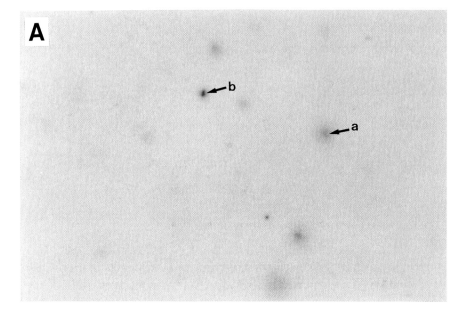

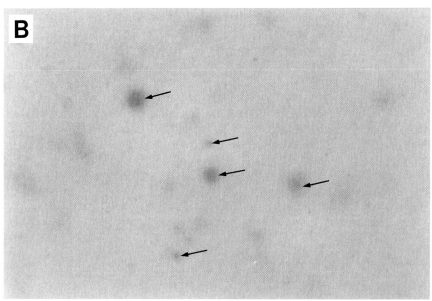

Fig. 4. Typical profile of the dual-color ELISPOT assay well. (**A**) Crude spleen cells of normal BALB/c mice were stimulated with 1 μg/mL Concanavalin A for 18 h. The cells were added to wells coated with the mixture of anti-IL-2 and IL-4 antibody, and subsequently spots were developed by the enzyme-substrate system shown in **Fig. 3.** IL-2-secreting cell is indicated by arrow a, and IL-4-secreting cell is indicated by arrow b (original magnification ×40). (**B**) The ideal spots of Th0 cells. The mixed

mixture including 5-bromo-4-chloro-3-indoryl phosphate (BCIP) and nitro blue tetrazolium (NBT) is commonly used. This enzyme-substrate system develops purple-colored spots in the presence of the cytokine-secreting cell.

7. The color depth or size of spots depends on the amount of secreted cytokines. The strong and well-defined spots should be counted; any small or faint spots are likely to be artifacts and should not be counted.

8. The developed spots would be kept for several weeks if the plates are stored at 4°C under light protection.

9. To confirm specificity of the assay, the experiment using the wells coated with an irrelevant antibody (e.g., in the case of detection of IL-6-secreting cells, an anti-IL-4 antibody coated well should be used) as a negative control should be included.

10. To detect the cells secreting both kinds of cytokines precisely, a reference profile of the double-stained spots (indigo) should be provided in the plate. To obtain the ideal spots corresponding to the cells secreting both kinds of cytokines, the plate was incubated with biotinylated monoclonal antibody for IL-4 and followed by the two kinds of chromogenic system; the mixture of the HRP-labeled and the AP-labeled streptavidin was added to the well after incubation with the biotinylated monoclonal antibody for IL-4. By this procedure, we obtained a typical profile corresponding to the cells secreting both cytokines (*see* **Fig. 4B**).

References

1. Czerkinsky, C., Nilsson, L.-A., Nygren, H., Ouchtarony, O., and Tarkowski, A. (1983) A solid-phase enzyme-linked immunospot assay for enumeration of specific antibody-secreting cells. *J. Immunol. Methods* **65,** 109–121.
2. Czerkinsky, C., Andersson, G., Ekre, H.-P., Nilsson, L.-Å., Klarenskog, L., and Ouchterlony, Ö. (1988) Reverse ELISPOT assay for clonal analysis of cytokine production. I. Enumeration of gamma-interferon-secreting cells. *J. Immunol. Methods* **110,** 29–36.
3. Sedgwick, J. D. and Czerkinsky, C. (1992) Detection of cell-surface molecules, secreted products of single cells and cellular proliferation by enzyme immunoassay. *J. Immunol. Methods* **150,** 159–175.
4. Skidmore, B., Stamnes, S., Townsend, K., Glasebrook, A., Sheehan, K., Schreiber, R., et al. (1989) Enumeration of cytokine-secreting cells at the single-cell level. *Eur. J. Immunol.* **19,** 1591–1597.
5. Taguchi, T., McGhee, J. R., Coffman, R. L., Beagley, K. W., Eldridge, J. H., Takatsu, K., et al. (1990) Detection of individual mouse splenic T cells producing IFN-γ and IL-5 using the enzyme-linked immunospot (ELISPOT) assay. *J. Immunol. Methods* **128,** 65–73.

---

colored spots (indigo) are shown as the ideal profile of the spots corresponding to a Th0 cell (arrows) (original magnification ×40). Reprinted from *Immunopharmacology*, **39**, Okamoto, Y., et al., Development of a dual color enzyme-linked immunospot assay for simultaneous detection of murine T helper type-1- and T helper type 2-cells, pp. 107–116. Copyright 1998, with permission from Elsevier Science (*20*).

6. Versteegen, J., Logtenberg, T., and Ballieux, R. (1988) Enumeration of IFN-gamma-producing human lymphocytes by spot-ELISA. A method to detect lymphokine-producing lymphocytes at the single-cell level. *J. Immunol. Methods* **111,** 25–29.

7. Hutchings, P. R., Cambridge, G., Tite, J. P., Meager, T., and Cooke, A. (1989) The detection and enumeration of cytokine-secreting cells in mice and man and the clinical application of these assays. *J. Immunol. Methods* **120,** 1–8.

8. Fujihashi, K., McGhee, J. R., Beagley, K. W., McPherson, D. T., McPherson, S. A., Huang, C.-M., et al. (1993) Cytokine-specific ELISPOT assay, single cell analysis of IL-2, IL-4 and IL-6 producing cells. *J. Immunol. Methods* **160,** 181–189.

9. Doncarli, A., Stasiuk, L. M., Fournier, C., and Abehsira-Amar, O. (1997) Conversion in vivo from an early dominant Th0/Th1 response to a Th2 phenotype during the development of collagen-induced arthritis. *Eur. J. Immunol.* **27,** 1451–1458.

10. Gabrielsson, S., Soderlund, A., Paulie, S., Rak, S., van der Pouw Kraan, T., and Troye-Blomberg, M. (1998) Increased frequencies of allergen-induced interleukin-13-producing cells in atopic individuals during the pollen season. *Scand. J. Immunol.* **48,** 429–435.

11. Hauer, A., Bajaj-Elliott, M., Williams, C., Walker-Smith, J., and MacDonald, T. (1998) An analysis of interferon gamma, IL-4, IL-5 and IL-10 production by ELISPOT and quantitative reverse transcriptase-PCR in human Peyer's patches. *Cytokine* **10,** 627–634.

12. Hiroi, T., Fujihashi, K., McGhee, J., and Kiyono, H. (1994) Characterization of cytokine-producing cells in mucosal effector sites: CD3$^+$ T cells of Th1 and Th2 type in salivary gland-associated tissues. *Eur. J. Immunol.* **24,** 2653–2658.

13. Okamoto, Y., Nagai, T., Abe, T., Ishikawa, S., Ishizuka, H., and Nishida, M. (1998) Unchanged cytokine production under exposure of excess manganese. *Biomed. Res.* **9,** 179–185.

14. Shirai, A., Holmes, K., and Klinman, D. (1993) Detection and quantitation of cells secreting IL-6 under physiologic conditions in BALB/c mice. *J. Immunol.* **150,** 793–799.

15. Shirai, A., Conover, J., and Klinman, D. M. (1995) Increased activation and altered ratio of interferon-gamma: interleukin-4 secreting cells in MRL-lpr/lpr mice. *Autoimmunity* **21,** 107–116.

16. Stallmach, A., Schafer, F., Hoffmann, S., Weber, S., Muller-Molaian, I., Schneider, T., et al. (1998) Increased state of activation of CD4 positive T cells and elevated interferon gamma production in pouchitis. *Gut* **43,** 499–505.

17. van der Meide, P. H., Joosten, A. M., Hermans, P., Kloosterman, T. C., Olsson, T., and de Labie, M. C. D. C. (1991) Assesment of the inhibitory effect of immunosuppressive agents on rat T cell interferon-γ production using an ELISPOT assay. *J. Immunol. Methods* **144,** 203–213.

18. Okamoto, Y., Murakami, H., and Nishida, M. (1997) Detection of interleukin-6 producing cells among the various organs in normal mice with an improved enzyme-linked immunospot (ELISPOT) assay. *Endocrine J.* **44,** 349–355.

19. Nordstrom, I. and Ferrua, B. (1992) Reverse ELISPOT assay for clonal analysis of cytokine production. II. Enumeration of interleukin-1-secreting cells by amplified (avidin-biotin anti-peroxidase) assay. *J. Immunol. Methods* **150,** 199–206.

20. Okamoto, Y., Abe, T., Niwa, T., Mizuhashi, S., and Nishida, M. (1998) Development of a dual color enzyme-linked immunospot (ELISPOT) assay for murine T helper type I (Th1)- and T helper type II (Th2)-cells. *Immunopharmacology* **39,** 107–116.

21. Shirai, A., Sierra, V., Kelly, C. I., and Klimman, D. M. (1994) Individual cells simultaneously produce both IL-4 and IL-6 in vivo. *Cytokine* **6,** 329–336.

22. Tanguay, S. and Killion, J. J. (1994) Direct comparison of ELISPOT and ELISA-based assays for detection of individual cytokine-secreting cells. *Lymphokine Cytokine Res.* **13,** 259–263.

23. Vaquerano, J., Peng, M., Chang, J., Zhou, Y., and Leong, S. (1998) Digital quantification of the enzyme-linked immunospot (ELISPOT). *Biotechniques* **25,** 830–836.

24. Ronnelid, J. and Klareskog, L. (1997) A comparison between ELISPOT methods for the detection of cytokine producing cells: greater sensitivity and specificity using ELISA plates as compared to nitrocellulose membranes. *J. Immunol. Methods* **200,** 17–26.

25. Mosmann, T. R., Cherwinski, H., Bond, M. W., Giedlin, M. A., and Coffman, R. L. (1986) Two types of murine helper T-cell clone. I. Definition according to profiles of lymphokine activities and secreted proteins. *J. Immunol.* **136,** 2348–2357.

26. Street, N. E., Schumacher, J. H., Fong, T. A. T., Bass, H., Fiorentino, D. F., Leverah, J. A., et al. (1990) Heterogeneity of mouse helper T cell: evidence from bulk cultures and limiting dilution cloning for precursors of Th1 and Th2 cells. *J. Immunol.* **144,** 1629–1639.

27. Firestein, G. S., Roeder, W. D., Laxer, J. A., Townsend, K. S., Weaver, C. T., Hom, J. T., et al. (1989) A new murine CD4+ T cell subset with an unrestricted cytokine profile. *J. Immunol.* **143,** 518–525.

28. Abbas, A. K., Murphy, K. M., and Sher, A. (1996) Functional diversity of helper T lymphocytes. *Nature* **383,** 787–793.

4

Assaying Interleukins Intracellularly by FACS

Liam O'Mahony and Maurice O'Donoghue

1. Introduction

From their genesis as instruments designed to count and size particles, flow cytometers have, over the last 40 years, evolved into a range of sophisticated instruments. These instruments are now used widely in all branches of biologic science. Originally, the preserve of the research laboratory, flow cytometers are now playing an increasingly important role in both clinical and industrial laboratories.

Flow cytometry is the measurement of chemical and/or physical properties of particles as they flow through a detector in a controlled manner. These characteristics, in the case of biologic specimens, include cell size, granularity, RNA and DNA content, cell surface and intracellular antigens, intracellular pH and Ca^{2+} ion levels, receptors, and cellular enzyme activity. Flow cytometry is a powerful technique because it allows the measurement of several parameters from large numbers of single cells in a short time. Typical analyses are performed at between 100 and 300 cells/s. Flow cytometric analysis is based on fluorescence and the light scattering properties of the cells being analyzed. This analysis is performed in an instrument that combines lasers, fluidics, filters and light detectors, electronics, computers, and associated software. The analysis also relies on the use of monoclonal antibodies, dye chemistry, and, in more recent times, molecular biology.

The flow cytometer consists of a number of integrated components. These include a light source or sources, flow cell, optical elements to detect light of different wavelengths, detectors/signal amplifiers, signal processing, and data analysis systems including computers and software. The most commonly used laser light source is the Argon ion laser, which emits light at 488 nm. This laser emits light in the blue region of the spectrum and excites many of the dyes

From: *Methods in Molecular Medicine, vol. 60: Interleukin Protocols*
Edited by: L. A. J. O'Neill and A. Bowie © Humana Press Inc., Totowa, NJ

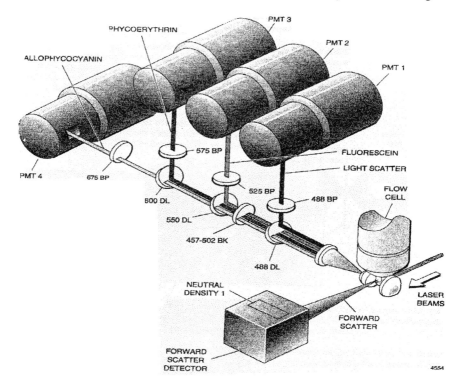

Fig. 1. Diagrammatic illustration of a typical optical arrangement of a flow cytometer comprising filters, PMTs, and a flow cell.

routinely used in flow cytometry. These dyes include fluorescein, phycoerythrein, tandem dyes such as Cy-5, all of which are used in immunofluorescence applications, and other dyes such as the DNA binding dye propidium iodide. Because of the range of dyes excited by this laser, it allows multiparametric analyses to be performed on a single laser instrument. The most commonly used flow cell is a quartz chamber, containing a channel of 100–250 μm. The flow cell is usually positioned at right angles to the laser beam. Placing the flow cell in this position allows the measurement of fluorescence and scattered light over a wide angle and also allows the measurement of forward light scatter.

In a flow cytometer, cells labeled with a fluorescent compound pass through the laser beam, causing light to be scattered in a particular manner and the fluorescent compound to be excited, with the concomitant production of light of a particular wavelength. This scattered light and fluorescence are then collected by photomultiplier tubes (PMTs) or photodiode detectors. These signals are amplified and converted to digital signals, which can be captured and analyzed by computer (**Fig. 1**).

Table 1
Useful Flow Cytometry Websites[a]

http://www.wiley.com
http://pingu.salk.edu/fcm.html
http://www.bio.umass.edu/mcbfacs/flowhome.html
http://www.isac-net.org/-isac
http://www.probes.com

[a]Many Internet sites contain useful information about flow cytometry and intracellular staining. These are examples of some useful sites.

The computer captures the data generated by the cytometer, which can be analyzed in various ways using the appropriate software. Individual populations of cells can be selected for analysis by electronic gating. A single experiment can therefore yield a substantial amount of data.

The currently available and still expanding range of monoclonal antibodies to leukocyte antigens, referred to as CD (cluster designation) markers, allows extensive analysis of lymphocytes and lymphocyte subsets. The simultaneous measurement of these markers (with monoclonal antibodies coupled to different fluorescent tags) by flow cytometry allows for the rapid, accurate identification of different cellular subsets and their activation status. In addition to these cell surface markers, intracellular processes, such as cytokine production, are critical to cellular activation. Furthermore, the cytokine profile of the cells in question is critical to the type of immune response being induced, e.g., T helper (Th)1/Th2.

Cytokines are small-molecular-weight proteins that exert powerful biologic effects. A large number of cytokines, and their corresponding receptors, have been characterized, and their study has relevance to normal body homeostasis and many disease pathologies. Therefore, methods for accurate measurement of cytokine levels and the cell types responsible for their production are continuously under development. The application of flow cytometry to this field of study is a recent one. However, the exploitation of this technology for cytokine measurement has yielded more than 400 peer-reviewed published articles and enormous commercial success for companies marketing these antibodies and staining systems. A number of useful web sites can be examined for further information on intracellular staining techniques, monoclonal antibodies, and flow cytometers (**Table 1**).

The bulk of previously published work on quantification of cytokine levels has concentrated on measuring cytokine production using cytokine-sensitive cell lines as biosensors or by bulk release assays, such as enzyme-linked immunoassays (ELISAs) and radioimmunoassays (*1–3*). Although these assay systems are useful in determining the total amount of cytokine being produced, they are prone to interference from naturally occurring biologic inhibitors, which can mask the amount of cytokine that is present *(4,5)*. Quantification of pooled cytokine levels using ELISAs can be misleading, as many complicating factors influence detection with this assay system. Specific binding proteins exist for a number of cytokines, including autoantibodies, α_2-macroglobulin, heterophilic antibodies, and soluble cytokine receptors, all of which interfere with cytokine detection. Furthermore, many of the methods employed in the quantification of cytokine levels in body fluids and culture supernatants do not allow identification of the cytokine-producing cell type, without prior separation of the different subpopulations.

Intracellular cytokine detection, using flow cytometry, avoids the influence of the extracellular milieu, and monoclonal antibodies to cell surface markers (such as CD3 for T cells and CD14 for monocytes) can be used to identify the cellular origin of cytokine production. Both qualitative and quantitative analysis can be performed. Qualitative intracellular proinflammatory cytokine methods examine the percentage of cells producing a specific cytokine *(6,7)*. Quantitative intracellular cytokine staining involves measuring the amount of cytokine being produced per cellular population (using median fluorescence intensity [MFI]). The primary difference between these two methods is the use of artificial inhibitors of cytokine export such as monensin and brefeldin A *(8,9)*. Preincubation of cells with these inhibitors results in accumulation of intracellular cytokine levels, thus facilitating detection. However, this methodology does not allow quantification of intracellular cytokine levels as the amount of cytokine present has been artificially amplified. By avoiding the use of export inhibitors, the levels of intracellular cytokine at a given time point, rather than the accumulated product, are measured.

A number of essential steps are necessary for intracellular cytokine staining by flow cytometry. Cells need to be fixed initially and then permeabilized to allow access to the intracellular space. Paraformaldehyde is the fixative of choice, as membrane stability and cell morphology are preserved, thus retaining the light-scattering properties required for the flow cytometric identification of different cell types. The most common agent used for permeabilization is saponin. Saponins are plant glycosides that replace cholesterol in cell membranes forming ring-shaped structures with central pores, thus allowing access to the intracellular compartment. Antibodies to cytoskeletal components normally expressed by the cell type in question, such as vimentin, can be utilized to confirm cellular permeabilization.

2. Materials

1. Brefeldin A (Sigma): Store aliquots of reconstituted brefeldin A at –20°C.
2. Monensin (Sigma): Extremely toxic; store aliquots of reconstituted monensin at –20°C.
3. Monoclonal antibodies (R&D Systems, Dako, etc.): All monoclonal antibodies have to be handled with care. Antibodies must be stored in the dark at 4°C.

4. Normal human serum (NHS): This was routinely generated in-house. Briefly, 10 mL of serum from 10 healthy adult volunteers were heat inactivated at 56°C for 30 min. Serum was pooled from all volunteers, aliquoted, and stored at –20°C until required.
5. Phosphate-buffered saline (PBS), pH 7.4: Dissolve 80 g NaCl, 2.0 g KCl, 11.5 g Na_2HPO_4, and 2.0 g KH_2PO_4 in 900 mL distilled water. Adjust pH to 7.4 with 1 M NaOH if necessary. Make volume up to 1 L with distilled water. Store at room temperature. Dilute 1 in 10 with distilled water for use.
6. Paraformaldehyde (PFA; Sigma): Powdered form is irritating upon inhalation. When reconstituting in PBS, make up a stock solution (10% [w/v]) and incubate in a 37°C waterbath overnight to ensure complete reconstitution.
7. 0.05% (w/v) saponin (Sigma) in PBS: Extremely unstable and should only be used on the day of reconstitution in PBS. Keep on ice.
8. Goat anti-mouse fluorescein isothiocyanate (FITC; Dako): Use 2.0 µg/test.
9. Normal mouse serum (Dako).
10. Phycoerythrin (PE)-labeled cell surface antibodies (R&D Systems).

3. Methods

A typical qualitative intracellular cytokine staining method for peripheral blood mononuclear cells is provided below. For quantitative analysis, do not incubate the cells with cytokine export inhibitors prior to staining. **Step 6** is omitted when the intracellular antibodies have been preconjugated to the appropriate fluorochrome.

1. Lymphocytes are stained for cytokine levels following culture with 25 ng/mL PMA. Four hours prior to staining, the cells are incubated with cytokine export blockers such as brefeldin A (10 µg/mL) or monensin (*see* **Note 1**).
2. Cells (1 mL of 1×10^6 cells/mL) are harvested by centrifugation (1200 rpm, 10 min, 4°C) fixed with 5 mL of 2% PFA in PBS, and incubated for 15 min at room temperature (RT). These cells are washed with saponin and centrifuged as above (*see* **Note 2**).
3. Supernatants are decanted and the cells are gently resuspended. The saponin wash is repeated.
4. The cells are resuspended in 1.8 mL saponin/0.2 L NHS, to block nonspecific binding sites, and incubated for 30 min at 4°C.
5. Cells (100 µL) are transferred into fluorescence-activated cell sorting (FACS) tubes, which already contain the relevant anticytokine antibodies (0.2 µg/test), mixed, and incubated for 15 min at RT.
6. Cells are washed by centrifugation with 1 mL saponin and resuspended in 100 µL of a 1/50 dilution of goat anti-mouse FITC, made up in saponin/10% NHS, and incubated for 15 min at RT in the dark.
7. Following another washing step with 1 mL saponin, the cells are resuspended in 100 µL of a 1/50 dilution of normal mouse serum in saponin and incubated for 10 min at RT in the dark.
8. The cells are washed again, and 5 µL of the PE-labeled cell surface antibodies are pipetted into each tube and incubated for 15 min at RT in the dark.

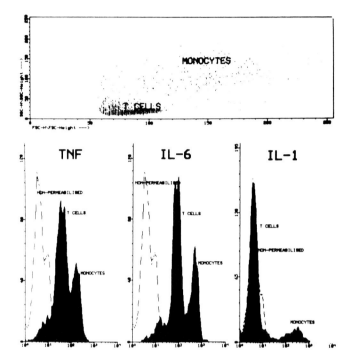

Fig. 2. Dot plots and histograms representing intracellular cytokine levels in T cells and monocytes. The distinct populations were gated in dot plots using the cell surface markers CD3 and CD14, respectively. Using the histograms, intracellular fluorescence was measured. The ordinate relates to the relative cell number, and fluorescence intensity can be seen on the abscissa, representing the amount of intracellular cytokine. A shift to the right demonstrates an increase in the amount of cytokine within a cell. Peaks can be observed for nonpermeabilized cells, T cells, and monocytes.

9. The cells are washed with 1 mL saponin and resuspended in 0.5 mL 0.5% PFA, which facilitates storage for up to 5 d in the dark at 4°C. Specific intracellular and cell surface fluorescence is measured using a flow cytometer.
10. Dot plots and histograms are generated using the T-cell (CD3-positive) or monocyte (CD14-positive) regions (**Fig. 2**). The percentage of cytokine-producing cells is estimated from these dot plots; single parameter histograms allow measurement of intracellular cytokine levels using median fluorescent intensity (*see* **Note 3**).

Owing to the development and availability of increasing numbers of dyes to measure various internal cellular processes and monoclonal antibodies directed against internal and cell surface antigens, the applications for flow cytometry are increasing rapidly. Indeed, active research is directed toward developing flow cytometers that are portable and capable of performing varied analyses, for near-patient use. Accurate measurement of cytokine production is becoming

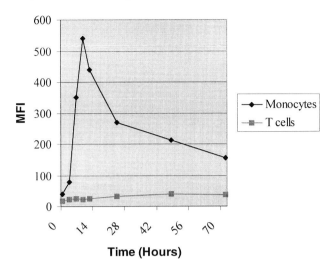

Fig. 3. The intracellular production of cytokines is temporally regulated in different cell types. Intracellular monocyte TNF production, following PMA stimulation, increases rapidly up to 9 h and decreases thereafter. Intracellular T-cell TNF levels increase slowly over the 72-h culture period. Thus, measurement of intracellular cytokine production must be examined at a number of different time points to ensure optimal staining.

increasingly important in understanding the genesis of chronic inflammatory disease, allergies, and the increased pathologies associated with certain infections. Using flow cytometry to monitor cytokine receptor expression, particularly intracellular cytokine expression in lymphocytes involved in an immune response, the Th1/Th2 path being taken by the lymphocytes can be determined. Knowing this, specific immunomodulators may be selected as therapeutic agents.

4. Notes

1. The specific length of time that cells are stimulated to produce cytokines prior to intracellular staining depends on a number of factors. The cell type, manner of stimulation, and specific cytokine in question should all be considered. For example, an experiment covering many different time points for both intracellular and extracellular production should be performed. We have examined intracellular cytokine levels over a 72-h culture period (*10*). Tumor necrosis factor-α (TNF-α) was used as the model cytokine due to its potent proinflammatory role. A rapid increase in intracellular monocyte TNF-α was observed following PMA stimulation (**Fig. 3**). After 9 h, intracellular monocyte cytokine levels began to fall. A modest increase in intracellular T-cell TNF-α levels was also observed, and this occurred later than in monocytes. Thus, time-course studies must be undertaken when initially examining intracellular cytokine levels in order to determine the optimal staining time points.

2. It is important to note that saponin must be included in all steps, as permeabilization with saponin is reversible. In addition, gentle handling of saponin-permeabilized cells is essential as prolonged agitation results in cell lysis.

3. A number of steps are necessary to authenticate the validity of this methodology. To confirm the intracellular origin of cytokine production, the specific cytokine in question should be added to culture supernatants 30 min prior to staining. Addition of extracellular cytokines should not interfere with intracellular cytokine staining. Antibody specificity is determined by preincubating these antibodies with their respective cytokine. A significant decrease in fluorescence intensity should be observed following preincubation with the appropriate cytokine.

References

1. Balkwill, F., Osborne, R., Burke, F., Naylor, S., Talbot, D., Durbin, H., et al. (1987) Evidence for tumor necrosis factor/cachectin production in cancer. *Lancet* **28,** 1229–1232.

2. Nakazaki, H. (1992) Preoperative and postoperative cytokines in patients with cancer. *Cancer* **70,** 709–713.

3. Oka, M., Yamamoto, K., Takahashi, M., Hakozaki, M., Abe, T., Iizuka, N., et al. (1996) Relationship between serum levels of interleukin 6, various disease parameters and malnutrition in patients with esophageal squamous cell carcinoma. *Cancer Res.* **56,** 2776–2780.

4. Cannon, J. G., Nerad, J. L., Poutsiaka, D. D., and Dinarello, C. A. (1993) Measuring circulating cytokines. *J. Appl. Physiol.* **75,** 1897–1902.

5. de Kossodo, S., Houba, V., and Grau, G. E. (1995) Assaying tumor necrosis factor concentrations in human serum. A WHO International Collaborative study. *J. Immunol. Methods* **182,** 107–114.

6. Hallden, G., Andersson, U., Hed, J., and Johansson, S. G. (1989) A new membrane permeabilization method for the detection of intracellular antigens by flow cytometry. *J. Immunol. Methods* **124,** 103–109.

7. Jung, T., Schauer, U., Heusser, C., Neumann, C., and Rieger, C. (1993) Detection of intracellular cytokines by flow cytometry. *J. Immunol. Methods* **159,** 197–207.

8. Ferrick, D. A., Schrenzel, M. D., Mulvania, T., Hsieh, B., Ferlin, W. G., and Lepper, H. (1995) Differential production of interferon-gamma and interleukin-4 in response to Th1- and Th2-stimulating pathogens by gamma delta T cells in vivo. *Nature* **373,** 255–257.

9. North, M. E., Ivory, K., Funauchi, M., Webster, A. D., Lane, A. C., and Farrant, J. (1996) Intracellular cytokine production by human CD4+ and CD8+ T cells from normal and immunodeficient donors using directly conjugated anti-cytokine antibodies and three-colour flow cytometry. *Clin. Exp. Immunol.* **105,** 517–522.

10. O'Mahony, L., Holland, J., Jackson, J., Feighery, C., Hennessy, T. P., and Mealy, K. (1998) Quantitative intracellular cytokine measurement: age-related changes in proinflammatory cytokine production. *Clin. Exp. Immunol.* **113,** 213–219.

5

Basic RT-PCR for Measurement of Cytokine Expression

Mona Bajaj-Elliott and Almuth Christine Hauer

1. Introduction

As an alternative to the ELISPOT assay described in previous chapters, the expression of known cytokines can be analyzed at the mRNA level. Although expression of mRNA for a particular cytokine does not imply corresponding expression of the protein, both techniques in combination provide important, specific information in a short time. Since the late 1980s, the polymerase chain reaction (PCR), a powerful and exquisitely sensitive technique, has revolutionized studies of rare mRNA molecules including analyses of cytokines in immune-mediated diseases.

As originally developed, the PCR process amplified short segments (approx 100–500 bp) of a longer DNA molecule; since the enzymes catalyzing this process require a DNA template, the technique was limited to the analysis of DNA samples (1). However, in many instances amplification of the mRNA is preferred, especially in analyses of differential expression of genes in tissues, e.g., during development or inflammation (2,3). In order to apply PCR technology to the study of mRNA expression, the RNA must therefore first be transcribed to its complementary DNA (cDNA) sequence to provide the essential template for the polymerase enzymes. This process is called reverse transcription (RT), hence the name RT-PCR.

The process of RT-PCR may be divided into three general steps. Initially, good-quality RNA must be obtained from the tissue of interest (biopsies, cell lines in culture, blood lymphocytes). Isolation of intact full-length total RNA is the most crucial step in the whole procedure as it is the quality of RNA that dictates the outcome of the analysis. We routinely use a simple, one-step procedure that allows processing of multiple samples in a short period, mak-

From: *Methods in Molecular Medicine, vol. 60: Interleukin Protocols*
Edited by: L. A. J. O'Neill and A. Bowie © Humana Press Inc., Totowa, NJ

ing the protocol feasible when dealing with large number of clinical samples. In our experience further isolation of the mRNA from the total RNA preparation is generally not required for the analysis of cytokine mRNA expression by RT-PCR.

The second step is production of DNA copies of the RNA template by viral reverse transcriptases. This process requires a primer (which may be sequence specific for a particular molecule of interest or nonspecific, such as random hexamers or oligo dT, the latter binding to the polyA tail of all mRNA molecules) for initial annealing to the RNA, appropriate buffer, deoxynucleotide triphosphates (dNTPs; the building blocks of the newly synthesized DNA copies), and the enzyme. The resulting cDNA is subsequently amplified in a PCR reaction.

The PCR reaction itself can be subdivided into three stages (**Fig. 1**). Initially, the two strands of the DNA molecules must be denatured and separated to allow recognition by and subsequent binding of the two sequence-specific primers on the two opposite strands of DNA. This *denaturation* occurs by incubating the reaction mix at high temperature (approx 94°C), followed by *annealing* of the primers at an optimum temperature (generally between 55 and 72°C, as dictated by the base composition of the primers and the ionic strength of the reaction mix). Once specific annealing has occurred, the *extension* of the strand is generally carried out at 72°C, the optimum temperature for the thermostable polymerases. This series of different temperature reactions is referred to as a cycle of amplification. As theoretically each PCR cycle doubles the amount of targeted template sequence, 10 cycles should multiply the target sequence by a factor of a 1000; and 20 cycles by a 1,000,000, leading to the synthesis of enough PCR product that it can be visualized by gel electrophoresis either by staining or blotting techniques.

The major advantage of the technique is the speed and the sensitivity, which allows detection of rare mRNA species in cells provided the sequence of the target RNA is known. Although great advances have been made in recent years, the major disadvantage still lies in the quantitation of the PCR product. Because of limitations of space, it is beyond the scope of this chapter to discuss the latest advances in the field; however, technical tips published regularly in journals such as *Trends in Biochemical Sciences* are recommended to the reader.

2. Materials

The success of any RNA preparation is critically dependent on the elimination of ribonuclease (RNase) contamination. RNases, especially of pancreatic origin, are extremely stable enzymes resistant to pH changes and heating. Although the amount of RNases will differ between different cell types, they are present in virtually all cell types. Thus, when isolating and working with RNA, the solutions and glassware should be rendered RNase free. Whenever possible, sterile disposable plasticware should be used. For RNA

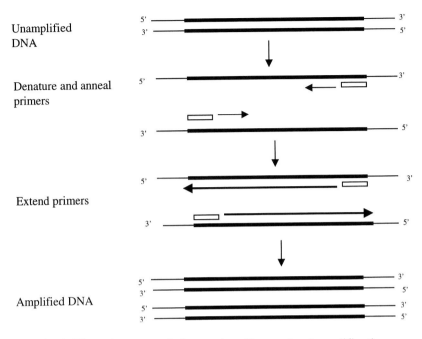

Unamplified
DNA

Denature and anneal
primers

Extend primers

Amplified DNA

Fig. 1. The polymerase chain reaction. One cycle of amplification.

work, all Eppendorf tubes (1.0 mL/0.5 mL, blue/yellow tips) should be removed from a new unopened bag (as delivered from the manufacturer) and autoclaved. Changing tips between each sample and each manipulation is *necessary* to avoid cross-contamination and false positives.

Most of the solutions in our protocol are received from the manufacturers ready to be used directly, so no pretreatment to inhibit RNAses is required. If any nonsterile solution or buffer requires RNAase inhibition, we follow the established method of incubating the solution in 0.1% diethylpyrocarbonate (DEPC) overnight and autoclaving the solution to inactivate completely any remaining DEPC (for details, *see* **refs. *4* and *5***). The reagents required for RNA isolation and RT-PCR are as follows:

2.1. Total RNA Extraction

1. TriZOL (Life Technologies, Paisley, UK).
2. Molecular biology grade chloroform and isopropanol (Sigma, Poole, UK).
3. Mini-Pestles (BDH, UK).
4. DEPC-treated RNase-free water (treated in the lab) or nuclease-free water available commercially (BDH, UK).
5. TE buffer: 1 mM EDTA, 10 mM Tris-HCl, pH 8.0. Both reagents can be made as individual stock solutions, e.g., 1 M Tris-HCl, pH 8.0, and 0.5 M EDTA, pH 8.0, autoclaved and stored at room temperature. Molecular biology grade Tris-base and EDTA are widely available (e.g., Sigma).

2.2. Reverse Transcription

1. Oligo dT (Amersham-Pharmacia, Bucks, UK): Dissolve the lyophilized oligo dT in RNase-free water to a concentration of 0.5 μg/μL and store in small aliquots at –20°C until use.
2. 10 mM dNTPs (Amersham-Pharmacia): The 100 mM stock of the four individual dNTPs is thawed on ice, and a 10 mM working stock is made as follows: 100 μL of each dNTP (dCTP, dATP, dGTP, dTTP) plus 600 μL of RNase-free water. This 10 mM working stock should be stored at –20°C in small aliquots (20–50 μL) until required. dNTPs are relatively unstable and repeated freeze-thawing is not recommended.
3. Moloney Murine Leukemia Virus (M-MMLV) reverse transcriptase (Life Technologies): The enzyme uses single-stranded RNA or DNA in the presence of a primer (e.g., oligo dT) to synthesize a complementary DNA strand. For general purpose PCR, this is our enzyme of choice, taking cost into account. For more stringent experiments such as cloning of the PCR products, superscript II RNase H-reverse transcriptase, which generally gives higher yields of cDNA and more full-length products, may be the enzyme of choice. The buffer required is provided with the enzyme by the manufacturer.

2.3. Polymerase Chain Reaction

Although the basic principle of the reaction is elegantly simple and straightforward, the reaction itself involves complex kinetic interactions among template, product, primer, nucleotide triphosphates, and the enzyme. Despite this complexity, PCR is a robust technique and will yield amplified products at the end of the reaction. However, adjustments may be required for individual reaction parameters, which may dramatically alter the specificity and yield of the PCR product (basic methodology and applications are detailed in **refs. 6** and **7**).

1. Primer selection: For selection of primers, a number of criteria have to be taken into account. A 20–30-bp unique sequence with a 50–60% GC content is acceptable. Complementary sequences at the end of each primer should be avoided as this may lead to loop and secondary structure formation within the primer or between the primers, encouraging monomer-dimer formation. GC residues at the end of the primers will form stronger H-bonds on annealing (three bonds in contrast to two on an A-T base pairing) with the template, thus increasing specificity, but runs of GCs should be avoided. Also, it is helpful if both primers have similar melting temperatures, which will result in a similar annealing temperature and thus greater specificity. The concentration of primers should range between 0.1 and 1 μM; higher concentration will lead to mispriming and an increase in nonspecific binding. In our laboratory, lyophilized primers are dissolved in RNAse/DNAse-free water at a concentration of 1 μg/μL and stored in aliquots. Working concentrations are 20 pmol/μL (approx 150–200 ng), and this dilution is done in water just prior to use. Repeated freeze thawing of primers is not recommended.

2. Nucleotide triphosphates (dNTPs): Use the same stock as for the RT reactions described in the above section. The working concentration of dNTPs in the PCR reaction is 200 μM, which is sufficient to synthesize 10 μg of DNA in a 100-μL reaction. It is accepted that dNTPs do not seem to affect specificity, but lowering concentration may substantially improve the fidelity of the enzyme.

3. Reaction buffer: There are several buffers available for PCR. The most common buffer used with Taq polymerase contains 50 mM KCl, 10 mM Tris-HCl (pH 8.4), 1.5 mM MgCl$_2$, and 100 μg/mL gelatin. The buffer is usually supplied in a 10 times concentrated form, which needs to be diluted before use. The component with the most dramatic effect on specificity is MgCl$_2$; optimal levels can vary from 0.5 to 5.0 mM. The ion has a dual role in the reaction: first it is required by the enzyme for its activity and second, the concentration of free Mg^{2+} greatly influences the annealing of the primers to the template (sequence dependence). Generally, insufficient Mg^{2+} leads to low yields, and excess Mg^{2+} will result in the accumulation of nonspecific products. Optimal concentration of MgCl$_2$ needs to be determined empiricially for each template primer pair.

4. Enzyme choice: Before the introduction of thermostable enzymes, DNA polymerases such as the Klenow fragment of *E. coli* DNA polymerase 1 and T4 DNA polymerase were the enzymes used. As these enzymes are heat labile, fresh enzyme addition was required after each temperature change in the PCR reaction. In contrast, thermostable enzymes, which require only a single addition, dramatically enhanced the viability of the PCR reaction to be used on a routine basis. Several thermostable enymes, including *Taq, Amplitaq,* Vent™, *Pfu, Tth,* (Amersham-Pharmacia) *UL*Tma DNA polymerase (Perkin-Elmer), and AccuTaq™ DNA polymerase (Sigma), are commercially available. Each enzyme has different advantages, such as synthesis of longer PCR products, greater thermostability, and 3' to 5' exonuclease proofreading ability; the reader is advised to choose an enzyme tailored to a particular application. Most of our studies have included analysis of cytokine-specific PCR products for quantitation; for this purpose, we find *Taq* polymerase to be the most cost effective. We routinely use 1 U of enzyme/50 μL PCR reaction volume (the product size varying from 150 to 600 bp). For larger predicted sizes, the amount of enzyme may be increased. For reproducible amplification of template DNA, preformulated, predispensed single-dose reaction beads are also available (Amersham-Pharmacia). The formulation ensures greater reproducibilty between reactions, minimizing pipeting steps, and reduces the potential for pipeting errors and contamination. However, the PCR beads are optimized for standard PCR, and individual template/primer combination may require further finer tuning of the reaction conditions.

2.4. Agarose-Gel Electrophoresis

Commonly used buffers contain EDTA, pH 8.0, and Tris-acetate (TAE) or Tris-borate (TBE) at a concentration of approx 50 mM. Buffers are generally made up in a concentrated form and stored at room temperature.

1. TAE 50 times concentrated stock/L is made of 242g Tris-base, 57.1 mL glacial acetic acid, and 100 mL 0.5 M EDTA, pH 8.0.

2. TBE 10 times concentrated stock/L is made of 108 g Tris-base, 55 g boric acid, and 40 mL 0.5 M EDTA, pH 8.0.

We routinely use 0.5X TBE as it provides enough buffering power. If any precipitate appears in your TBE stock, it should be discarded. Historically, TAE is the most commonly used buffer. However, its buffering capacity is rather low, and it is not recommended for long electrophoresis runs.

3. Methods

3.1. Total RNA Extraction

1. RNA can be extracted from whole biopsies or blood samples using a monophasic solution of phenol and guanidine isothiocycanate (TriZOL). Approximately 50–100 mg of tissue (100 µL of blood) are mixed with 1 mL of TriZOL reagent and homogenized thoroughly by using minipestles (ideal for homogenization in 1.5-mL Eppendorf tubes). Further single cell suspension can also be achieved by passing the solution up and down using syringe needles of decreasing diameters (19–23 g). Using syringe needles with human tissue is best avoided to limit chances of infection through needlestick injury.
2. At this stage, the solution is incubated at room temperature for 5 min to dissociate protein further from RNA-protein complexes.
3. After complete homogenization, 200 µL of molecular biology grade chloroform is added and the mixture vortexed thoroughly to mix the two phases (*see* **Note 1**). The mixture is allowed to stand at room temperature for 2 min before centrifugation at 14,000*g* at 4°C for 15 min.
4. Following this step, the mixture separates into a lower (organic) phase and an upper (aqueous) phase containing RNA. Carefully transfer the upper layer into a fresh tube (*see* **Note 2**). The RNA is precipitated by the addition of an equal volume of ice-cold isopropanol. If time is limited, the RNA can be precipitated at –20°C in 20–30 min, but preferably overnight, before being pelleted by centrifugation at 14,000*g* for 15–20 min (*see* **Note 3**).
5. The supernatant is discarded carefully and washed with ice-cold 70% ethanol (14,000*g* for 5–10 min). This wash allows the removal of excess salts, which may interfere with the reactions at later stages. The ethanol supernatant is discarded and the RNA pellet dried under vacuum and resuspended in RNAse-free water or TE buffer (*see* **Note 4**).
6. We generally dissolve our RNA pellet in 10–20 µL of nuclease-free water and keep the solution as concentrated as possible. Once the concentration is known, it is easy to dilute further if required.

3.2. DNase Digestion of RNA Samples

1. Generally DNA contamination in the above RNA extraction is minimal and does not require any special treatment; however, if it is a problem in your study, treat

the RNA with an enzyme such as (3–5 U) RQ1 DNase (Promega), and incubate the sample at 37°C for 1 h.

2. Following DNA digestion, the RNA has to be purified by a phenol/chloroform extraction (Sigma). As before the RNA will be in the upper aqueous layer and needs to be reprecipitated using salt and absolute ethanol. This can be achieved as follows: To 1 vol (100 µL) RNA aqueous layer, add 1/10th (10 µL) vol of 3 *M* sodium acetate and 2.5–3 vol (250–300 µL) of absolute ethanol. As described earlier, the precipitated RNA is washed in 70% ethanol, vacuum-dried, and resuspended in water or TE buffer before use.

3.3. Measurement of RNA

1. Total RNA concentration is measured routinely by UV spectroscopy utilizing the fact that a pure RNA solution at a concentration of 40 µg/mL has an optical density (OD) of 1.0 at 260 nm. As an example, remove 2 µL from your 20 µL RNA solution and add it to a quartz cuvet containing 498 µL of water (mix well). As these reagents are not sterile, we routinely discard the RNA used for measuring concentration. The reading at 260 nm = OD × 250 × 40 = RNA µg/mL (250 is the dilution factor; 40 is the known concentration at a known OD reading).
2. In addition, the purity of an RNA solution can be assessed by the ratio of its optical density at 260/280 nm, this ratio being 2.0 for a pure RNA solution.

3.4. First-Strand Synthesis Using M-MMLV Reverse Trancriptase

1. For a typical reaction, 1–5 µg (depending on availability) of total RNA is required as template. To 11 µL of total RNA (1–5 µg), add 1 µL of oligo dT, mix, and incubate the mixture at 70°C for at least 10 min to encourage complete denaturation of the template.
2. Place the tube immediately on ice for a few minutes. The temperature change allows for more specific annealing of the primer to the template.
3. Centrifuge the sample briefly to collect the contents at the bottom of the centrifuge tube.
4. Add the following components to the above mix:
   4 µL of 5X first strand buffer.
   2 µL of 0.1 *M* DTT (both reagents provided by the manufacturer with the enzyme).
   1 µL 10 m*M* dNTPs.
5. Mix contents of the tube gently before adding 100 U of the enzyme and mix gently by pipetting up and down (no vortex mixing, *see* **Note 5**). Incubate the reaction mix at 42°C for 50 min. Inactivate the enzyme by heating at 70°C for 15 min. The cDNA can now be used as a template for amplification in PCR.

3.5. PCR Reaction

1. Use only 10% of the first-strand reaction for PCR. Adding larger amounts of the first-strand reaction may not increase amplification and may result in decreased

amounts of PCR product. We routinely use 5 µL of cDNA in a typical 50-µL PCR reaction. The components of the reaction are as follows:

5 µL cDNA.
5 µL 10X reaction buffer.
2 µL primer mix (20 pmol/µL; approx 150–200 ng of each primer).
1 µL 10 mM dNTP.
x µL of $MgCl_2$ (0.5–5 mM; optional).
y µL nuclease-free water.
49 µL total volume.

2. Mix gently and layer 2–3 drops (approx 70 µL) of mineral oil (Sigma) over the reaction (*see* **Note 6**).
3. Heat reaction to 94°C for 5 min to denature before the addition of the enzyme (1 U/µL) (*see* **Note 7**).
4. Perform 25–35 cycles of PCR. Annealing and extension conditions are primer and template dependent and must be determined empirically.

3.6. Agarose-Gel Electrophoresis

1. PCR products are generally electrophoresed in 1–2% agarose (Sigma) gels. For a 100-mL gel, weigh 1 g of agarose, add 100 mL of 1X TAE or TBE, and boil the mixture in a microwave for a few minutes until the agarose has completely dissolved.
2. Cool the gel and add 1 µL of ethidium bromide (10 mg/mL stock; Sigma) to the gel mixture before casting the gel. Ethidium bromide can also be added to the running buffer; however, disposing of carcinogenic liquid waste is more tedious than treating the gel itself as solid clinical waste (*see* **Note 8**).
3. Run the gel at 80–150 V as required.
4. As ethidium bromide intercalates within the major groove of the double helix of DNA, the fluorescent PCR product can be visualized on a UV transilluminator and quantified densitometrically. Several gel scanning packages are now commercially available for this purpose, if they are not already installed in your laboratory.

3.7. Quantitative Competitive RT-PCR

In the last few years, modifications in the basic RT-PCR methodology have resulted in more sensitive and quantitative analysis of mRNA expression. In 1995, Jung and colleagues *(2)* constructed a synthetic RNA molecule that allowed the simultaneous quantitation of a range of human cytokine molecules from a single sample. Since then several papers have appeared in the literature utilizing the same principle. Commercial kits are also becoming increasing available from companies such as R&D systems and Endogen for quantitative measurement of mouse and human cytokines. As the field is developing at a very rapid pace, the reader is encouraged to scan the scientific journals and websites of companies regularly for the availability of new reagents.

4. Notes

1. As described above for 1 mL TRIzol solution, 200 µL of chloroform was added to achieve phase separation for total RNA isolation. If you need to use more TRIzol to dissolve your tissue, proportionately increase the amount of chloroform, always maintaining the ratio of 5:1 (TRIzol/chloroform).
2. TRIzol/chloroform centrifugation results in two-phase separation, with the total RNA in the upper aqueous phase. Extra care should be taken in removing the upper layer to avoid uptake of any TRIzol, as the phenolic content of this reagent is a potent denaturant of proteins and will affect enzymatic activity at later stages.
3. The amount of starting clinical specimen is generally very limited; therefore, if time allows, overnight precipitation of RNA is recommended to ensure maximum yield.
4. We routinely dissolve the RNA pellet in nuclease-free water and immediately proceed to reverse transcription. It is useful to store the sample as a cDNA template, as the latter is more stable and the opportunity of RNA degradation by RNAses is minimized. Any remaining resuspended RNA should be stored at –70°C to reduce the possibility of degradation.
5. For most reactions the enzyme should be the last addition to the reaction mix. Two important points to note are, first, to mix the enzyme by gentle pipeting as fierce vortexing would lead to denaturing of the enzyme. Second, glycerol is present in the enzyme stock and at high concentrations can inhibit the reaction rate. Therefore, it is advisable that the enzyme volume added not exceed more than 5% of the total reaction volume.
6. The addition of mineral oil is unnecessary in thermal cyclers equipped with a heated lid.
7. Hot Start: To increase the "specificity" of primer binding, most PCR reactions are subjected to a hot start. The PCR reaction is heated to 94°C for 3–5 min and the enzyme added at the end of this incubation and then cooled to the annealing temperature. This ensures that gene-specific primers will bind to target DNA at a higher annealing temperature and begin synthesis of the PCR product before nonspecific binding of the primers can occur.
8. Ethidium bromide is carcinogenic, and great care should be taken in its usage and disposal.

References

1. Saiki, R. K., Schauf, S., Faloona, F., Mullis, K. B., Horn, G. T., Erlich, H. A., et al. (1985) Enzymatic amplification of beta-globin genomic sequences and restriction site analysis for diagonsis of sickle cell anemia. *Science* **230,** 1350–1354.
2. Jung, H. C., Eckmann, L., Yang, S.-K., Panja, A., Fierer, J., Morzycka-Wroblewska, E., et al. (1995) A distinct array of proinflammatory cytokines is expressed in human colon epithelial cells in response to bacterial invasion. *J. Clin. Invest.* **95,** 55–65.

3. Pender, S. L. F., Tickle, S. P., Docherty, A. J. P., Howie, D., Wathen, N. C., and MacDonald, T. T. (1997) A p55 TNF receptor immunoadhesion prevents T cell mediated intestinal injury by inhibiting matrix-metalloproteinase production. *J. Immunol.* **158,** 1582–1590.
4. Sambrook, J., Fritsch, E. F., and Maniatis, T. (1989) *Molecular Cloning: A Laboratory Manual,* Cold Spring Harbor Laboratory, Cold Spring Harbor, NY.
5. Promega Corporation (1996) *Protocols and Application Guide,* 3rd ed., cat. no. P1610, Promega, Madison, WI.
6. Erlich, H. A. (1989) *PCR Technology—Principles and Applications for DNA Amplifications.* Stockton Press, NY.
7. Newton, C. R. and Graham, A. (1994) *PCR—Introduction to Biotechniques* (Graham, J. M. and Billington, D., eds). Alden, Oxford, UK.

6

Quantitative PCR for Measurement of Cytokine Expression

Ellen M. Nilsen, Finn-Eirik Johansen, and Per Brandtzaeg

1. Introduction

Cytokines play a crucial role in innate and adaptive immunity. The onset or progression of immunopathology in various diseases is often associated with aberrant production of one or more cytokines. It is therefore of considerable interest to characterize cytokine "profiles" associated with disease processes. However, the minute amounts of cytokine protein often produced in autocrine or paracrine microenvironments may not be easily detectable, especially when tissue samples or cells are available in only small quantities *(1)*.

As an alternative (or adjunct) to cytokine protein measurement, an indication of cytokine production can be obtained by quantification of mRNA for the actual product. To this end, quantitative polymerase chain reaction (PCR) has proved to be the molecular technique of choice. RNA cannot serve as a template for PCR, so amplification of RNA molecules is performed by a method that combines reverse transcription (RT), to turn RNA into a complementary DNA (cDNA) strand, with PCR (RT-PCR). RT-PCR is simple, reproducible, specific, and highly sensitive. However, its extreme sensitivity also explains the main weakness of PCR, namely, its tendency to produce false-positive results due to exogenous contamination, particularly from the product of previous reactions *(2–4)*. Moreover, it should be realized that quantitative RT-PCR is usually labor intensive and costly because many reactions have to be performed and analyzed for one measurement.

PCR is an in vitro method for enzymatically driven synthesis of defined sequences of DNA. Basic PCR consists of three steps: denaturation of the target DNA, primer annealing of synthetic oligonucleotide primers, and extension of

From: *Methods in Molecular Medicine, vol. 60: Interleukin Protocols*
Edited by: L. A. J. O'Neill and A. Bowie © Humana Press Inc., Totowa, NJ

the annealed primers by a thermostable DNA polymerase. This three-step cycle is then repeated a number of times, each time approximately doubling the number of product molecules. The length of the products generated during PCR is equal to the sum of the lengths of the two primers plus the distance in the target DNA between the primers. One inherent problem in RT-PCR is that this method is at best semiquantitative and can only be used to provide qualitative results. Because amplification is (at least initially) an exponential process, small differences in any of the variables that control the reaction rate will dramatically affect the yield of the PCR product. We describe here a technique that obviates these problems and allows precise quantitation of mRNA from small samples or small numbers of cells.

The major steps involved in quantitative RT-PCR are illustrated in **Fig. 1**. By this approach, an exogenous RNA standard is added to the target RNA sample and amplified simultaneously with the target transcript in a single PCR reaction mixture. The standard and target sequences compete for the same primers and, therefore, for the amplification. The relative amount of target RNA vs competitor RNA can be measured by direct scanning of ethidium-stained agarose gels. Because the starting concentration of the standard is known, the initial concentration of the target RNA can be determined. This method allows compensation for tube-to-tube variation in amplification efficiency. The internal control RNA used in our laboratory consists of linearly connected sequences of the 5' primers of multiple cytokine genes followed by the complementary sequences to their 3' primers in the same order. This structure of the internal standard permits use of the same internal standard for quantification of several cytokine mRNAs.

We describe the rapid and accurate detection of cytokine mRNA in biopsy specimens taken from the small intestinal mucosa of celiac disease patients, or gluten-specific mucosal T-cell clones; the method can be applied to the quantification of cytokines expressed at low levels ($\geq$1000 transcripts/μg total RNA). This competitive PCR approach has been shown to be highly sensitive and specific when compared with Northern blot analysis or dot blot analysis *(5,6)*, and it is considered to be the best method for determination of gene expression at low levels. The application of this approach has extended the use of PCR to, for example, analysis of mRNA induction in response to exogenous cellular stimuli.

2. Materials

2.1. Patient Material/Cell Culture Preparation

1. Mucosal specimens obtained by use of an Olympus endoscope (GIF IT20) with biopsy forceps (Olympus FB13K).
2. Gluten-specific mucosal T-cell clones *(7,8)*.

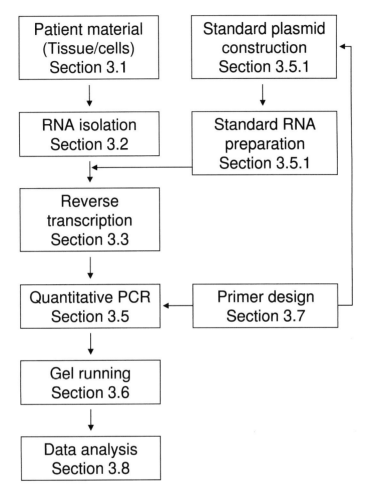

Fig.1. Overview of the RT-PCR method with reference to sections in the text. Total RNA prepared (for example) from an intestinal biopsy specimen is added to a dilution series of an exogenous RNA standard, and both samples are reverse-transcribed and then coamplified in a single PCR reaction mixture. Following gel electrophoresis, the relative amount of target RNA vs standard RNA is measured by direct scanning of an ethidium-stained agarose gel. When target and standard RNAs are present at equal concentrations, coamplification results in equal amounts of both products with bands of equal density. Because the concentration of the standard is known, this gives the concentration of the target (unknown) RNA.

2.2. RNA Isolation

1. 5.7 M CsCl, 0.01 M EDTA in a final volume of 50 mL autoclaved deionized H_2O. Store at room temperature.

2. Guanidine isothiocyanate (GTC) with β-mercaptoethanol (5 *M* GTC, 25 m*M* sodium citrate, 0.5% sodium lauroyl sarcosine, 0.1 *M* β-mercaptoethanol added fresh). Store at 4°C.

2.3. Reverse Transcription

1. 5X first-strand buffer: 250 m*M* Tris-HCl, pH 8.3, 375 m*M* KCl, 15 m*M* MgCl$_2$ (Gibco, Paisley, UK). Store at –20°C.
2. Superscript™ in storage buffer: 20 m*M* Tris-HCl, pH 7.5, 100 m*M* NaCl, 0.1 m*M* EDTA, 1 m*M* dithiothreitol (DTT), 0.01% (v/v) NP-40, 50% (v/v) glycerol (Gibco). 200 U/µL. Store at –20°C.
3. RNase inhibitor (RNasin) (Promega, Madison, WI) at 40 U/µL. Store at –20°C.
4. DTT, 100 m*M* stock (Gibco). Store at –20°C.
5. Oligo dT$_{16}$, 100 pmol/µL in TE (Gibco). Store at –20°C.
6. dNTP mixture (Pharmacia, Uppsala, Sweden): A 10X stock solution of 10 m*M* each of dATP, dCTP, dGTP, and dTTP is prepared. Store in aliquots at –20°C.

2.4. Polymerase Chain Reaction

1. 10X *Taq* DNA polymerase reaction buffer: 100 m*M* Tris-HCl, pH 8.3, 500 m*M* KCl (Perkin Elmer, Branchburg, NJ). Store at –20°C.
2. MgCl$_2$, 25 mM (Perkin Elmer). Store at –20°C.
3. *Taq* DNA polymerase in storage buffer: 20 m*M* Tris-HCl, pH 8.0, 100 m*M* KCl, 0.1 m*M* EDTA, 1 m*M* DTT, 50% (v/v) glycerol, 0.5% Tween-20, 0.5% Nonidet P-40 (Perkin Elmer) at 5 U/µL. Store at –20°C.
4. PCR primers: 18–25 bases in length, 100 pmol/µL in TE (Gibco). Store at –20°C (*see* **Subheading 2.7.**).
5. Light white mineral oil (Sigma, St. Louis, MO).
6. Microfuge tubes: Use only tubes specified for use in the thermal cycler, because ill-fitting tubes will result in inconsistent and inefficient amplifications.
7. Pipets and cotton-plugged pipet tips.

2.5. Quantitative Polymerase Chain Reaction

1. To quantify the amounts of different cytokine transcripts, we use standard RNA generated from the plasmids pHCQ1, pHCQ2, and pHCQ3 (courtesy of Dr. M. F. Kagnoff, University of California, San Diego, CA). The construction of these plasmids has been described *(9)*.

2.6. Gel Running and Data Analysis

1. 6X loading buffer: 0.25% xylene cyanol and 30% glycerol in a final volume of 20 mL autoclaved deionized H$_2$O. Store at room temperature.
2. Seakem LE agarose (FMC, Rockland, MD).
3. DNA marker: 123-bp ladder (Gibco). Store at 4°C.
4. 1X TBE buffer: 0.045 *M* Tris-borate, 0.001 *M* EDTA, pH 8.3. A 5X stock is prepared. Store at room temerature.
5. Gel apparatus: Horizontal slab gel casting/electrophoresis chamber/power supply.

2.7. Selection of Primers (Primer Design)

Primer selection for PCR is most often undertaken by computer programs designed to take into account variables such as G/C ratio, sequence homology, the probability of primer-dimer or "hairpin" formation, and anchor sequence characteristics. There are many PCR primer sequences available from published sources; in most cases these can be used with confidence. Alternatively, suitable primers and primer pairs may be designed with the aid of commercially available computer software (e.g., Primer Designer 1.0). Many national molecular biology nodes on the World Wide Web have available software, e.g., embnet.no.PRIMER. Primers that are used in combination should have a similar Tm value.

3. Methods
3.1. Patient Material/Cell Culture Preparation

1. Obtain mucosal specimens by the use of an Olympus endoscope (GIF IT20) with biopsy forceps (Olympus FB13K). Snap-freeze the biopsy specimens in liquid nitrogen, and store at –70°C (*see* **Note 1**).
2. T cells (5×10^5) are incubated with antigen and antigen-presenting cells (1.5×10^6). After appropriate stimulation, collect the cells by centrifugation. Snap-freeze the cells in liquid nitrogen, and store at –70°C.

3.2. RNA Isolation

RNA is less stable and very prone to degradation by ribonucleases from tissues and cells. RNases are also present in the environment so that appropriate precautions (wearing and changing gloves, working on ice, RNase-free plasticware and glassware) must be taken.

The best sources for good quality (undegraded) and quantity of RNA are fresh tissues or cells. If adequately stored (best in liquid nitrogen), RNA extracted from tissues or cells will be equally suitable for subsequent analysis. The most frequently used types of RNA for PCR amplification are total RNA or messenger RNA (polyA+ RNA). RNA may be prepared from tissue or cells in several ways. Here, we have isolated total RNA by the guanidium thiocyanate (GTC) method *(10)*. *Please follow the instructions that are provided with the RNA isolation method you choose.* Numerous commercial kits are available, and we have used RNAzol (Biogenesis, UK) and RNAesy (Qiagen, Hilden, Germany) with succes.

1. Remove frozen biopsy specimens or cell pellets from liquid nitrogen and homogenize in GTC by the stroke of a tightly fitting pestle in a glass Dounce homogenizer (Kontes, Vineland, NJ). We use 3.5 mL GTC to one biopsy specimen with a size corresponding to 25–35 mg wet weight. The same amount of GTC was used for the cell pellet, which consists of approx 2×10^6 cells.
2. Isolate total RNA. We most often isolate RNA according to MacDonald et al. *(10)*.
3. The precipitated RNA is dissolved in 10–20 µL diethyl pyrocarbonate (DEPC)-treated water (*see* **Note 2**).

4. The yield and purity of the RNA are determined by measuring the OD 260/OD 280 ratio. RNA purified by this method should result in an OD 260/OD 280 ratio of >1.7 (*see* **Note 3**).

5. At this point the isolated RNA should be kept on ice when being handled, or stored at –70°C.

3.3. Reverse Transcription

Because RNA cannot serve as a template for PCR, reverse transcription is first performed to make RNA into cDNA suitable for PCR. As defined above, the combination of both techniques is referred to as RT-PCR. Here, total RNA (0.5–1 µg) is reverse transcribed into cDNA according to a standard protocol (Gibco). *Please follow the instructions that are provided with the protocol and for the solutions you choose.*

1. Synthesize cDNA by reverse transcriptase in a 20-µL reaction mixture at 42°C.
2. Centrifuge all reagents briefly (≥ 8000*g* for 5–10 s) before beginning the procedure.
3. Keep all solutions and the reaction mixture on ice during the preparation.
4. For each reverse transcription, mix the following components in a sterile microfuge tube (*see* **Note 4**): 4.0 µL 5X first-strand buffer; 2.0 µL 0.1 *M* DTT; 1.0 µL 10 m*M* dNTP mix; 1.0 µL 20 pmol/µL oligo dT$_{16}$ (*see* **Note 5**); 0.5 µL RNasin (40 U/µL); 9.0 µL autoclaved deionized H_2O; 0.5 µL Superscript™ (200 U/µL; *see* **Note 6**), and 2.0 µL total RNA (500 ng/µL).
5. Gently tap the tubes to mix all the reagents.
6. After a brief centrifugation (8000*g* for 5–10 s) to deposit all of the liquid at the bottom of the reaction tube, place tubes into PCR thermal cycler.
7. Incubate at 42°C for 60 min, followed by heat inactivation at 99°C for 10 min (*see* **Note 7**).
8. Store cDNA at –20°C until required for use.

3.4. Polymerase Chain Reaction

PCR is carried out in a 25-µL reaction mixture according to a standard protocol (Perkin Elmer) (*see* **Notes 8–10**). *Please follow the instructions that are provided with the protocol and for the solutions you choose.*

1. Centrifuge all reagents briefly (8000*g* for 5–10 s) (*see* **Subheading 2.4.**) before beginning the procedure.
2. Keep all solutions on ice during the preparation of reaction mixtures.
3. For each reaction, mix the following components in a sterile microfuge tube: 2.5 µL 10X buffer; 1.5 µL 25 m*M* $MgCl_2$ (*see* **Note 11**); 0.5 µL 10 m*M* dNTP (*see* **Note 12**); 1.0 µL 10 pmol/µL of forward primer; 1.0 µL 10 pmol/µL of reverse primer (*see* **Note 13**); 16.5 µL autoclaved deionized H_2O; 1.0 µL *Taq* DNA polymerase (5 U/µL, diluted 1/8) (*see* **Note 14**) and 1.0 µL cDNA (*see* **Note 15**).
4. Gently tap the tubes to mix all the reagents. Layer 25 µL of mineral oil on top of the PCR solution to prevent evaporation of liquid during thermal cycling.

5. After brief centrifugation (8000*g* for 5–10 s) to deposit all the liquid at the bottom of the reaction tube, place tubes into PCR thermal cycler. Follow the manufacturer's instructions for programming.
6. For an initial denaturing step, incubate at 95°C for 4 min.
7. A typical temperature profile is: denaturation (95°C for 1 min), annealing (50–72°C for 30 s), and elongation (72°C for 1 min) (*see* **Notes 16** and **17**).
8. Repeat these steps for 25–35 cycles (*see* **Notes 18,19**, and **20**).
9. For the final step, incubate at 72°C for 10 min to promote completion of partial extension products and annealing of single-stranded complementary products.
10. Keep PCR products at 4°C until they are analyzed.

3.5. Quantitative Polymerase Chain Reaction

One drawback of RT-PCR is that this method at best is semiquantitative (*see* **Notes 21**, **22**, and **23**). In an attempt to correct for tube-to-tube variations in both the cDNA synthesis and PCR amplification efficiency, it is recommended that internal RNA standards are used (*see* **Note 24**). By this approach, an exogenous RNA standard is added to the target sample and amplified simultaneously with the target transcript in a single PCR reaction mixture. The standard and target sequences compete for the same primers and, therefore, for amplification. A dilution series is made of either the target sequence or the standard sequence, and a constant amount of the other component is added to each of the reactions. Quantification is performed after competitive amplification of the entire series of reactions and is achieved by distinguishing the two PCR products in each tube by differences in size.

1. Quantitative PCR is carried out in a 25-µL reaction mixture (*see* **Subheading 3.4.**). A constant amount of total RNA (we use 500 ng to 1 µg) from each sample is reverse-transcribed into cDNA together with serial dilutions (i.e., two- or threefold dilutions) of standard RNA transcripts in the same reaction volume and coamplified by PCR. We typically begin at 2–10 pg standard/µg total RNA.

3.5.1. RNA Standards for Quantification of Cytokines

Since the first study by Wang et al. *(5)* was published, several reports have described the construction of exogenous RNA and DNA internal standards that differ from target sequences only by the presence or absence of small introns or restriction sites *(9,11–13)*. In these cases, there is little doubt that the amplification efficiencies of the standard and target sequences will be the same. To quantify the amounts of different cytokine transcripts, we used standard RNA generated from the plasmids pHCQ1, pHCQ2, and pHCQ3 (courtesy of Dr. M. F. Kagnoff, University of California, San Diego, CA). The construction of these plasmids has been described *(9)*. The arrangements of priming sites are designed to yield PCR products that differ in size from those of the target RNA. Because the same primer set is used in the PCR amplification on both templates, differences in primer annealing efficiency and hence PCR efficiency are minimized.

3.6. Gel Running

After amplification, separate the PCR products generated by standard and target RNA by agarose gel electrophoresis and visualize the bands by ethidium bromide staining. Horizontal agarose gels are usually run in an electrical field at constant strength and direction. Prepare the gel for loading as follows:

1. Seal the open ends of the plastic tray supplied with the electrophoresis apparatus (or a glass plate) with autoclave tape to form a mold.
2. Add the correct amount of powdered agarose (*see* **Notes 25** and **26**) to a measured quantity of electrophoresis buffer in a glass bottle. Heat in a microwave oven until the agarose dissolves. Heat the solution for the minimum time required to allow all grains of agarose to dissolve. Swirl the bottle from time to time. Check that the volume of the solution has not decreased by evaporation during boiling; replenish with water if necessary.
3. Cool the solution to 60°C, add ethidium bromide to a final concentration of 0.5 µg/mL, and mix thoroughly (*see* **Notes 27** and **28**).
4. Pour the agarose solution into the mold and position the comb 0.5–1.0 mm above the plate so that a complete well is formed when the agarose is added. The gel should be between 3 and 5 mm thick. Check to see that no air bubbles are retained under or between the teeth of the comb.
5. After the gel is completely set (20–30 min at room temperature), carefully remove the autoclave tape and mount the gel in the electrophoresis tank.
6. Add just enough electrophoresis buffer to cover the gel, and remove the comb carefully.
7. Mix the sample of DNA with the gel-loading buffer. Slowly load the mixture (15–25 µL is used for analysis) into the slots of the submerged gel by use of a pipet.
8. A DNA marker (123-bp ladder) is loaded into one slot of the gel. This ladder allows verification of predicted size of PCR products and makes it easier to determine the sizes of unknown DNAs if any systematic distortion of the gel should occur during electrophoresis (*see* **Note 29**).
9. Close the lid of the gel tank and attach the electrical leads so that the DNA will migrate toward the anode (red lead). Apply a voltage of 1–5 V/cm.
10. Run the gel until the bands have migrated the appropriate distance, or until the bands for standard and target are appropriately separated.
11. Turn off the electric current and remove the leads and lid from the gel tank. If ethidium bromide was present in the gel, examine the gel by ultraviolet light (*see* **Note 27**).

3.7. Primer Design

1. A critical requirement in the selection of primers is that the extension products of each primer extend far enough through the target region to include the sequences of the other flanking primer. In this way, each extension product made in one cycle can serve as a template for extension in the next cycle; this results in an exponential increase in PCR product as a function of cycle number. After the first few cycles, the major product is a DNA fragment that is exactly equal in length to the sum of the lengths of the two primers and the intervening target DNA (*see* **Notes 30–35**).

3.8. Data Analysis

1. Take photographs of the gels with Polaroid 665 film, and use the negatives to quantify band intensities by a Nicon Scantouch 110 (Nikon, Japan).
2. Analyze the data. We use Phoretix Array Advanced (Phoretix, Newcastle upon Tyne, UK).

3.9. Applications: Use of Quantitative PCR for Detection of Cytokine Expression in Biopsy Specimens of Celiac Mucosa

In the experiment shown in **Fig. 2**, competitive RT-PCR was used to quantify interferon-γ (IFN-γ) transcripts in duodenal/jejunal biopsy specimens from untreated celiac disease by use of the HCQ1 competitive template as an internal standard.

1. Isolate RNA (*see* **Subheading 3.2.**) from biopsy specimens (*see* **Subheading 3.1.**).
2. Perform reverse transcription (*see* **Subheading 3.3.** and below).
3. Prepare the master mix (*see* **Note 4**), and add 17 μL of the master mix to each of seven (or more if necessary) marked tubes, for example, A–G (*see* **Note 36**).
4. Add 1 μL of standard RNA at known concentration in a dilution series (usually two- or threefold dilution) to each tube (*see* **Notes 36**, **37**, and **38**).
5. Add 1–2 μL (1 μg RNA) of the sample to each tube.
6. Perform reverse transcription (*see* **Subheading 3.3.**).
7. Perform PCR (*see* **Subheading 3.4.**).
8. Mix the sample of DNA with the gel-loading buffer, and load 25 μL/well on a 1.6% ethidium-stained Seakem LE agarose gel.
9. Photograph and analyze the gel as described (*see* **Subheading 3.8.**).
10. Plot standard mRNA per target mRNA as a function of the amount of standard mRNA. The point of equivalence is where target mRNA equals standard mRNA (i.e., ratio 1:1) and thus represents the concentration of RNA in the unknown sample (**Fig. 2B**) (*see* **Note 39**).

As shown by the broken line in **Fig. 2B**, the unknown sample contains 0.25 pg mRNA/μg total RNA. To convert this pg value into the number of transcripts (often a more useful figure), we apply the following equation:

$$(\text{g RNA} \times 6 \times 10^{23}) \text{ divided by } [350 \text{ (MW/base)} \times \text{number of nucleotides}]$$
$$0.25 \text{ pg} \times 10^{-12} \text{ g/pg} \times 6 \times 10^{23}: 350 \times 840 = 5 \times 10^5 \text{ transcripts/μg total RNA.}$$

The unknown RNA sample is then found to contain 5×10^5 IFN-γ transcripts/μg total RNA (*see* **Note 40**).

4. Notes
4.1. Patient Material

1. The critical factor in isolating RNA from eukaryotic tissues is inactivation of endogenous RNases and avoidance of RNases from external sources. RNA is highly unstable in samples once removed from the body, so it is critical to quick-freeze the tissue in liquid nitrogen.

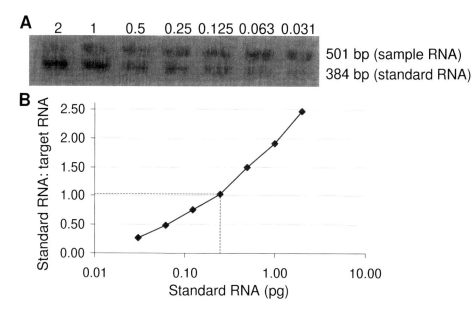

A 2   1   0.5   0.25 0.125 0.063 0.031

501 bp (sample RNA)
384 bp (standard RNA)

B

Fig. 2. **(A)** Competitive quantitative analysis of IFN-γ transcripts in RNA extracted from a duodenal biopsy specimen isolated from an untreated celiac disease patient. A master mixture was prepared containing IFN-γ primers, and 17 μL of the master mixtures was aliquoted into each of seven tubes. Sample RNA (2 μL, 1 μg) was added together with a serial dilutions of the standard (competitor). The final concentrations of standard RNA in each tube were 2, 1, 0.5, 0.25, 0.125, 0.063, and 0.031 pg, respectively. After reverse transcription and 30 cycles of PCR on 1 μL cDNA, the PCR products generated by standard (384 bp) and sample (501 bp) were electrophoresed on an agarose gel. Polaroid 665 negatives were scanned by a Nicon Scantouch and analyzed by Phoretix Array Advanced. **(B)** Quantitative analysis of amplified IFN-γ mRNA products. The ratio of standard IFN-γ mRNA per target IFN-γ mRNA was plotted as a function of the amount of known standard IFN-γ mRNA. The level of IFN-γ mRNA was determined by calculating how much of the standard was required to achieve equal amounts of products. The point of equivalence (1:1 ratio marked with broken line), indicates where target IFN-γ mRNA equals standard IFN-γ mRNA and represents the concentration of RNA in the unknown sample.

4.2. RNA Isolation

2. For RNA isolation, extreme care must be taken to avoid RNases. All solutions should be prepared by use of RNase-free glassware, autoclaved DEPC-treated water, and chemicals reserved for work with RNA. Nondisposable glassware should be baked at 150°C for 4 h to destroy RNases. RNA is extremely liable to degradation by endogenous RNases after cell lysis and before cDNA synthesis.

3. Total RNA can be used directly for production of cDNA without the need of mRNA isolation, and this may be an advantage because the low amounts of available mRNA (5–10% of total RNA) are difficult to quantify. If the starting material consists of isolated cells, cell counting is a convenient means of quantification. A solution whose OD 260 = 1 contains approx 40 μg/mL of RNA.

4.3. Reverse Transcription

4. When multiple samples are to be analyzed for content of a given mRNA, a master mix may be prepared containing all the components except the RNA source. Use of such mixtures will minimize reagent loss during pipetting, increase accuracy, and reduce the number of reagent transfers. Preparation of this master mix will eliminate the need for repeated pipetting of small volumes and will increase consistency among samples.

5. Three types of primers may be used for reverse transcription:
   a. Oligo dT_{12-18} binds to the endogenous poly(A) tail at the 3' end of mammalian mRNA. This primer most frequently produces a full-length cDNA product, but the 5' end of some mRNAs may be reverse transcribed inefficiently due to the secondary structure of the mRNA.
   b. Random hexanucleotides can bind to mRNA templates at any complementary site and will give partial length (short) cDNAs.
   c. Specific oligonucleotide sequences can be used to prime the RNA of interest selectively.

6. Superscript reverse transcriptase is a DNA polymerase that synthesizes cDNA from single-stranded RNA or DNA. We have also used the enzyme murine leukemia virus (MuLV) reverse transcriptase (Perkin Elmer) for cDNA synthesis with succesful results.

7. Reverse transcriptase binds to cDNA and is thereby inhibitory to PCR amplification. Under the conditions provided (12.5 U/μL), incubation at 99°C for 10 min inactivates the reverse transcriptase and removes the inhibitory effect.

4.4. Polymerase Chain Reaction

8. For most PCR applications, it is essential that the only DNA entering the reaction is the added template. The ideal way to ensure that PCR is performed only with the desired template is to maintain a DNA-free clean environment. It is suggested that a selected laboratory area, preferably a laminar flow hood, be dedicated to performance of PCRs. No amplified product should ever be brought into this hood. A set of pipetors, racks, tubes, cotton-plugged pipet tips, etc. should be confined to the preparation hood and used only to mix the reactions. Autoclaved deionized water, sterile mineral oil, and buffers should be aliquoted and stored in small amounts, enough for an average single preparation. Use autoclaved tubes and solutions whenever possible. Always wear gloves to avoid nuclease contamination from fingers. It is recommended to prepare your own sets of reagents and store them in small aliquots. Do not apply these reagents for other purposes. Use new glasswares, plasticwares, and pipets that have not been exposed to DNAs in the laboratory. After use, discard aliquots of reagents; do not return them to storage.

9. RT-PCR is a very powerful technique for the detection of small amounts of mRNA; it appears ideally suited for use on cells that cannot be grown in large numbers, or tissue that is available in only minute quantities. However, it is at the same time important to be aware of the fact that the high sensitivity of mRNA transcript detection may lead to false conclusions regarding protein translation. Even detection of large amounts of mRNA is no proof of protein translation. Several examples of posttranscriptional regulation of protein expression have been described in the literature *(14,15)*.

10. Each new PCR application is likely to require optimization. Some problems often encountered include the following: no detectable product or low yield of the desired product; the presence of nonspecific background bands due to mispriming or misextension of the primers; the formation of "primer-dimers" that compete for amplification with the desired product; and mutations or heterogeneity due to misincorporation.

11. It is beneficial to optimize the magnesium ion concentration. The magnesium concentration may affect all of the following: primer annealing; strand dissociation temperatures of both template and PCR product; product specificity; formation of primer-dimer artifacts; and enzyme activity and fidelity. *Taq* DNA polymerase requires free magnesium on top of that bound by template DNA, primers and dNTPs. Accordingly, PCRs should contain 0.5–2.5 m*M* magnesium *(16)*.

12. The nucleotide concentration must be sufficient to saturate the enzyme, but not so high or imbalanced as to promote misincorporation. The primer concentration must be high enough to anneal rapidly to the single-stranded target and, in later stages of the reaction, faster than target-target reassociation.

13. Too low primer concentrations will result in little or no PCR product, and too high concentrations may result in amplification of nontarget sequences. Primer concentrations in the range of 0.1–0.5 μ*M* will work for most PCR amplifications *(16)*.

14. The isolation of a heat-resistant DNA polymerase from *Thermus aquaticus (Taq)* allows primer annealing and extension to be carried out at an elevated temperature *(17)*, thereby reducing mismatched annealing to nontarget sequences. This added selectivity results in the production of large amounts of virtually pure target DNA. Another important advantage of *Taq* polymerase is that it escapes inactivation during each cycle, unlike the Klenow enzyme, which has to be added after every denaturation step. This has allowed automation of PCR in machines that have controlled heating and cooling capability. The *Taq* polymerase has measurable activity at room temperature and at almost all of the temperatures up to the DNA denaturation temperature *(16)*. For optimal specificity, the highest possible annealing temperature should be used to reduce nonspecific primer extension. We have also used other thermostable polymerases such as Vent (New England Biolabs, Beverly, MA), Dynazyme (Finnzyme, Espoo, Finland), and Amplitaq Gold (Perkin Elmer) with success.

15. Always include a control that contains all the components of the PCR reaction except the template DNA. A negative control tube is necessary to monitor possible DNA contamination and to estimate background levels. A cDNA synthesis reaction with all components including RNA except reverse transcriptase is a good negative control. Whenever possible, include a positive control.

16. Temperature control and timing are important. The temperatures used must maximize specific primer annealing and polymerase elongation but not sacrifice yield by reducing primer-template hybridization. Denaturation must be efficient, but the temperature should neither be too high nor be kept for too long because the *Taq* polymerase, although heat resistant, is not indefinitely stable. The range of enzyme activity varies by two orders of magnitude between 20 and 85°C *(16)*. The temperature and length of time required for primer annealing depends on the base composition, length, and concentration of the amplification primers. An applicable annealing temperature is 5°C below the true Tm of the amplification primers. Annealing temperatures in the range of 55–70°C generally yield the best results. Increasing the annealing temperature enhances discrimination against incorrectly annealed primers and reduces misextension of incorrect nucleotides at the 3' end of primers. Therefore, stringent annealing temperatures will help to increase specificity.

17. For some primer-template pairs, two-temperature rather than three-temperature cycles may work when the annealing temperature is above 60°C; the extension is then completed at the annealing temperature. The slower extension rate at lower temperatures may require optimization of the time for such combined anneal-extend steps. We have often used a two-step reaction in which the annealing and extension steps are carried out at the same temperature, with successful results, as has also been reported by other laboratories *(9)*.

18. The number of PCR cycles required depends on the level of the target. Usually, 20–40 cycles are used, but the optimal number should be determined for each reaction (*see* **Note 19**). Use the smallest number of PCR cycles that provides the "cleanest" result. Increasing the number of cycles often produces more nonspecific amplification. Also, with a large number of amplification cycles, contamination problems are more likely to occur.

19. Optimizing the number of PCR cycles is the best way to avoid the problems in reaching the plateau phase. This can be performed by preparing a master mix, with trace radioactive dCTP. PCR is then performed for different numbers of cycles (e.g., between 15 and 40 cycles). After separation on an 5% acrylamide gel (approx 30 mL of 5% acrylamide gel solution with 300 µL 10% ammonium persulfate [APS] and 20 µL *N,N,N',N'*-tetramethylenediamine [TEMED] are used for a 14-well gel), the radioactivity is quantified as described above (*see* **Subheading 3.8.**). Calculate the PCR product yield as a function of cycle numbers. Always use cycle numbers below the plateau phase.

20. Limiting amplification to the desired target can also be enhanced with a nesting strategy that involves two different rounds of PCR. After amplification with one set of primers, a small aliquot is taken and amplified in a second round, either with two new primers internal to those used in the first round (nesting) *(18)* or with one new internal primer and one of the original primers ("heminesting") *(19)*. This strategy works because, unlike the desired target, any nontarget sequences amplified in the first round cannot be further amplified with the internal target-specific primer(s) used in the second round.

4.5. Quantitative Polymerase Chain Reaction

21. If every template molecule in the sample is completely extended at each cycle, then the amplification efficiency is 100%. In practice, efficiencies can vary quite significantly throughout the course of amplification. For example, the amount of product produced at each cycle eventually levels off. This plateau can be explained by two phenomena. First, as the concentration of double-stranded product reaches high levels, competition increases between annealing of template (PCR product) to primer and reannealing of the complementary template strands. Second, the amount of enzyme is finite, and eventually there is not enough to extend all the primer-template complexes during the allotted time. The efficiency may also depend on the amount of original target and on properties of the target that are not well understood, such as the likelihood of secondary structure in the single-stranded template. In general, long targets are less efficiently amplified than shorter ones, but there are exceptions to this rule, which could be due to the actual sequence involved.

22. It is often useful to include an endogenous mRNA sequence, e.g., for β-actin or glyceraldehyde phosphate dehydrogenase (GAPDH), known to be present at constant levels throughout a series of samples as an internal control for a semiquantitative analysis. To ensure reliability, the level of expression of this control gene must be the same in each sample to be compared and must not change as a result of the experimental treatment. Unfortunately, few if any genes are expressed in a strictly constitutive manner. This is even the case for many "housekeeping" genes, including β-actin *(6,20)*. Therefore, such data must be examined very carefully for constancy among all experimental conditions studied. Because the amplification is initially exponential, any tube-to-tube variation or differences in the rate of amplification of the different templates will be magnified over the course of the reaction. Furthermore, this method does not allow comparison of mRNA levels for two different genes (e.g., IFN-γ and IL-4) to be made, because the efficiency of each reaction may vary significantly. Consequently, the amount of the unknown template may be over- or underestimated.

23. To account for cytokine differences caused by a varying number of T cells in the tissue samples, T-cell-derived mRNA can be quantified by the use of T-cell receptor (TCR)α-chain-specific primers. This is particularly important when the specimens in question contain variable proportions of different cell types with presumably variable amounts of the transcripts of interest.

24. It is a clear advantage to use RNA standards instead of DNA standards. In this way, the efficiency of reverse transcription is controlled.

4.6. Gel Running and Data Analysis

25. Agarose gels have a lower resolving power than polyacrylamide gels but have a greater range of separation. DNAs from 200 bp to approx 50 kb in length can be separated on agarose gels of various concentrations *(21)*. We generally use SeaKem LE agarose to separate the PCR products. This is an agarose often used for routine nucleic acid electrophoresis of fragments between 100 and 23,000 bp.

In addition, we have also used the NuSieve GTG agarose (FMC Corporation) with success (*see* **Note 26**). We recommend 1.6% ethidium-stained Seakem LE agarose gel made in 1X TBE buffer.

26. To obtain a better resolution (separation) of the PCR products (between standard and template) and sharper gel bands, we have used the NuSieve GTG Agarose with success.

27. During electrophoresis, ethidium bromide migrates toward the cathode (in the direction opposite to that of DNA). Extended electrophoresis can remove much of the ethidium bromide from the gel, making detection of small fragments difficult. If this occurs, restain the gel by soaking it for 30–45 min in a solution of ethidium bromide. The presence of ethidium bromide allows the gel to be examined by ultraviolet illumination at any stage during electrophoresis. However, some researchers feel that sharper bands of DNA are obtained when the gel is run in the absence of this dye. In that case, stain the gel after electrophoresis.

28. Ethidium bromide is a carcinogen and should be handled with care.

29. Primary confirmation of PCR product identity is obtained by the anticipated molecular weight. A single band of the expected size will most likely be the appropriate product. To confirm the identity of the PCR product, one method is restriction fragment mapping. The sequence of the PCR product can be examined for the presence of single sites of restriction enzyme activity, leading to the generation of digestion products of specific size that can then be resolved on an agarose gel. Other techniques include sequencing the PCR product, thereby directly confirming the identity of the band, or transferring the PCR product to a suitable membrane via Southern blotting and probing the product(s) by use of an oligo-probe.

4.7. Selection of Primers (Primer Design)

30. The length of the primers (usually 15–30 bases) must be sufficient to overcome the statistical likelihood that their sequence would occur randomly in the overwhelmingly large number of nontarget DNA sequences present in the sample.

31. The G + C percentage of primers should be near 50%, to maximize annealing efficiency.

32. Primers should not be self-complementary, complementary to each other, or have secondary structure, as this will inhibit the specific PCR reaction.

33. Whenever possible, primers used for amplifying cDNAs of RNAs should be derived from separate exons, thus spanning one or more introns; amplification products of genomic DNA can then easily be distinguished from those of reverse-transcribed mRNA; only minute amounts of contaminating genomic DNA may give a false-positive signal in this type of assay. It is often useful to test the primers with genomic DNA as template.

34. Optimization of reactions for each primer-template pair is necessary and can be achieved by varying $MgCl_2$ concentration, primer concentration, and anneal-extend temperature. The effect of these variations can be monitored by examining the intensity and distribution of product samples electrophoresed on agarose gels. It may be

necessary to lower or raise (in the range of 37–75°C) the anneal-extend temperature for the primer-template pairs. Higher anneal-extend temperatures generally result in a much more specific product *(22)*.

35. Various DNAs differ in purity, GC content, chemical modification, secondary structure, or other variables that can inhibit PCR. Certain primer-template combinations have characteristics that cause poor PCR amplification in the "standard" buffer supplied with *Taq* DNA polymerase. The Opti-Prime PCR optimization kit (Stratagene, La Jolla, CA) provides a convenient method for determining which PCR buffers and adjuncts are most effective for a specific template and primer set. The kit consists of a matrix of 12 buffers that vary in pH and final concentrations of $MgCl_2$ and potassium. Six different adjuncts or cosolvents known to affect PCR are also included. We have used this kit with succesful results.

4.8. Applications

36. An example of a reaction mixture typically used to quantify IFN-γ mRNA is shown below.

Tube	Standard/sample
a	2 pg/1 µg
b	1 pg/1 µg
c	0.5 pg/1 µg
d	0.25 pg/1 µg
e	0.125 pg/1 µg
f	0.063 pg/1 µg
g	0.031 pg/1 µg

37. The ratio of competitive template per unknown template plotted against competitive template is a hyperbolic relationship that approaches an asymptote when one species is present in vast excess. For this reason, the most accurate results are obtained when competitive template and unknown template are amplified at nearly equivalent concentrations.

38. It is often advantageous to perform an initial titration in log increments to determine the approximate concentration of the unknown RNA. Then perform a finer titration to obtain the most accurate results.

39. When target and standard RNA are at equal concentrations, coamplification results in equal amounts of both products with bands of equal density. Because the concentration of the standard is known, this gives the concentration of the target (unknown) RNA **(Fig. 2A)**. A point is determined where the starting number of standard RNA transcripts is equal to the starting number of target RNA transcripts. To determine this point, the ratios of the band intensities of the PCR products from the standard RNA and target RNA (i.e., ratio standard RNA/target RNA band intensity) is plotted against the starting number of standard RNA molecules on a semilogarithmic scale **(Fig. 2B)**.

40. Although we found that all transcripts examined for could be detected at a level even below 10^3 transcripts/µg total RNA, this value was chosen as a lower limit for the quantitative PCR analysis.

Acknowledgments

We thank Erik Kulø Hagen for help with the drawings. Studies in the authors' laboratory have been supported by the Norwegian Cancer Society, the Research Council of Norway, Anders Jahre's Fund, the Norwegian Coeliac Disease Association, and the Medinnova Governmental Research Organization, Rikshospitalet.

References

1. Nilsen, E. M., Jahnsen, F. L., Lundin, K. E. A., Johansen, F.-E., Fausa, O., Sollid, L. M., et al. (1998) Gluten induces an intestinal cytokine response strongly dominated by interferon-gamma in patients with celiac disease. *Gastroenterology* **115,** 551–563.
2. Lo, Y.-M. D., Mehal, W. Z., and Fleming, K. A. (1988) False-positive results and the polymerase chain reaction. *Lancet* **2,** 679.
3. Kwok, S. and Higuchi, R. (1989) Avoiding false positives with PCR. *Nature* **339,** 237–238.
4. Erlich, H. A., Gelfand, D., and Sninsky, J. J. (1991) Recent advances in the polymerase chain reaction. *Science* **252,** 1643–1651.
5. Wang, A. M., Doyle, M. V., and Mark, D. F. (1989) Quantitation of mRNA by the polymerase chain reaction. *Proc. Natl. Acad. Sci. USA* **86,** 9717–9721.
6. Siebert, P. D. and Larrick, J. W. (1992) Competitive PCR. *Nature* **359,** 557–558.
7. Lundin, K. E. A., Scott, H., Hansen, T., Paulsen, G., Halstensen, T. S., Fausa, O., et al. (1993) Gliadin-specific, HLA-DQ (α1*0501,β1*0201) restricted T cells isolated from the small intestinal mucosa of celiac disease patients. *J. Exp. Med.* **178,** 187–196.
8. Lundin, K. E. A., Scott, H., Fausa, O., Thorsby, E., and Sollid, L. M. (1994) T cells from the small intestinal mucosa of a DR4, DQ7/DR4, DQ8 celiac disease patient preferentially recognize gliadin when presented by DQ8. *Hum. Immunol.* **41,** 285–291.
9. Jung, H. C., Eckmann, L., Yang, S. K., Panja, A., Fierer, J., Morzycka-Wroblewska, E., and Kagnoff, M. F. (1995) A distinct array of proinflammatory cytokines is expressed in human colon epithelial cells in response to bacterial invasion. *J. Clin. Invest.* **95,** 55–65.
10. MacDonald, R. J., Swift, G. H., Przybyla, A. E., Rutters, W. J., and Chirgwin, J. M. (1979) Isolation of RNA using guanidium salts. *Methods Enzymol.* **152,** 219–234.
11. Kanangat, S., Solomon, A., and Rouse, B. T. (1992) Use of quantitative polymerase chain reaction to quantitate cytokine messenger RNA molecules. *Mol. Immunol.* **29,** 1229–1236.
12. Huang, S. K., Essayan, D. M., Krishnaswamy, G., Yi, M., Kumai, M., Su, S. N., et al. (1994) Detection of allergen- and mitogen-induced human cytokine transcripts using a competitive polymerase chain reaction. *J. Immunol. Methods* **168,** 167–181.
13. Sun, B., Wells, J., Goldmuntz, E., Silver, P., Remmers, E. F., Wilder, R. L., et al. (1996) A simplified, competitive RT-PCR method for measuring rat IFN-γ mRNA expression. *J. Immunol. Methods* **195,** 139–148.

14. Neel, H., Gondran, P., Weil, D., and Dautry, F. (1995) Regulation of pre-mRNA processing by src. *Curr. Biol.* **5,** 413–422.
15. Bamford, R. N., Tagaya, Y., and Waldmann, T. A. (1997) Interleukin 15—what it does and how it is controlled. *Immunologist* **5,** 52–56.
16. Innis, M. A. and Gelfand, D. H. (1990) Optimization of PCRs, in *PCR Protocols. A Guide to Methods and Applications* (Innis, M. A., Gelfand, D. H., Sninsky, J. J., and White, T. J., eds.), Academic, San Diego, pp. 3–12.
17. Saiki, R. K., Gelfand, D. H., Stoffel, S., Scharf, S. J., Higuchi, R., Horn, G. T., et al. (1988) Primer-directed enzymatic amplification of DNA with a thermostable DNA polymerase. *Science* **239,** 487–491.
18. Mullis, K. B. and Faloona, F. A. (1987) Specific synthesis of DNA in vitro via a polymerase-catalyzed chain reaction. *Methods Enzymol.* **155,** 335–350.
19. Li, H., Cui, X., and Arnheim, N. (1990) Direct electrophoretic detection of the allelic state of single DNA molecules in human sperm by using the polymerase chain reaction. *Proc. Natl. Acad. Sci. USA* **87,** 4580–4584.
20. Elder, P. K., French, C. L., Subramaniam, M., Schmidt, L. J., and Getz, M. J. (1988) Evidence that the functional β-actin gene is single copy in most mice and is associated with 5' sequences capable of conferring serum- and cycloheximide-dependent regulation. *Mol. Cell. Biol.* **8,** 480–485.
21. Sambrook, J., Fritsch, E. F., and Maniatis, T. (1989) Gel electrophoresis of DNA, in *Molecular Cloning. A Laboratory Manual* (Ford, N., Nolan, C., and Ferguson, M., eds.), Cold Spring Harbor Laboratory Press, Cold Spring Harbor, NY, pp. 6.1–6.19.
22. Sambrook, J., Fritsch, E. F., and Maniatis, T. (1989) In vitro amplification of DNA by the polymerase chain reaction, in *Molecular Cloning: A Laboratory Manual* (Ford, N., Nolan, C., and Ferguson, M., eds.), Cold Spring Harbor Laboratory Press, Cold Spring Harbor, NY, pp. 14.1–14.35.

7

Single Cell RT-PCR for the Detection of Cytokine mRNA

Moshe Ligumsky, Hovav Nechushtan, and Ehud Razin

1. Introduction

The introduction of the polymerase chain reaction (PCR) methodology has dramatically revolutionized basic and clinical molecular biology research in the recent decade. Accurate detection and identification of tiny and limited amounts of DNA are now possible *(1)*.

The PCR method, in combination with cell isolation and purification techniques has promoted the identification and characterization of specific mRNA types and the equivalent proteins produced in these single cells, which differ from those expressed by the other cells in their vicinity. Following this development, it was shortly demonstrated that this method is applicable and valid for identifying mRNA expressed by an individual cell *(2)*.

Single cell reverse transcription (RT-PCR) is advantageous in assessing the pattern of a specific mRNA expression by cells that are widely distributed and intermingled with other tissue cells and are not easily identified by their morphology or histology.

We modified the single cell RT-PCR approach previously described *(2)* into a reproducible and friendly technique, for studying and characterization of certain biochemical events in mast cells cocultured with fibroblasts *(3)*. This original work clearly showed enhancement of interleukin (IL)-3 accumulation in connective tissue mast cells cocultured with fibroblasts. This may explain the physiologic role of IL-3 in maintaining the survival of mast cell subpopulations and probably other cells. This new approach has promoted studies examining the regulation of various stimulatory and inhibitory cytokines in cell systems derived from different tissues. Moreover, the RT-PCR approach was also used by our group to detect acetylcholine esterase mRNA expression in single mast cells derived from human colonic mucosa *(4)*, supporting the notion of a physiologic neuronal-mast cell interaction. We have recently summarized our use of single cell RT-PCR *(5)*.

From: *Methods in Molecular Medicine, vol. 60: Interleukin Protocols*
Edited by: L. A. J. O'Neill and A. Bowie © Humana Press Inc., Totowa, NJ

Using RT-PCR, accurate determination of mRNA linearly may be difficult even at relatively high amounts of RNA, and until now it has not been used for quantitative assessment of specific mRNAs in single cells. Although this approach may seem counterintuitive to the notion that the increase of mRNA in the tissue reflects stimulated expression of each cell, there is good evidence that at least in some instances *(6,7)* the increased tissue mRNA expression results from the increase in the numbers of the expressing cells rather than increased expression by each cell.

Fiering et al. *(6)* studied NF-AT-regulated expression in activated T cells. Plasmids expressing the β-Galactosidase *(β-Gal)* gene, regulated by NF-AT, were transfected into T cells, and β-Gal activity was measured in single cells of the activated T-cell population. The β-Gal activity was enhanced in the total cell population as a result of the increased percentage of the cells expressing β-Gal, but beyond a certain threshold there was no increased activity in the individual cell. Thus, it may well be that in certain circumstances, the increased expression of tissue mRNA may reflect the increasing percentage of cells expressing the gene rather than stimulation of gene expression by each cell.

An important and original use of the RT-PCR method was to study the profile of various cytokines expressed by colonic mucosal mast cells in inflammatory bowel disease (IBD) *(8)*. Mast cells are one of the main sources of cytokines; they have a distinct histologic pattern and play a role in inflammatory/immunologic reactions. However, in the tissue they are distributed among other cell types, and their isolation and identification may be difficult. Following dispersion and isolation of the cells from mucosal biopsies (obtained from patients during colonoscopy), we measured c-kit expression and IgE receptor α-G-chain expression in the isolated-single cells for the verification of mast cells. Following enrichment and short-term culture, the estimated yield of purification was 15–20%. IL-3 was clearly expressed in cells derived from untreated patients, whereas it was almost totally abolished in mast cells derived from steroid-treated patients. In this work, we thus used the combination of isolation, identification, and functional activity (cytokine expression) to study the characteristics of a single mucosal mast cell derived from patients with IBD *(8)*.

A differentiation and maturation study of lymphocytes also used a similar approach *(9)*, as did a study characterizating odor receptors on single cells, which may play a role in the mechanism of olfaction *(10)*.

An additional important use of the single cell RT-PCR method was in evaluating the allele-specific expression of genes. Recent cumulative data indicate that expression of one allele occurs only in a specific cell (even in genes whose control is unrelated to imprinting) and may turn out to be an important biologic regulatory mechanism. T-cell studies indicate that an allele-specific regulation of IL-4 is operative *(11)*. Moreover, *Pax5*, a gene that is essential for controlling and regulating B cells and midbrain development was found to be predominantly transcribed from one allele only in early progenitors and mature B cells, whereas it switches to a biallelic transcription mode in immature B cells *(12)*. Thus, by using the single cell RT-PCR method in such instances, vital information regarding the function of special genes expressed by specific cells could be recruited.

2. Materials

1. Inverted microscope programmable thermal controller table-top microfuge.
2. Sterile pipet tips, gloves, Terasaki plates, sterile (RNAase-free) 1.5-mL microfuge tubes.
3. Lysis buffer: 10 mM Tris-HCl, pH 8.0, 100 mM NaCl, 1 mM EDTA, and 0.5% sodium dodecyl sulfate (SDS) supplemented with 100 µg proteinase K/100 µL solution.
4. OligodT-cellulose solution: 50 mg oligodT-cellulose in sterile 3 M NaCl.
5. Binding buffer: 0.5 M NaCl, 10 mM Tris-HCl, pH 8.0, 1 mM EDTA, and 0.1% SDS.
6. Washing buffer: 0.1 M NaCl, 10 mM Tris-HCl, pH 8.0, 1 mM EDTA, and 0.1% SDS; sterilize in autoclave.
7. 10 mM Tris-HCl, pH 8.3.
8. tRNA: 5 g/1 µL in sterile distilled water.
9. 70% Ethanol made with RNAase-free water.
10. Reverse transcriptase.
11. RNAase inhibitor.
12. Reverse transcription buffer from the company that supplied the reverse transcriptase or, alternatively, 50 mM Tris-HCl, pH 7.6, 60 mM KCl, 1 mM dithiothreitol (Sigma).
13. 10 mM MgCl$_2$.
14. dNTP Li salt at 2.5 mM solution.
15. Oligodeoxynucleotide primers (around 20 bp long) at a concentration of 100 mM.
16. *Taq* DNA polymerase.
17. *Taq* DNA polymerase buffer is supplied by the company or, alternatively, 100 mM Tris-HCl, pH 8.0, 15 mM MgCl$_2$, 500 mM KCl, and 1% (w/v) gelatin is used.
18. αFcεRI oligonucleotide primers:
    Sense: 5'-ATG GCT CCT GCC ATG GAA TCC CCT ACT-3'.
    Antisense: 5'-GGT TCC ACT GTC TTC AAC TGT GGC AAT-3' corresponding to bases 106–519.
    IL-4 primers:
    Sense: 5'-ATG GGT CTC ACC TCC CAA CTG CTT CCC-3'.
    Antisense: 5'-ATT TCT CTC TCA TGA TCG TCT TTA GCC-3' corresponding to bases 64–505.
    IL-3 primers:
    Sense: 5'-GCT CCC ATG ACC CAG ACA ACG TCC TTG-3' .
    Antisense: 5'-GTC CTT GAT ATG GAT TGG ATG TCG CGT-3' corresponding to bases 67–360.
    IL-8 primers:
    Sense: 5'-ATG ACT TCC AAG CTG GCC GTG GCT CTC-3'.
    Antisense: 5'-ATG AAT TCT CAG CCC TCT TCA AAA ACT-3' corresponding to bases 1–295.

TNFα primers:
    Sense: 5'-CTG CGC CAG GCA ACG GGT CCT GCG CCT-3'
    Antisense: 5'-CAG CTT CAG GTC CCT CAA AGC GCT GCG GGG-3'.
c-Kit primers:
    Sense: 5'- TCA CAG CTT GGC AGC CAG -3' and antisense: 5'- GGG GAT
    CTG CAT CCC AGC AAG-3' corresponding to 2384-2754.

3. Methods

1. To separate single cells, serial dilution of the cells is performed in Terasaki microtiter plates until single cells are visualized in each well by inverted microscope.
2. For mRNA production (the reverse transcriptase step), it is essential to wear gloves to avoid possible RNAse contamination.
3. Each cell is to be transferred from its well into a 1.5-mL microfuge tube containing 100 mL of lysis buffer with a sterile tip and than incubated for 10 min at 37°C.
4. 2.5 µL from the oligodT-cellulose solution is then to be added.
5. The solution is incubated overnight, with rotation, at room temperature.
6. It is then centrifuged for 30 s in a microfuge and the oligodT-cellulose pellet is washed three times with binding buffer followed by one wash with a washing buffer.
7. The RNA is eluted by incubating the oligodT-cellulose pellet for 10 min at room temperature with 50 µL of 10 mM Tris-HCl, pH 8.3.
8. The mRNA is ethanol-precipitated in the presence of 5 µg tRNA, spun, and then washed with 70% ethanol.
9. Dried mRNA pellets are redissolved in 4 µL of reverse transcription buffer, 5 U RNAase inhibitor, 4 µL dNTP, primers 2 µL each, RT (200 U). Final volume should be 20 µL (*see* **Notes 1–6**).
10. Incubation is for 60 min.
11. A solution containing 2.5 U of *Taq* DNA polymerase should be added to the RT reaction, 6 µL dNTP, 3 µL of the primer from each primer pair to a final volume of 100 µL.
12. Amplification in the usual three-temperature cycles in a programmable thermal controller. The temperature used in the annealing cycle should be determined according to the G + C content of the primers. Most of our experiments were carried out at 55°C.
13. Analysis of the PCR reaction products by electrophoresis, Southern blot, and hybridization with the appropriate DNA probe.

4. Notes

1. One method that has been used to enhance the sensitivity of the PCR reaction is the use of a nested set of primers. We had no need for this method, perhaps because there is high enough expression of cytokines in mast cells under the condition checked.
2. We routinely coamplified up to four different genes together; however, we never used a nested set in these conditions, which might have been more problematic in an assay of several different genes together.
3. Kits for performing single tube RT and amplification are now available (i.e., Titan from Boehringer Manheim). We used those kits successfully for quantitative RT-PCR. We have not used this kit for single cell PCR, although it might have been useful.

4. The primers are chosen from sequences in different exons spanning an intron so that fragments amplified from cDNA generated from mRNA could be readily distinguished by their much smaller size from those predicted to be generated from any contaminating genomic DNA

5. Further verification as to the nature of the amplified fragment can be obtained by a small 25-mer oligonucleotide from the amplified segment labeled by γ-ATP using the regular α-labeled NTP (usually dCTP) available by terminal deoxytransferase.

6. Since results also depend on the success of the amplification and hybridization step, it is preferable to collect RT samples than to amplify and analyze as many samples as possible at the same time, if a semiquantitative assessment is required.

References

1. Ausubel, F. M., Kingstone, R. E., Moore, D. D., Seidman, J. G., Smith, J. A., and Struhl, K., eds. (1994) *Current Protocols in Molecular Biology*. Greene, Wiley Interscience, Brooklyn, NY.
2. Rappolee., D. A., Wang, A., Mark, D., and Werb, Z. (1989) Novel method for studying mRNA phenotypes in single or small numbers of cells. *J. Cell Biochem.* **39,** 1–7.
3. Razin, E., Leslie, K. B., and Schrader, J. W. (1991) Connective tissue mast cells in contact with fibroblasts express IL-3 mRNA. Analysis of single cells by polymerase chain reaction. *J. Immunol.* **146,** 981–987.
4. Nechashtan, H., Soreq, H., Kuperstein, V., Tshori, S., and Razin, E. (1996) Murine and human mast cells express acetylcholinesterase. *FEBS Lett.* **379,** 1–6.
5. Nechushtan, H. and Razin, E. (1997) cDNA PCR amplification of RNA from single mast cells, in *Immunology Methods Manual*, Academic Press, Ltd., pp. 1429–1433.
6. Fiering, S., Northrop, J. P., Nolan, G. P., Mattila, P. S., Crabtree, G. R., and Herzenberg, L. A. (1990) Single cell assay of a transcription factor reveals a threshold in transcription activated by signals emanating from the T-cell antigen receptor. *Genes Dev.* **4,** 1823–1834.
7. Karttunen, J. and Shastri, N. (1991) Measurement of ligand-induced activation in single viable T cell using the lacZ reporter gene. *Proc. Natl. Acad. Sci. USA* **88,** 3972–3976.
8. Ligumsky, M., Kuperstein, V., Nechushtan, H., Zhang, Z., and Razin, E. (1997) Analysis of cytokine profile in human colonic mucosal FceRI-positive cells by single cell PCR: inhibition of IL-3 expression in steroid-treated IBD patients. *FEBS Lett.* **413,** 436–440.
9. Mostoslavsky, N., Singh, A., Kirilov, A., et al. (1998)*k* Chain monoallelic demethylation and the establishment of allelic exclusion. *Genes Dev.* **12,** 1801–1811.
10. Malnic, B., Hirono, J., Sato, T., and Buck, L. B. (1999). Combinatorial receptor codes for odors. *Cell* **96,** 713–723.
11. Bix, M. and Locksley, R. M. (1998) Independent and epigenetic regulation of the interleukin-4 alleles in CD4+ T cells. *Science* **281,** 1352–1354.
12. Nutt, S. L., Vambrie, S., Steinlein, P., et al. (1999) Independent regulation of the two *Pax5* alleles during B-cell development. *Nat. Genet.* **21,** 390–395.

8

Quantitation of Cytokine mRNA by Flash-Type Bioluminescence

Jeffrey K. Actor

1. Introduction

Cytokines produced by a variety of cells in response to stimuli are important in the regulation of physiologic and immunologic processes; tremendous efforts have been made to study cytokine profiles in various physiologic and disease conditions. Bioluminescent reverse transcription polymerase chain reaction (BL RT-PCR) has been especially useful for the quantitation of cytokine mRNA during parasitic infections (1–8). RT-PCR has the advantage of target amplification, requiring only small amounts of RNA (9). By combining the advantages of RT-PCR with the sensitivity, stability, and the unique properties of the photoprotein aequorin, the bioluminescent system becomes an obvious alternate choice for analytic applications of cytokine RT-PCR.

The need to replace radioisotopes and maintain sensitivity of analyte detection has been a major factor in the development of new technologies for measurement of RT-PCR products. Although fluorescence applications are intrinsically more sensitive than absorption measurements, the background signals resulting from inefficient separation of incidence and emitted light and the presence of nonspecific fluorescence from many biologic materials has limited fluorescence applications in classical enzyme-linked immunosorbent assay (ELISA) formats for ultrasensitive, quantitative measurements. For quantitative analyses of analytes in microplate formats, the enzyme-induced chemiluminescence systems also have severe limitations. Background light from nonspecific hydrolysis or oxidation of the substrates results in background signals in relative light units (RLU) that can be one or more logs above the dark current background of photon counting instruments. The high background is difficult to distinguish from low signals, and this situation is exacerbated if this background is amplified during long integration times.

From: *Methods in Molecular Medicine, vol. 60: Interleukin Protocols*
Edited by: L. A. J. O'Neill and A. Bowie © Humana Press Inc., Totowa, NJ

Bioluminescence-based detection protocols for cytokine messages have been developed that are sensitive into the attomolar range *(10,11)*. This allows fewer cycles of PCR and avoids the plateau effect traditionally associated with other noncompetitive RT-PCR techniques. These assays are based on use of a recombinant form of the photoprotein aequorin, the calcium-dependent bioluminescent protein isolated from the jellyfish *Aequorea victoria*. The photoprotein is uniquely suited as a detection system because it is not an enzyme. It is a "self-contained," triggerable, light-generating protein *(12–14)* that is perhaps better described as a stable enzyme-substrate complex. Signals that produce a rapid flash reaction with little or no background light from substrates are potentially more useful for sensitive, quantitative applications. The signal-to-noise ratio for the Aequorin-based formats is very high because of the stability of aequorin, resulting in little or no background noise from reagent decomposition. Bioluminescence, which can be defined as the production of light by the direct enzymatic oxidation of a luciferin to an intermediate that produces light, is generally more efficient than chemiluminescent reactions and has relatively high quantum yields. Upon addition of calcium ions ($K_d = 1.4 \times 10^{-7}$) the AquaLite catalyzes the oxidation of the bound coelenterazine by the bound oxygen. The oxidized substrate decays to a ground state, which is accompanied by the emission of a flash of blue light ($\lambda_{max} = 469$ nm) at a quantum efficiency of 25–30% and a half-life of about 0.5 s *(15)*. AquaLite is used as the raw material for the manufacture of bioluminescent conjugates of antibodies, haptens, or oligonucleotides for applications in immunoassays and nucleic acid probe-based assays.

The bioluminescence produced by the aequorin conjugate covers more than 7 logs of concentration, of which approx 5 logs produces a linear relationship between product and bioluminescence signal *(10,16)*. Direct comparison with electrochemiluminescence and with radiometric readouts revealed that the flash-type aequorin-based bioluminescence has greater sensitivity *(2,10)*, especially when amplicons are assayed in a PCR cycle range where broad-range, linear detection is most robust. An additional advantage of aequorin-based bioluminescent methods is their ease of automation and reduced cost. Aequorin tags generate rapid signals with high signal-to-noise ratios *(17)*. The assay is robust and flexible, allowing analysis of multiple messages. The use of AquaLite for the detection and quantification of nucleic acids in open architecture microplate formats represents the most exciting applications of this unique detection system.

2. Materials

1. Luminometer: A luminometer is required that can inject a calcium solution and simultaneously measure a flash of blue light (469 nm). Luminometers with positive displacement dispensers are acceptable and typically can accommodate

a number of applications (e.g., alkaline phosphatase glow reactions and enhanced glow luciferase reporter gene assays in addition to the flash aequorin assays). The machine should have nearly eight decades of dynamic range, the ability to read every 10 ms (100 readings per second), and minimal cross-talk between wells. The equipment is usually software driven, allowing readings to be averaged, summed, graphed and/or scaled depending on the options selected. (A scaling factor of 1–10,000 changes the magnitude of the RLU values.) The flash-type light reaction is relatively insensitive to temperature changes; therefore temperature control within the luminometer is not required.

2. Nucleic acid sequences: Nucleotide primer and probe sequences have been optimized for bioluminescent detection using the sequence parameters described below. Specific primer and probe sequences to measure human and mouse cytokine messages have been published elsewhere *(2,3)*.
   a. Optimized sequences should be 18–22 nucleotides in length, with melting temperatures of 60°C.
   b. Amplicons produced should be between 150 and 400 bp. Larger amplicons may be used, but assay sensitivity decreases with increased amplicon size.
   c. Probes may be labeled on either the 5' or 3' terminal nucleotide. Reversal of label from one end to the other has been known to reduce background (reasons unknown, empirical testing).
   d. Relative to RT-PCR and message specificity: Primers should cross exons to limit detection of genomic sequences. Ideally, probes that span exon junctions practically eliminate background hybridization to genomic sequences.

2.1. Bioluminescent Hybridization ImmunoAssay

1. Streptavidin-coated Microplates: Manufactured by many commercial entities, including Boehringer Mannheim (Indianapolis, IN), Dynex (Chantilly, VA), and MicroCoat (Penzberg, Germany). Microtiter plates in these assays are white, opaque plates. It is recommended that each laboratory evaluate streptavidin-coated microplates for amplicon binding capacity, background, and consistency under their operating conditions. The optimal plate should have a high capacity for PCR product capture, low nonspecific binding, and a 12–24 mo shelf life at 4°C.
2. Denaturation buffer: 1 M NaOH, 200 mM EDTA.
3. Neutralization buffer: 0.15 M Na$_2$HPO$_4$, pH 6.0.
4. Hybridization buffer: 62.5 mM Na$_2$HPO$_4$, 94 mM citric acid, 10 mM MgCl$_2$, 0.0125% Tween-20, 0.0625% bovine serum albumin (BSA), 15 mM NaN$_3$, pH 7.0.
5. Wash buffer: 20 mM Tris-HCl, 5mM EDTA, 0.15 M NaCl, 0.05% Tween-20, 15 mM NaN$_3$, pH 7.5.
6. Assay buffer: 25 mM Tris-HCl, 10 mM EDTA, 2 mg/mL BSA, 0.15 M KCl, 0.05% Tween-20, 15 mM NaN$_3$, pH 7.5.
7. Trigger solution: 50 mM Tris-HCl, 10 mM calcium acetate, 15 mM NaN$_3$, pH 7.5.
8. Aequorin-conjugated anti-hapten Fab: Aequorin-conjugated antibodies may be obtained from Chemicon (Temecula, CA). Chemicon distributes the ChemFLASH™ Universal Detection Assay, which contains AquaLite® anti-fluorescein isothiocyanate

(FITC) and buffers for use in the bioluminescent hybridization immunoassay (*see* **Note 1**). Custom aequorin conjugates to antibodies with other specificities may also be obtained.

2.2. Bioluminescent Hybridization Assay

1. Streptavidin-coated microplates, denaturation buffer, neutralization buffer, and trigger solution as in **Subheading 2.1.**
2. Direct-label oligonucleotide hybridization buffer: 125 mM Na$_2$HPO$_4$, 188 mM citric acid, 50 mM MgCl$_2$, 40 mM EGTA, 4 mM EDTA, 0.125% BSA, 15 mM NaN$_3$, pH 7.0.
3. Conjugate diluent: 25 mM HEPES, 0.15 M KCl, 10 mM EDTA, 2 mg/mL BSA, 0.05% Tween-20, 15 mM NaN$_3$, pH 7.0.
4. Direct aequorin-conjugated nucleic acid sequences (*see* **Note 1**): Custom aequorin-conjugated nucleic acids are obtained from Chemicon.

2.3. Bioluminescent Capture Assay

1. Hybridization buffer, denaturization buffer, and neutralization buffer as in **Subheading 2.1.**
2. Specific amine-modified oligonucleotides capture probes.
3. Microplates: Corning (Corning, NY) has developed a white, opaque microplate surface-derivatized with N-oxysuccinimide that can be used to attach an aminated DNA probe covalently.
4. Oligo binding buffer: 0.1 M HEPES, 0.8 M sodium citrate, 1 mM EDTA, pH 8.0.
5. Oligo block buffer: 3% BSA in oligo binding buffer.
6. Oligo plate rinse: 2X standard sodium citrate (SSC), 0.5% sodium dodecyl sulfate (SDS).
7. Aequorin-conjugated streptavidin: Aequorin-conjugated streptavidin may be obtained from Chemicon, which distributes the ChemFLASH™ AquaLite® Streptavidin Kit containing buffers and aequorin conjugates for use in the bioluminescent hybridization immunoassay (*see* **Note 1**)

3. Methods
3.1. Reverse Transcriptase Polymerase Chain Reaction

RT-PCR was done like published methods (*18*), modified for bioluminescent quantitation of PCR products (*1,10*). RNA isolation may be accomplished through standard techniques or commercial kits. The bioluminescent quantitation of RT-PCR products described here has been optimized for analysis using 1 µg RNA starting material. The methods described here for cDNA production and PCR amplification may be modified; the example given is typical for our laboratory, using SuperScript II for reverse transcription and *Taq* DNA polymerase for amplification (GIBCO BRL, Grand Island, NY). Cycle number will vary according to parameters described (*see* **Note 2** and **Subheading 3.5.**). A more detailed explanation of PCR and its parameters may be found in the literature (*19,20*).

1. Combine 1 µg total RNA together with 1X Superscript II reverse transcriptase (RT) buffer (GIBCO BRL), 0.1 M dithiothreitol , 2.5 mM deoxynucleotidestriphosphate (dNTPs; Boehringer Mannheim), 80 U random hexamer oligonucleotides (Boehringer Mannheim), 20 U RNase inhibitor (RNasin; Promega, Madison, WI) in a 25-µL volume.
4. Heat for 5 min at 70°C, then chill on ice for 5 min.
5. Add 1 µL (200 U) SuperScript II RT and incubate for 60 min at 37°C.
6. To inactivate the enzyme, heat to 90°C for 5 min.
7. Dilute the sample 1:8 using distilled water prior to PCR amplification.
8. Combine 5 µL cDNA, 0.2 U GIBCO *Taq* DNA polymerase (GIBCO BRL), 1X *Taq* polymerase assay buffer (20 mM Tris-HCl, pH 8.4, 50 mM KCl), 1.73 mM MgCl$_2$, 200 mM dNTPs, 0.2 µM sense and antisense primers.
9. Perform 15–40 cycles of amplification. Denaturate, anneal, and elongate at 94°C, 54°C, and 72°C for 30 s, 30 s, and 40 s, respectively, in a standard thermal cycler (e.g., PTC-100-96V thermal cycler; MJ Research, Waltham, MA).

3.2. Bioluminescent Hybridization Immunoassay

The current approach to aequorin-based assays to detect and quantify PCR products uses a biotin-labeled primer to generate biotinylated amplicons that are captured on streptavidin-coated plates for detection. In these experiments, one of the two primers is 5'-labeled with biotin for later capture onto a streptavidin matrix. The biotinylated amplicons are detected using solid phase techniques according to a modified version of published methods as depicted in **Fig. 1** *(21)*.

1. Denature 25 µL of the biotinylated PCR product by addition of 6.25 µL denaturation buffer for 5 min at room temperature.
2. Add 31.25 µL neutralization buffer.
3. Add 12.5 µL of denatured and neutralized product to wells of streptavidin-coated microtiter plates, which already contain 2 ng hapten (e.g., FITC)-labeled probe in 100 µL hybridization buffer.
4. Cover the wells and incubate for 1–2 h at 42°C, shaking.
5. Wash the wells 4 times with 200 µL wash buffer.
6. Add 5 ng of aequorin-conjugated anti-hapten Fab diluted in 100 µL assay buffer to the wells. Incubate for 30 min with agitation (180 rpm) at room temperature.
7. Wash the wells 4 times with 200 µL wash buffer.
8. Detect the conjugate by measuring the flash reaction in a microplate luminometer, after injection of trigger solution, integrating for 2 s with a 0.2-s delay.

3.3. Bioluminescent Hybridization Assay

The bioluminescent hybridization assay (BHA) eliminates necessity of the F(ab) conjugate by attaching aequorin directly to a nucleic acid probe sequence *(22)*. These are available as custom conjugates (Chemicon). Following incubation with direct labeled probes, the wells are covered and incubated for only 1 h. The conjugate is then immediately ready for detection by measuring integrated flash (469 nm) on a luminometer (**Fig. 2**).

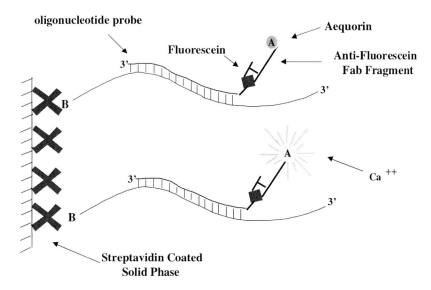

Fig. 1. Diagrammatic representation of the Bioluminescence hybridization immunoassay (BHIA) for detection of cytokine RT-PCR amplicons. Amplicons are generated using a biotinylated primer, denatured, neutralized, and captured onto streptavidin-coated microplates. Captured amplicons are probed with hapten-labeled probes, and aequorin-conjugated anti-hapten is added (*top*). Addition of calcium acetate triggers release of a flash of light detectable at 469 nm (*bottom*).

1. Denature the biotinylated PCR product (25 µL) by addition of 1/4 vol denaturation buffer for 5 min at room temperature and neutralize by equal volume of neutralization buffer.
2. Add 12.5 µL of denatured and neutralized product directly to wells of streptavidin microtiter plates, which already contain 100 µL direct label oligonucleotide hybridization buffer.
3. Add 5–10 ng aequorin-conjugated probe diluted in 100 µL conjugate diluent to each well. It should be emphasized that the optimal concentration of probe must be determined empirically.
4. Cover the wells and incubate the plates for 1 h at 37°C, shaking (180 rpm).
5. Wash the wells are washed 4 times with 300 µL wash buffer.
6. Detect the conjugate by measuring the flash reaction in a microplate luminometer, after injection of trigger solution, integrating for 2 s, with a 0.2-s delay.

3.4. Bioluminescent Capture Assay

Another approach is to capture the PCR product with a microplate that has been covalently derivatized with a unique capture probe. In this format, the NH2-5'-oligonucleotide probe derivatized surface of the microplate provides the definition of the assay and specificity of capture, and the detection utilizes an

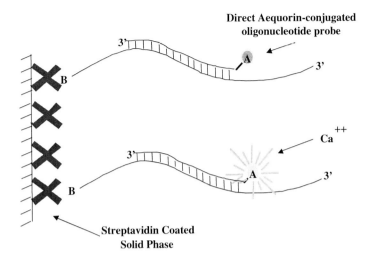

Fig. 2. Bioluminescence hybridization assay (BHA) for detection of RT-PCR amplicons. Amplicons are generated using a biotinylated primer, denatured, neutralized, and captured onto streptavidin-coated microplates. Captured amplicons are probed directly with aequorin-conjugated nucleic acid sequences (*top*). Addition of calcium acetate triggers release of a flash of light detectable at 469 nm (*bottom*).

aequorin-streptavidin universal reagent. Using this format, cytokine RT-PCR capture assays have been developed (*23*). The microplate wells, derivatized with the specific capture probe, provide the specificity of detection, and a universal bioluminescent reagent such as aequorin-streptavidin can be used for all assays. The product capture assay provides a versatile format for nucleic acid detection and quantification **(Fig. 3)**.

1. Immobilize amine-modified oligonucleotide capture sequences onto capture plates according to the manufacturer's instructions. When using the DNA-BIND™ plate (Costar, Cambridge, MA), dilute 0.05–5 μ*M* NH2-capture sequences in 100 μL oligo binding buffer. Incubate the plates overnight at 4°C, or for 1 h at 37°C.
2. Remove unbound capture sequences, and block wells with 200 μL oligo block buffer for 30 min at 37°C.
3. Wash plates 3× with oligo plate rinse (let plate stand for 5 min with liquid in wells between rinses).
4. Add 100 μL BHIA hybridization buffer to wells (*see* **Note 3**); use plates immediately.
5. Prepare amplicons for addition to wells: Denature 25 μL biotinylated PCR product by addition of 1/4 vol denaturation buffer for 5 min at room temperature.
6. Equal volume neutralization buffer is added to the denatured amplicon.
7. Add 12.5 μL of denatured and neutralized product to wells coated with the capture sequence.

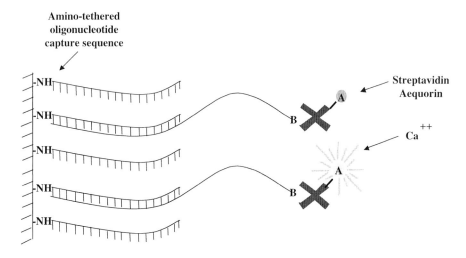

Fig. 3. Bioluminescent capture assay. Amplicons are generated using a biotinylated primer, denatured, neutralized, and captured onto microplates containing amino-tethered capture nucleic acid sequences. Captured amplicons are probed with aequorin-conjugated streptavidin (*top*). Addition of calcium acetate triggers release of a flash of light detectable at 469 nm (*bottom*).

8. Cover the wells and incubate for 1 h at 42°C, shaking at 180 rpm.
9. Wash the wells 4 times with 200 µL wash buffer.
10. Add 5–15 ng of aequorin-conjugated streptavidin in 100 µL assay buffer to the wells. Incubate for 30 min with agitation (180 rpm) at room temperature.
11. Wash the wells 4 times with 200 µL wash buffer.
12. Detect the conjugate by measuring the flash reaction in a microplate luminometer, after injection of trigger solution, integrating for 2 s with a 0.2-s delay.

3.5. Application of Bioluminescence Assay and Data Analysis

Analysis of relative changes in cytokine mRNA using bioluminescent RT-PCR is most accurate when amplicons are assayed in a PCR cycle range where linear detection is most robust. To illustrate this concept, RNA was prepared from mouse splenocytes following a 4-h in vitro ConA stimulation. Following reverse transcription of 1 µg RNA, cDNA was diluted and subjected to increasing amplification, from 2 through 40 cycles using interleukin-2 (IL-2) primer sequences *(10)*. BL immunoassay was able to detect IL-2 RT-PCR product in the stimulated population above 15 cycles (**Fig. 4**).

When compared with cDNA from unstimulated cells, a relative increase in IL-2 cDNA, and thus an increase in corresponding RNA, was demonstrated. At 20 cycles of amplification, there was significant increase in signal generated from the stimulated cells over levels in the unstimulated population. By 30

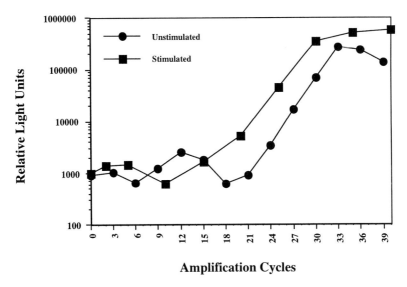

Amplification Cycles

Fig. 4. Effect of PCR cycle number on IL-2 RT-PCR amplicon detection using BL. cDNA derived from mouse splenocytes stimulated for 4 h with ConA (■), or unstimulated (●), was amplified through 40 cycles using a 5'-biotin-labeled sense primer sequence for mouse IL-2. Captured biotinylated RT-PCR amplicons were probed with an FITC-labeled sequence and detected using an aequorin-conjugated anti-FITC antibody. Background light registered less than 600 RLU.

cycles of amplification, the stimulated population had just entered the product plateau phase; the PCR reaction had produced a maximal amount of detectable RT-PCR amplicons. For the unstimulated cells, detection of presumably constitutive RT-PCR signal began above 21 cycles, with increasing signal through 33 cycles of amplification.

For clarity of analysis, the linear portion for our above amplification example is depicted in **Fig. 5** (*see* **Note 4**). Accurate quantitation of RNA may be calculated as the ordinal difference between the linear portions of the curves (the difference in their *x*-intercepts) derived from RT-PCR linear regression. By this analysis, 4.3 additional amplification cycles are necessary to achieve similar quantities of product from the unstimulated than for the stimulated group. This translates into a 20.3-fold difference (equivalent to 4.3 doublings) in IL-2 cDNA between the two populations. These data exemplify the importance of comparing both populations during the linear phase of RT-PCR expansion. The relative difference in signals generated between stimulated and unstimulated groups decreased as cycles increased, due to the plateau phase of RT-PCR product generated at higher cycle sets. At 30 cycles of amplification, the stimulated population had a relative difference in signal generated that was only

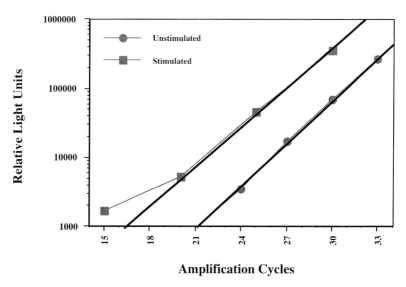

Amplification Cycles

Fig. 5. Comparative quantitation of IL-2 RT-PCR amplicons using BL. cDNA from mouse splenocytes stimulated for 4 h with ConA (■), or unstimulated (●), was amplified through 40 cycles using a 5'-biotin-labeled sense primer sequence for mouse IL-2. Captured biotinylated RT-PCR amplicons were probed with an FITC-labeled sequence and detected using AquaLite anti-FITC conjugate. Regression analysis of signal generated during the linear growth phase of PCR amplification allowed quantitation of differences between cDNA derived from either unstimulated (●, $r = 0.977$) or mitogen-stimulated (■, $r = 0.975$) mouse splenocytes. Evaluation was performed on duplicate samples using linear regression analysis in Excel, Version 5.0 (Microsoft, Redmond, WA). The standard deviation for duplicate samples was less than 5%.

5.0-fold. By 35 cycles of amplification, the RLUs generated were nearly identical. Conversely, comparisons in signals generated at the low amplification cycles (prior to signal detection from both populations) also do not properly reflect amplicon levels; at 20 cycles, the unstimulated group was below detectable levels.

A simplified analysis is valid at single points along the linear portions of the curve, provided linear curves have a slope equivalent approaching a value of 1.0. In this instance, the fold-difference in RLU values obtained directly equals the value obtained through linear regression analysis. Therefore, it is imperative that the RT-PCR analysis be performed along the linear portion of the amplification phase. Proper controls must be included to ensure location along the linear amplification portion of the curve (*see* **Note 5**). A more detailed explanation of analyses may be found in the literature (*2*).

Finally, bioluminescent detection analysis may be applied when using competitive sequences to quantitate accurately the initial copy number of the molecules amplified. The extreme sensitivity of the bioluminescent assay, combined with the competition of primers for template sequences in the PCR, places additional constraints on the amplification procedure. In this type of procedure, standard concentrations of reagents (dNTPs, $MgCl_2$, and primer concentrations) must be adapted to fit the constraints of the reaction occurring at low cycle number. A detailed explanation of the changes in these parameters has been published *(3)*.

The bioluminescent assay is an alternative method for evaluating RT-PCR products and quantifying changes in cytokine mRNA. This technique offers exceptional sensitivity and has been developed in an automated open architecture format. The assay is versatile, operates with a broad linear range of product detection, and has favorable signal-to-noise ratios compared with standard methodologies.

Flash-type bioluminescence has a capacity for high throughput, because of microtiter analysis, therefore increasing the number of samples that can be assayed concurrently. The time necessary for signal detection after amplification of PCR product is reduced to less than 4 h, compared with 24 or more hours for radioactive detection, mostly due to reduced manipulations of product prior to detection. The open architecture format lends itself to detection of any given message; suitable primers and probes can be readily generated using known sequences and software available to most laboratories.

Bioluminescence is offered as an attractive alternative to radioactivity methodology. Although radioactive tags have traditionally been successful in applications involving detection of nucleic acids on membranes, sensitivity is limited by the film threshold and binding capacity of the binding matrix. Thus, for quantitative measurements, radioactively based systems normally present high backgrounds and (because of excess manipulations from gels to membranes) lowered precision attributes that limit sensitivity *(25,26)*. Additional complications with radioactive probes involve disposal of waste and compliance with ever increasing regulations for use of these material. With flash-type bioluminescence, signal-to-noise ratios are dramatically increased *(16,17)*, in essence allowing for linear quantitation over a broad range of amplification cycles. Moreover, there are no waste disposal concerns, and sample manipulations are considerably reduced.

The flexibility in design of primers and probes has allowed the BHIA to be successfully applied toward the understanding of immunoregulation during disease pathogenesis. In summary, use of the flash-type bioluminescence, aequorin-based immunoassay has allowed quantitative comparisons between RNA populations and as such is a viable and sensitive analytic tool for a more accurate, rapid assessment of biologic responses during infectious disease.

4. Notes

1. Concerns over aequorin instability have been perhaps the greatest arguments against the commercialization of bioluminescence for in vitro testing; however, this issue was a greater impediment for aequorin-based assays. The simple solution to this perceived obstacle was the addition of a chelator like EDTA and/or EGTA. The concentrations of these chelators at 5–10 times the endogenous calcium concentration in the sample is sufficient to protect the AquaLite conjugates during incubation times of up to 10 h at 37°C. Thus, in the absence of calcium ions, AquaLite conjugates are stable in solutions that contain calcium chelators such as EDTA or EGTA. In addition to calcium-selective chelators like EDTA, it is possible to include Mg^{2+} in assay buffers containing AquaLite to enhance solution stability. Mg^{2+} binds the calcium binding sites of aequorin but does not trigger the reaction. The bound Mg^{2+} competes for any trace Ca^{2+} and may inhibit the calcium-independent bioluminescence of aequorin.

   The stability of the protein under many different storage and assay conditions has been evaluated *(21,24)*. The recombinant protein and its antibody conjugates are remarkably stable under normal conditions for immunoassays. Although AquaLite conjugates of oligonucleotides cannot survive stringent hybridization conditions and the high temperature of thermocycling, they are sufficiently stable to survive conventional hybridization conditions of 45°C for 1.5 h and thus make excellent bioluminescent reagents for detection and quantification of PCR products. In solutions, buffered between pH 6.5 and 8.5 and containing appropriate chelators, 5–10 mM Mg^{2+}, and bovine serum albumin, AquaLite conjugates are stable (less than 15% loss of light activity) for 1 mo when stored at 2–8°C. Such solutions are stable for over a year at –20°C and can be subjected to three freeze-thaw cycles without significant loss of light activity. At room temperature these preparations are stable for 24 h. For preparation of commercial reagents, AquaLite conjugates are lyophilized and sealed under dry nitrogen or argon where they are stable for 18–24 mo at 2–8 °C and lose less than 20% of their light activity when stored at 35°C for 1 mo.

   AquaLite and its conjugates are stable in the presence of sodium azide at 0.1%. However, preservatives such as thimerosal, isothiazolinones, and other compounds that react with the sensitive sulfhydryl groups at the active site of AquaLite rapidly inactivate the photoprotein at concentrations less than 0.01%. Additives commonly used in immunoassays like washing buffers that eliminate nonspecific reagent binding have little affect on the stability of AquaLite and its conjugates. For example, low levels of nonionic detergents like Triton X-100 at 0.1% have a slightly stabilizing effect at 4°C, whereas Tween-20 must be maintained at concentrations less than 0.05% to prevent inactivation. Proteins and protein cocktails commonly used to eliminate nonspecific backgrounds in immunoassays have no affect on AquaLite stability.

2. We observed that bioluminescence detection is optimal for measurement of PCR products derived from the early phase of log amplification. This property of

detecting product during the early amplification phase translates into quantitative advantages; high sensitivity for low copy number and increased range in product detection maximize accurate quantitation of product. True quantitation requires comparison of RT-PCR products during the linear phase of amplification (*see* **Subheading 3.5.**). As each cDNA may be differently represented in each sample, unique sets of cycles of PCR are required to represent the linear phase of amplification.

3. Sensitivity is related to efficiency of hybridization *(23)*. In a tumor necrosis factor-α (TNF-α) capture assay, four probes were tested; each probe differed in relation to sequences exposed to theoretical internal folding structures of the PCR amplicon. Inclusion of 2.5 *M* TMACl (tetramethylammonium chloride) into the hybridization buffer (*see* **Subheading 3.4.4.**) improved signal strength for each of the probes, with sensitivities achieved between 10 and 40 amol.

4. In these studies, for one cytokine, using two culture conditions and duplicate sample sets, we generated nearly 50 samples for analysis. Overall, this represented half the microtiter plates, the signal from which can be analyzed at 2 s/sample. Although the sample size may at first appear daunting, with BL this is quite feasible. Although linear regression is the most accurate way to quantitate fold differences, a single comparison can be made by choosing one overlapping cycle set in which both populations are undergoing equivalent rates of linear amplification. In our studies, the relative differences in signals generated between groups decreased as cycles increased, because of the plateau phase inherent to PCR at the higher cycle sets, resulting from reactant depletion *(9,11)*. The data generated for IL-2 would allow selection of one overlapping cycle number for further studies of similar experimental populations, reducing the number of samples to be examined per condition. These evaluations exemplify the importance of identifying proper experimental comparisons for the quantitative evaluation of RT-PCR amplicons.

5. Detection of signal from resulting amplicons has also been compared with plasmid standard curves, allowing quantitation of the cDNA, as demonstrated by Xiao et al. *(6)*. In these examples, mRNA was isolated from phytohemagglutinin-stimulated splenocytes, and cDNA was prepared and amplified. Parameters were established to detect plasmids containing mouse cDNA message inserts, detecting as little as 40 amol of amplified cytokine products, or 500 copies of templates when 27 PCR cycles were used. Their sensitivity extended nearly 6 logs dilution of plasmid DNA template.

Acknowledgments

This work was supported by NIH-NHLBI grant RO1HL55969-01 and completed at the University of Texas-Houston Medical School, Houston, TX. We thank Cari Leonard for technical assistance, and David F. Smith, Ph.D., of Chemicon International, Inc. for kind contribution of bioluminescent reagents.

References

1. Actor, J. K., Olsen, M., Boven, L. A., Werner, N., Stults, N. L., Hunter, R. L., and Smith, D. F. (1996) A bioluminescent assay using AquaLite for RT-PCR Amplified RNA from mouse lung. *J. NIH Res.* **8,** 62.
2. Actor, J. K., Kuffner, T., Dezzutti, C. S., Hunter, R. L., and McNicholl, J. M. (1998) A flash-type bioluminescence immunoassay that is more sensitive than radioimaging: quantitative detection of cytokine cDNA in activated and resting human cells. *J. Immunol. Methods* **211,** 65–77.
3. Actor, J. K., Limor, J. R., and Hunter, R. L. (1999) A flexible bioluminescent-quantitative polymerase chain reaction assay for analysis of competitive PCR amplicons. *J. Clin. Lab. Anal.* **13,** 40–47.
4. Jagannath, C., Actor, J. K., and Hunter, R. L. (1998) Induction of nitric oxide in human monocytes and monocyte cell lines by *Mycobacterium tuberculosis. Nitric Oxide* **2,** 174–186.
5. Jagannath, C., Pai, S., Actor, J. K., and Hunter, R. L., Jr. (1999) CRL-1072 enhances antimycobacterial activity of human macrophages through interleukin-8. *J. Interferon Cytokine Res.* **19,** 67–76.
6. Xiao, L., Yang, C., Nelson, C. O., Holloway, B. P., Udhayakumar, V., and Lal, A. A. (1996) Quantitation of RT-PCR amplified cytokine mRNA by aequorin-based bioluminescence immunoassay. *J. Immunol. Methods* **199,** 139–147.
7. Xiao, L., Owen, S. M., Rudolph, D. L., Lal, R. B., and Lal, A. A. (1998) *Plasmodium falciparum* antigen-induced human immunodeficiency virus type 1 replication is mediated through induction of tumor necrosis factor-alpha. *J. Infect. Dis.* **177,** 437–445.
8. Jennings, V. M., Actor, J. K., and Hunter, R. L. (1997) Cytokine profile suggesting that cerebral malaria is an encephalitis. *Infect. Immun.* **65,** 4883–4887.
9. Babu, J. S., Kanangat, S., and Rouse, B. T. (1993) Limitations and modifications of quantitative polymerase chain reaction. Application to measurement of multiple mRNAs present in small amounts of sample RNA. *J. Immunol. Methods* **165,** 207–216.
10. Siddiqi, A., Jennings, V. M., Kidd, M. R., Actor, J. K., and Hunter, R. L. (1996) Evaluation of electrochemiluminescence and bioluminescence based assays for quantitating specific DNA. *J. Clin. Lab. Anal.* **10,** 423–431.
11. Yang, B., Yolken, R., and Viscidi, R. (1993) Quantitative polymerase chain reaction by monitoring enzymatic activity of DNA polymerase. *Anal. Biochem.* **208,** 110–116.
12. Shimomura, O. and Johnson, F. H. (1962) Extraction, purification and properties of aequorin, a bioluminescent protein from the luminous hydromedusan, *Aequorea. J. Cell. Comp. Physiol.* **59,** 223–240.
13. Shimomura, O. and Johnson, F. H. (1969) Properties of the bioluminescent protein aequorin. *Biochemistry* **8,** 3991–3997.
14. Shimomura, O. and Johnson, F. H. (1975) Regeneration of the photoprotein aequorin. *Nature* **256,** 236–238.
15. Cormier, M. J., Prasher, D. C., Longiaru, M., and McCann, R. (1989) The enzymology and molecular biology of the Ca^{2+}-activated photoprotein, aequorin. *Photochem. Photobiol.* **49,** 509–512.

16. Stults, N. L., Rivera, H. N., Ball, R. T., and Smith, D. F. (1995) Bioluminescent hybridization immunoassays for digoxigenin-labeled PCR products based on AquaLite, a calcium- activated photoprotein. *J. NIH Res.* **7,** 74.

17. Smith, D. F., Stults, N. L., and Mercer, W. D. (1995) Bioluminescent immunoassays using streptavidin and biotin conjugates of recombinant Aequorin. *Am. Biotechnol. Lab.* **14,** 17–18.

18. Wynn, T.A., Eltoum, I., Cheever, A. W., Lewis, F. A., Gause, W. C., and Sher, A. (1993) Analysis of cytokine mRNA expression during primary granuloma formation induced by eggs of Schistosoma mansoni. *J. Immunol.* **151,** 1430–1440.

19. Innis, M. A., Felfand, D. H., Sninsky, J. J., and White, T.J., eds. (1990) *PCR Protocols: A Guide to Methods and Applications*, Academic, San Diego, CA.

20. White, B. A. (1993) PCR protocols: current methods and applications, in *Methods in Molecular Biology,* vol. 15. Humana, Totowa, NJ, pp. 1–392.

21. Stults, N. L., Stocks, N. F., Rivera, H. N., Gray, J., McCann, R. O., O'Kane, D., et al. (1992) Use of recombinant biotinylated Aequorin in microtiter and membrane-based assays: purification of recombinant apoaequorin from Escherichia coli. *Biochemistry* **31,** 1432–1442.

22. Stults, N. L., Rivera, H. N., Burke-Payne J., Ball, R. T., and Smith, D. F. (1997) Preparation of stable conjugates of recombinant aequorin with proteins and nucleic acids, in *Bioluminescence and Chemiluminescence: Molecular Reporting with Photons* (Hastings, J. W., Kricka, L. J., and Stanley, P. E., eds.), John Wiley & Sons, Chichester, UK, pp. 423–426.

23. Smith, D. F., Stults, N. L., Cormier, M. J., and Actor, J. K. (1999) Recombinant Aequorin, A Bioluminescent Signal for Molecular Diagnostics. *J. Clin. Ligand Assay* **22,** 158–172.

24. Flannagan, K., Sanchez-Brambila, G., Barnes, C., Rivera, H., Scheuer, B., Stults, N. L., et al. (1993) A study of the stability of AquaLite (recombinant aequorin) lyophilized and in solution in various buffers, in *Bioluminescence and Chemiluminescence: Current Status* (Stanley P. and Kricka, L., eds.), John Wiley & Sons, Chichester, UK, pp. 60–63.

25. Kricka, L. J. (1991) Chemiluminescent and bioluminescent techniques. *Clin. Chem.* **37,** 1472–1481.

26. Kricka, L. J. (1993) Ultrasensitive immunoassay techniques. *Clin. Biochem.* **26,** 325–331.

9

Measurement of Interleukin mRNA by Northern Blotting Using a Nonradioactive Detection Method

Ginette Tardif, John A. Di Battista, Jean-Pierre Pelletier, and Johanne Martel-Pelletier

1. Introduction

The regulation of gene activity plays a cardinal role, not only in the overall function of a cell, but also in the response of a given tissue to challenges by extracellular signals, amplifying the response well beyond stimulus-secretion coupling.

Cellular activity is largely defined by the amount and identity of the proteins synthesized. Although some proteins are turned over very slowly within a cell, most have half-lives of minutes to hours. This permits changes in the rate of synthesis of the proteins, governed almost exclusively by the levels of mRNA encoding them, to have profound effects on cellular physiology. Steady-state levels of mRNA in turn are dramatically affected by the rate of mRNA synthesis, or gene transcription, in which the rate of initiation of new RNA chains is the key regulated step (*1*).

Gene transcription results in the synthesis of a single-stranded linear unit of RNA, called heteronuclear RNA or hnRNA, which contains all the sequences encoding the exons and introns. The hnRNA precursor is then processed into mature mRNA within the nucleus. Introns are removed and the remaining exons joined together at defined base sequences by a process called splicing. Additional processing steps include the addition of a special nucleotide (7'-methylguanosine) called a "cap" at the 5'-end of the mRNA and the addition at the 3'-end of a string of continuous A residues called the poly-A tail. The transcription initiation site and the transcription stop site, which coincide with a signal to add the poly-A tail at defined sequences such as AUAAAA, are encoded directly within the gene. The "cap" site appears to play a role in the translational efficiency of the mRNA,

From: *Methods in Molecular Medicine, vol. 60: Interleukin Protocols*
Edited by: L. A. J. O'Neill and A. Bowie © Humana Press Inc., Totowa, NJ

whereas the poly-A tail is postulated to provide a measure of protection against cellular RNases. RNA processing proceeds within minutes inside the nucleus, with the mature mRNA rapidly transported to the cytoplasm. Some mRNAs have several possible polyadenylation sites, resulting in different sizes of mature mRNA encoding the same protein. The 3'UT has been postulated to play a role in mRNA stability *(1,2)*.

Our discussion is confined to the most common but least sensitive mRNA detection method, Northern blotting. Each detection procedure (e.g., reverse transcription-polymerase chain reaction [RT-PCR]) has its own advantages and may answer questions that cannot be addressed by other methods, so that no one technique is automatically best. However, Northern blotting allows the investigator to determine the number of mRNA species hybridizing to a given probe and the apparent molecular size. It is the only technique that provides sizing information for the entire mRNA molecule and is often the first experiment performed after sequencing to characterize a newly cloned mRNA (cDNA). Blotting can also give valuable information about the efficacy of the probe itself, to the extent that appropriate bands appear in the absence of any background. Therefore, *in situ* hybridization can only be properly performed once the probes have shown the necessary level of specificity. Although not considered ideally a quantitative technique, relative levels of a given mRNA can be assessed by Northern blotting under different experimental conditions. Also, the blots can be reprobed a number of times, which is especially convenient when quantitating genes of the same family (e.g., protooncogenes of the *c-jun* family) or for controlling for variations in RNA loading (e.g., glyceraldehyde-3-phosphate dehydrogenase [GAPDH], β-actin are constitutively expressed) *(1)*.

Cytokines are a family of protein mediators of both natural and acquired immunity. They are synthesized in response to inflammatory or antigenic stimuli and act locally, in an autocrine or paracrine fashion, by binding to high-affinity receptors on target cells. Cytokines serve many functions that are critical to host defense against pathogens and provide links between specific (lymphocytes) and natural (monocyte/macrophages) immunity. These molecules are also present in tissues, including those from articular joints, where they act as mediators of catabolic and/or anabolic processes.

The genes of most cytokines generally exist as single copies in the haploid genome and are generally organized in 4 or 5 exons and 3 or 4 introns. The 5'-flanking region of most cytokine genes (i.e., 300–500 bp upstream from the TATA box) are highly conserved between species, although there are considerable differences from one cytokine to another. Still, *cis*-acting elements that are recognizable as AP-1, CRE, NF-AT, NF-κB, and c/EBP have been described in the promoter region of many cytokine genes *(3)*.

Generally, cytokine mRNA reaches a maximum level of 0.01–2% of total mRNA 3–8 h after stimulation of leukocytic cells, with transcriptional activity declining quite rapidly thereafter. In other cell types (e.g., fibroblasts, chondrocytes), the levels of steady-state cytokine mRNA are much lower, but the kinetics of stimulation are similar to those of lymphocyte/macrophages. However, the kinetics of activation are unique to each cytokine gene. The time-course of cytokine mRNA production is also regulated at the posttranscriptional level; most cytokine mRNAs have canonical Shaw-Kamen instability sequences (i.e., UUAUUUA) in the 3' UTR region. The latter sequences are believed to promote rapid polyA tail shortening and possible decapping, leading to mRNA degradation *(3)*.

Thus, cytokine steady-state mRNA levels are influenced by both 5' and 3' UTR *cis*-acting elements, and one important goal for future work will be to identify those gene products that act at 5' and/or 3' and ultimately affect cytokine protein synthesis.

2. Materials

It is essential, when manipulating RNA, to avoid contamination with RNases. Most published protocols have stressed the importance of wearing gloves, using high-purity reagents, and distilled water that has been treated with the chemical diethylpyrocarbonate (DEPC). This compound binds to and inactivates RNases.

2.1. Total RNA Extraction from Eukaryotic Cells Grown in Monolayers or in Suspension

1. TRIzol® reagent: Gibco BRL (Gaithersburg, MD). Light-sensitive; store at 4°C. Toxic (contains phenol and guanidine isothiocyanate).
2. Chloroform.
3. Isopropyl alcohol.
4. 70% Ethanol.
5. RNase-free water: 0.1% DEPC in distilled water and autoclaved. The DEPC will break down to ethanol and CO_2. Wear gloves when handling DEPC.

2.2. RNA Extraction from Soft Tissues (Synovial Membranes)

1. TRIzol reagent: Gibco BRL. Light-sensitive; store at 4°C. Toxic (contains phenol and guanidine isothiocyanate).
2. Chloroform.
3. Acetate-saturated phenol: Mix 100 mL of melted redistilled phenol (Gibco BRL) with 100 mL of 0.02 *M* sodium acetate, pH 5.0; add 0.1 g hydroxyquinoline. Stir overnight at 4°C; let stand until the phases separate, remove most of the aqueous phase, and store at 4°C in the dark.
4. Isopropyl alcohol.
5. 70% Ethanol.
6. RNase-free water (*see* **Subheading 2.1.**).

2.3. RNA Extraction from Hard Tissues (Cartilage)

1. 6 *M* Guanidine HCl.
2. 3 *M* Sodium acetate, pH 5.0.
3. Acetate-saturated phenol (*see* **Subheading 2.2.**).
4. Chloroform-isoamyl alcohol (49:1 v/v).
5. Isopropyl alcohol.
6. RNeasy kit (QIAGEN, Chatsworth CA): Contains QIAshredder spin columns, RNeasy spin columns, lysis buffer RLT (contains guanidinium isothiocyanate), wash buffer RW1 (contains guanidinium salt), wash buffer RPE.
7. β-Mercaptoethanol.
8. 95% Ethanol.
9. RNase-free water (*see* **Subheading 2.1.**).

2.4. Preparation of Digoxigenin-Labeled RNA Probes

1. Column for DNA purification.
2. Nucleotide labeling mix (10X): Can be purchased from Boehringer Mannheim (Mannheim, Germany). 10 m*M* ATP, 10 m*M* CTP, 10 m*M* GTP, 6.5 m*M* UTP, 3.5 m*M* digoxigenin (DIG)-11-UTP, pH 7.5. Store at –20°C.
3. Transcription buffer (10X): 0.4 *M* Tris-HCl, pH 8.0, 0.06 *M* MgCl$_2$, 0.1 *M* dithiothreitol (DTT), 0.02 *M* spermidine.
4. RNA polymerase (SP6, T7, or T3).
5. Water (autoclaved).
6. DNase I, RNase-free.
7. 0.2 *M* EDTA, pH 8.0.
8. 4 *M* Lithium chloride.
9. 95% Ethanol.
10. 70% Ethanol.
11. RNase inhibitor.
12. Nylon membrane positively charged (Hybond-N, Amersham).
13. DIG-labeled control RNA (100 ng/μL; Boehringer Mannheim).
14. Maleate buffer: Mix 11.61 g maleic acid, 8.77 sodium chloride into 800 mL water. Adjust the pH to 7.5 and complete to 1000 mL with water. Autoclave and store at room temperature.
15. Washing buffer: 0.3% Tween-20 in maleate buffer.
16. Blocking reagent (10%): Dissolve 10 g blocking powder in 100 mL maleate buffer; it is important to heat the mixture on a heating plate or a water bath until the powder is completely dissolved. Autoclave and store at 4°C or –20°C.
17. Blocking buffer: Prepare 2% blocking reagent in maleate buffer.
18. Anti-DIG antibody: Can be purchased from Boehringer Mannheim. Conjugated to alkaline phosphatase. Store at 4°C.
19. Equilibration buffer: 100 m*M* Tris-HCl, 100 m*M* sodium chloride. Adjust to pH 9.5.
20. Nitroblue tetrazolium (NBT): Prepare 75 mg/mL in 70% dimethylformamide.
21. 5-Bromo-4-chloro-3-indolyl phosphate (BCIP): Prepare 50 mg/mL in 100% dimethylformamide.

2.5. Electrophoresis of RNA in Formaldehyde-Agarose Gels

1. 10X 3-(*N*-morpholino)propane sulfonic acid (MOPS) buffer: 0.2 *M* MOPS, 0.08 *M* sodium acetate, 0.01 *M* EDTA. Adjust pH to 7.0 and filter (0.45 µm). Store at room temperature and protect from light.
2. Agarose (ultrapure).
3. Formaldehyde (toxic; use under fume hood).
4. Formamide (ultrapure, distilled).
5. RNA sample buffer: Mix 2 mL of 10X MOPS buffer, 3.5 mL formaldehyde, 10 mL formamide, and 6.5 mL RNase-free water. It is better to prepare the buffer fresh, but it can be stored at room temperature or at –20°C.
6. Loading buffer: Mix 500 µL glycerol, 2 µL 0.5 *M* EDTA, and 498 µL RNase-free water. Add bromophenol blue *ad libitum*. Store at 4°C.
7. Ethidium bromide solution: 500 µg/mL in sterile water. Store at room temperature, protected from light. Mutagen.

2.6. Electrophoretic Transfer of RNA to Nylon Membranes

1. 20X Transfer buffer: Mix 96.9 g Tris, 54.44 g sodium acetate, and 40 mL of a 0.5 *M* EDTA solution into 800 mL water. Adjust pH to 7.8 with glacial acetic acid, complete to 1000 mL with water, and store at room temperature.
2. Nylon membrane, positively charged (Hybond-N, Amersham Pharmacia).
3. Filter paper, Whatman 3MM.
4. Electrophoretic transfer apparatus (Hoefer, Bio-Rad): Includes a transfer tank, transfer cassettes, and foam sponges.

2.7. Hybridization and Detection

1. SSC 20X: Add 88.2 g of sodium citrate and 175.3 g of sodium chloride to 800 mL water. Adjust to pH 7.0, and complete to 1000 mL with water. Sterilize by autoclaving and store at room temperature.
2. Prehybridization buffer: Mix 25 mL of 20X SSC stock, 50 mL formamide, 0.02 g sodium dodecyl sulfate (SDS), 1 mL 10% *N*-lauroylsarcosine stock solution, 20 mL 10% blocking reagent stock solution, 50 µL of a 20-mg/mL polyadenylic acid stock solution, and 500 µL of 10 mg/mL salmon testes DNA stock solution. Complete to 100 mL with sterile water, and store at –20°C.
3. Hybridization buffer: Denature the RNA probe (50 ng/mL) by heating at 65°C for 15 min. Cool on ice (5 min) and add the denatured probe to the prehybridization buffer just before use.
4. Maleate buffer (*see* **Subheading 2.4.**).
5. Washing buffer (*see* **Subheading 2.4.**).
6. Blocking reagent (10%) (*see* **Subheading 2.4.**).
7. Anti-DIG antibody (*see* **Subheading 2.4.**).
8. Blocking buffer (*see* **Subheading 2.4.**).
9. Equilibration buffer (*see* **Subheading 2.4.**).
10. CDP-star: Can be purchased from Boehringer Mannheim. Chloro-substituted 1,2-dioxetane chemiluminescence substrate for alkaline phosphatase. Store in the dark at 4°C.

3. Methods

Several protocols for RNA isolation, electrophoresis, and filter hybridization have been described *(4)*. The following methods have been optimized to obtain maximal recovery of good-quality total RNA as well as to get the most sensitive detection by filter hybridization (*see* **Note 1**).

3.1. Total RNA Extraction from Eukaryotic Cells Grown in Monolayers or in Suspension

1. RNA is extracted from the cells using the TRIzol reagent. Grow the cells in the appropriate medium in 3.5-cm-diameter dishes. Remove the culture medium, and lyse the cells directly in the plate by adding 1 mL of TRIzol; there is no need to wash the cells if the culture medium has been totally removed. For cells grown in suspension, centrifuge the cells and resuspend about 1 million cells in 1 mL of TRIzol (*see* **Note 2**).

2. Pass the cell lysate several times through a pipet until the lysate is homogeneous. A final viscous lysate indicates contamination with chromosomal DNA, and more TRIzol should be added to obtain a clear, nonviscous preparation. Incubate the lysate at room temperature for 5 min.

3. Add 0.2 mL of chloroform for each mL of TRIzol used to lyse the cells. Shake the tubes vigorously by hand for 15 s, and incubate at room temperature for another 3 min.

4. Centrifuge the tubes at 14,000g for 15 min at 4°C. Transfer the upper aqueous phase to a new tube. It is important not to disturb the interface when taking the aqueous phase because the quality of the RNA preparation will be affected. It is better to leave some of the upper phase near the interface.

5. To precipitate the RNA, add 0.5 mL of isopropyl alcohol for each mL of TRIzol reagent originally used. Incubate at room temperature for 10 min. Centrifuge at 14,000g for 10 min at 4°C, and wash the RNA pellet once with 70% ethanol (1 mL for each 1 mL of TRIzol originally used). Centrifuge at 8500g at 4°C for 5 min. Remove the supernatant, and air-dry the pellet for a few minutes.

6. Resuspend the RNA pellet in RNase-free water (usually 10–20 µL for 1 million cells), and quantitate by spectrophotometry (OD_{260}). Adjust the RNA concentration to 1 µg/µL, and store at –20°C in a frost-free freezer or at –70°C.

7. Depending on the cell type, one should recover from 15 to 30 µg of total RNA from 1 million cells.

3.2. RNA Extraction from Soft Tissues (Synovial Membranes)

1. RNA is also extracted from soft tissues with the TRIzol reagent. First cut the tissue (0.5 g) into small pieces with a sterile scalpel, add to it 10 vol of TRIzol and homogenize with a Polytron (1 min at full speed). Incubate the homogenate for 5 min at room temperature.

2. Add 0.2 mL of chloroform for each mL of TRIzol used to lyse the cells. Shake the tubes vigorously by hand for 15 s, and incubate at room temperature for another 3 min.

3. Centrifuge the tubes at 14,000*g* for 15 min at 4°C. Transfer the upper aqueous phase to a new tube. If the interface is thick, extract the aqueous phase one or two times at 65°C with acetate-saturated phenol.

4. To precipitate the RNA in the aqueous phase, add 0.5 mL of isopropyl alcohol for each mL of TRIzol reagent originally used. Incubate at room temperature for 10 min. Centrifuge at 14,000*g* for 10 min at 4°C, and wash the RNA pellet once with 70% ethanol (1 mL for each 1 mL of TRIzol originally used). Centrifuge at 8500*g* at 4°C for 5 min. Remove the supernatant, and air-dry the pellet for a few minutes.

5. Resuspend the RNA pellet in RNase-free water and quantitate by spectrophotometry (OD_{260}). Adjust the RNA concentration to 1 µg/µL, and store at –20°C in a frost-free freezer or at –70°C.

6. The amount of total RNA recovered from tissues depends on the type of tissue. For example, 1.0 g of synovial membrane will yield about 500 µg of total RNA.

3.3. RNA Extraction from Hard Tissues (Cartilage)

The extraction of RNA from hard tissues such as human articular cartilage is hampered by the fact that this tissue contains relatively few cells in a large amount of extracellular matrix. The expected total RNA yield will not be as much as that obtained from the same weight of soft tissues.

1. Remove pieces of articular cartilage with a sterile scalpel and cut into small pieces. Resuspend 1 g of cartilage pieces in 10 mL of 6 *M* guanidine HCl, and homogenize for 1 min at full speed with the Polytron.

2. To the homogenate, add 0.1 vol 3 *M* sodium acetate buffer, pH 5.0, 0.5 vol of acetate-saturated phenol and 0.25 vol of chloroform-isoamyl alcohol (49:1). Shake vigorously for 20 s, and then put on ice for 1 h.

3. Centrifuge for 2 h at 12,000*g* at 4°C. Transfer the aqueous phase to a new tube, and add 1 vol of ice-cold isopropyl alcohol. Mix well and let stand overnight at –20°C.

4. Centrifuge for 20 min at 12,000*g* at 4°C. Discard the supernatant and dissolve the pellet in 450 µL Qiagen Lysis buffer RLT and 4.5 µL of β-mercaptoethanol. If necessary, heat for 2–3 min at 56°C to dissolve the pellet completely.

5. Apply the lysate to a QIA shredder column and centrifuge for 2 min at full speed. Transfer the flowthrough fraction to a new centrifuge tube (be careful not to disturb the debris pellet), add 225 µL of 95% ethanol, and mix.

6. Apply the solution to an RNeasy spin column, and centrifuge for 15 s at 10,000*g*. Discard the flowthrough and wash the column with 700 µL of Wash buffer RW1 (15 s, 10,000*g*). Discard the flowthrough and wash with 500 µL of wash buffer RPE (15 s, 10,000*g*).

7. Wash again with 500 µL of wash buffer RPE and centrifuge for 2 min at full speed to dry the membrane of the spin column. Transfer the column to a new centrifuge tube.

8. Add 30 µL of RNase-free water to the column and centrifuge for 60 s at 10,000*g*. The RNA is in the collected fraction and can be further concentrated, if needed, by precipitation of the RNA with 3 vol of cold 95% ethanol and 1 vol of 3 *M*

sodium acetate, pH 5.0, and resuspending the pellet in a smaller volume. The RNA is quantitated by spectrophotometry (OD_{260}) and routinely used at 1 µg/µL.

9. Usually, 1 g of human cartilage will yield about 30 µg total RNA. If the cartilage is taken from young animals (rabbits, dogs), the yield can be increased to 60 µg.

3.4. Preparation of DIG-Labeled RNA Probes

Both RNA probes (riboprobes) and DNA probes can be used in Northern hybridization. When detecting mRNA present in small amounts, riboprobes are preferred because of increased sensitivity; because the RNA/RNA hybrids are very stable, the stringency of the hybridization and washing conditions can be increased, resulting in lower nonspecific background. The DNA to be transcribed into a riboprobe should be cloned into the multiple cloning site of a plasmid vector containing recognition sites for two RNA polymerases (SP6, T7, or T3) that flank the DNA of interest. The plasmid is linearized with a restriction enzyme, preferably one that leaves 5'-overhangs, so that transcription is started at one of the RNA polymerase transcription site, spans the cloned DNA, and ends at the restriction cut. The linearized plasmid is purified by passage through a column or, alternatively, by extraction with phenol/chloroform. The transcription is done so as to obtain an antisense RNA (from the 3'-to the 5'-end) that will hybridize to the specific sense mRNA extracted from the cells.

1. In a 0.5-mL sterile centrifuge tube, add on ice 2 µL linearized DNA (1 µg/µL), 2 µL nucleotide labeling mix, 2 µL transcription buffer 10X, 12 µL sterile water, and 2 µL RNA polymerase. Incubate at 37°C for 2 h.
2. Add 2 µL of DNase and incubate at 37°C for 15 min.
3. Add 2 µL of 0.2 *M* EDTA, pH 8.0, to stop the reaction.
4. Precipitate the DIG-labeled RNA with 2.5 µL of 4 *M* LiCl and 75 µL of 95% ethanol, and incubate at –20°C overnight.
5. Centrifuge for 15 min at 14,000g to pellet the RNA; wash the pellet with 50 µL of 70% ethanol (14,000g for 5 min).
6. Resuspend the RNA pellet in 100 µL of sterile water and 1 µL of RNase inhibitor. Store the labeled probe at –20°C. The probes synthesized by this method are stable for several months.
7. To quantitate the amount of labeled probe, compare the RNA probe with known amounts of control DIG-labeled RNA. Make 10-fold dilutions (1:10–1:1000) in sterile water of both the probe and the control labeled RNA (100 ng/µL).
8. Spot 1 µL of each dilution on a hydrated nylon membrane. Wrap the membrane in Saran Wrap™ and expose both sides (3 min each) to UV light to crosslink the RNA to the membrane.
9. The detection of the DIG-labeled probes can be done by colorimetry. All the incubation steps in the detection protocol are done at room temperature with agitation, and the volumes are given for a 100-cm^2 membrane.
10. Wash the membrane for 5 min in the washing buffer.
11. Transfer the membrane into 100 mL of 2% blocking buffer and incubate for 30 min.

12. Discard the blocking buffer and replace with 20 mL of the anti-DIG antibody solution (antibody diluted 1:10,000 in the blocking buffer and prepared just before use). Incubate for 30 min.
13. Wash the membrane 2× (15 min each time) with 50 mL of the washing buffer.
14. Incubate the membrane for 5 min in 20 mL of the equilibration buffer.
15. Mix 35 μL of BCIP and 45 μL of NBT in 10 mL of the equilibration buffer.
16. Incubate the membrane in the BCIP/NBT mixture in the dark without agitation until the spots appear, usually within 10 min.

3.5. Electrophoresis of RNA in Formaldehyde-Agarose Gels

1. Prepare a 1.2% agarose-formaldehyde gel: Dissolve 1.2 g of agarose in 82.5 mL MOPS buffer 1X by heating in a microwave oven (about 3 min) or by stirring on a heating plate. Let the agarose cool down to about 65°C, and add 17.5 mL of formaldehyde. Mix well and pour in the casting tray of the gel electrophoresis apparatus (*see* **Note 3**).
2. Load the RNA samples: Add 15 μL of sample buffer to 5 μL of the RNA preparation (1 μg/μL in RNase-free water), 2 μL of loading buffer, and 1 μL of ethidium bromide solution; mix and put at 65°C for 15 min. Cool on ice for 5 min, and load the whole mixture into the wells of the gel.
3. Run the electrophoresis in 1X MOPS, at 100 V for 2–4 h (*see* **Note 4**).
4. After the migration, rinse the gel in water for 30 min, and take a picture of the gel to check the quality of the RNA .

3.6. Electrophoretic Transfer of RNA to Nylon Membranes

The use of a nylon membrane as support for the UV-crosslinked RNA has the advantage of being more resistant than a nitrocellulose membrane. The increased resistance will allow the membrane to be stripped and reprobed; this is particularly useful when extracting RNA from cells or tissues that have a limited availability.

1. Cut a nylon membrane to the same dimension as the gel and two pieces of Whatman 3MM paper to the dimension of the sponges used in the transfer cassette. Identify the orientation of the membrane by cutting one corner of the membrane.
2. Equilibrate the gel, the nylon membrane, and the transfer cassette sponges into 0.5X transfer buffer for 20 min at room temperature (the filter papers can be soaked just before use); chill the transfer buffer that will be used in the transfer tank.
3. To prepare the transfer cassette add in the following order starting from the black side of the transfer cassette: one sponge, one filter paper, the gel (inverted), the nylon membrane, one filter paper, one sponge. Make sure that there are no air bubbles between the different layers of the cassette. Close the transfer cassette and put it in the transfer tank (the black side of the cassette at the cathode). Transfer at 4°C at 30 V overnight followed by 1 h at 60 V the next morning. The transfer voltage and length may vary depending on the transfer apparatus used; always make sure that the transfer buffer has not overheated during the transfer.
4. After the transfer, remove the gel and the membrane. Take a picture of the membrane and check the gel to make sure that all the RNA has been transferred. Put the membrane in Saran Wrap on a standard transilluminator, and fix the

RNA on the membrane by crosslinking with UV irradiation (3 min on each side). If the membrane is not to be used immediately in the hybridization reaction, place it between two sheets of filter paper, and store at room temperature in a plastic bag.

3.7. Hybridization and Detection

1. Place the membrane into a heat-sealable pouch, and add the prehybridization buffer (20 mL for a 100-cm^2 membrane). Seal the bag and incubate at 68°C for at least 6 h (overnight is acceptable).
2. Cut one corner of the bag and remove the prehybridization buffer. Add the preheated hybridization buffer (3–4 mL for a 100-cm^2 membrane). Reseal the bag and incubate at 68°C overnight between two glass plates. Make sure that the bag is flat and that there are no bubbles. Redistribute the buffer 2 or 3× during the incubation.
3. Remove the hybridization buffer, and store at –20°C for future use (*see* **Note 5**). Take the membrane and wash it successively at 68°C in 2X SSC (10 min), 0.5X SSC (15 min), and twice in 0.1X SSC (15 min). All the washing steps are done on a shaker in about 100 mL of buffer (for a 100-cm^2 membrane).
4. After the washing steps, prepare the membrane for detection of the hybridized probe (*see* **Note 6**). All the incubation steps in the detection protocol are done at room temperature with agitation, and the volumes are given for a 100-cm^2 membrane (*see* **Note 7**).
5. Wash the membrane for 5 min in the washing buffer.
6. Transfer the membrane into 100 mL of 2% blocking buffer and incubate for 60 min.
7. Discard the blocking buffer and replace with 20 mL of the anti-DIG antibody solution (antibody diluted 1:10,000 in the blocking buffer and prepared just before use). Incubate for 30 min.
8. Wash the membrane 3 times (15 min each time) with 50 mL of the washing buffer.
9. Incubate the membrane for 5 min in 20 mL of the equilibration buffer.
10. Dilute the CDP-star chemiluminescent substrate 1:100 with the equilibration buffer. This substrate is used to localize the alkaline phosphatase conjugated to the anti-DIG antibody. Incubate the membrane with the substrate for 5 min at room temperature.
11. Remove the substrate and put the membrane on a filter paper to absorb excess liquid. Seal the membrane (still wet) in a plastic pouch and expose to X-ray film (usually 1–20 min depending on the abundance of specific mRNA) (*see* **Note 8**).
12. If the membrane is to be reprobed, do not allow it to dry. After the detection steps, strip the membrane by washing it in water for 1 min, and incubating it at 75°C for 1 h in 60% formamide, 1% SDS, 0.05 M Tris, pH 8.0. Rinse again in water, and put it in 2X SSC until the prehybridization (*see* **Note 9**).

4. Notes

1. Although it is advisable to add DEPC to the water used for the RNA extraction as well as to decontaminate the gel electrophoresis apparatus for the elimination of RNases, it is possible to obtain nondegraded RNA of very good quality

without using DEPC. It is essential, however, to have all the water and plasticware sterilized by autoclaving, and to always wear gloves during the RNA extraction procedure.

2. The procedure is described for cells grown in 3.5-cm-diameter dishes but can be applied to cells grown in any other size dishes. Larger dishes will require a larger quantity of TRIzol (about 1 mL/10 cm^2).

3. We routinely use 1.2% agarose, but the percentage can vary from 1.0 to 1.6% depending on the expected size and the number of specific mRNAs to be detected.

4. The RNA should not migrate for too long in the gel (more than 9 cm from the wells); a long migration will result in "fuzzy" RNA bands.

5. The hybridization buffer can be reused up to five times. Keep the buffer stored at $-20°C$; when needed, heat the solution at 65°C for 10 min in order to redenature the probe.

6. Make sure that the membrane remains wet throughout the hybridization steps. Even a slightly dried membrane will result in a high background.

7. Always use gloves and handle the membranes with forceps; fingertips will leave smudges after detection.

8. If the amount of specific interleukin mRNA is low, such as in total RNA extracted from connective tissue cells, several nonspecific bands or a smear covering the lane will appear after the first use of the hybridization buffer. In this case, it is better to use a hybridization buffer that has already been used in order to reduce the nonspecific binding.

9. It is always better to do the first hybridization with a probe that will give a faint signal after several minutes of exposure to the film and do the second one with a probe (such as GAPDH or 28S) that will detect a very strong signal after only 1 or 2 min of exposure. This will minimize the background noise from the first hybridization if the stripping is not complete.

Acknowledgments

Several of these protocols have been adapted from those suggested by the Boehringer Mannheim company (experiments involving digoxigenin) and from Gibco BRL (extraction of total RNA from eukaryotic cells). We thank François Mineau and Changshan Geng, whose expertise has been invaluable in the optimization of these protocols.

References

1. Shupnik, M. A. (1995) Measurement of gene transcription and messenger RNA, in *Molecular Endrocrinology: Basic Concepts and Clinical Correlations* (Weintraub, B. D., ed.), Raven, NY, pp. 41–58.

2. Beelman, C. A. and Parker, R. (1995) Degradation of mRNA in eukaryotes. *Cell* **81,** 179–183.

3. Arai, K. I., Lee, F., Miyajima, A., Miyatake, S., Arai, N., and Yokota, T. (1990) Cytokines: coordinators of immune and inflammatory responses. *Annu. Rev. Biochem.* **59,** 783–836.

4. Sambrook, J. F., Fritsch, E. F., and Maniatis, T. (1989) *Molecular Cloning. A Laboratory Manual* (Ford, N., Nolan, C., and Ferguson, M. eds.), Cold Spring Harbor Laboratory Press, Cold Spring Harbor, NY.

10

Quantification of Mouse IL-6 and TNF-α mRNA Using Xplore Assays

Scott W. Van Arsdell, Kevin P. Murphy, Csaba Pazmany, Diane Erickson, and Mark D. Moody

1. Introduction

The production of cytokines can be controlled by the regulation of transcription, by the regulation of translation, and by post-translational mechanisms. Therefore, to understand better the control of cytokine production, it is important to measure both concentration of the free cytokine in solution and cytokine mRNA in the cytokine-expressing cells. Traditional methods of examining gene expression, such as as Northern blots, reverse transcriptase polymerase chain reaction (RT-PCR), and RPA, tend to be labor intensive and semiquantitative. To overcome these limitations, we have developed the Xplore® (Endogen, Woburn, MA) assay for the quantification of cytokine mRNA. These microtiter plate-based assays are rapid (under 6 h), quantitative over three orders of magnitude, and have no risk of false-positive values from contamination.

The Xplore assay is based on a novel signal amplification system for the quantitative detection of nucleic acids that utilizes the endonuclease activity of a Cleavase® (Third Wave Technologies, Madison, WI) enzyme to recognize a specific nucleic acid structure composed of two oligonucleotides that are hybridized to the mRNA target (1–4). The probes are designed so that the 3'-end of the upstream Invader™ (Third Wave Technologies) probe overlaps the 5'-end of the downstream Signal probe (**Fig. 1**). The endonuclease recognizes this complex and cuts the Signal probe. The reaction is incubated at a temperature near the T_m of the Signal probe to permit the rapid exchange of hybridized Signal probe. This turnover (hybridization, cleavage, dissociation of cleaved Signal probe, and replacement with an uncleaved Signal probe) occurs rapidly

From: *Methods in Molecular Medicine, vol. 60: Interleukin Protocols*
Edited by: L. A. J. O'Neill and A. Bowie © Humana Press Inc., Totowa, NJ

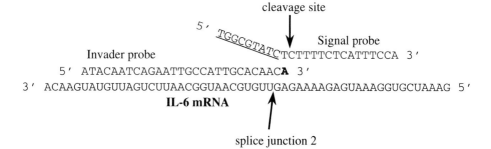

cleavage site

Fig. 1. Probe design for the mIL-6 Xplore mRNA assay. The 3' base of the Invader probe (designated in bold) "invades" the region where a base of the Signal probe hybridizes to the target sequence. The Cleavase enzyme recognizes this complex and cuts the Signal probe (the 5' arm of the Signal probe [underlined] is not complementary to the target).

so that multiple copies of the probe are cleaved for each copy of the target sequence without temperature cycling, thereby amplifying the signal from the reaction. The signal accumulates in a linear manner at a rate proportional to the amount of target in the original sample. The reaction products, or cleaved Signal probes, are distinguished from uncleaved probe molecules by the addition of modified bases, and subsequent detection by an alkaline phosphatase antibody conjugate *(2)* (**Fig. 2**).

We have designed Xplore assays to measure the concentration of a number of cytokines (interleukin [IL]-1β, IL-2, IL-4, IL-6, IL-10, interferon-γ [IFN-γ], and tumor necrosis factor-α [TNF-α]), and we describe here the development and performance of assays for the measurement of mouse (m) IL-6 and TNF-α mRNA.

2. Materials

1. DNA probe synthesis: DNA oligonucleotides used for the Invader and Signal probes were obtained as polyacrylamide gel electrophoresis (PAGE)-purified probes from Midland Certified Reagent Company (Midland, TX).
2. Xplore mRNA assay components: Xplore mRNA assays for mIL-6 and mTNF-α were developed and run using components (Cleavase enzyme, DNA polymerase, antibody-alkaline phosphatase conjugate, FdUTP, 96-well streptavidin-coated plate, and buffers) from the Xplore mouse IL-1β mRNA assay kit (available from Endogen).
3. Media and cells: J774 (ATCC TIB67) cells were grown in RPMI-1640 media supplemented with with 10% fetal calf serum (FCS), 1% Pen/Strep (cat. no. 1540-122, Gibco LTI, Gaithersburg, MD), 2 mM L-glutamic acid at 37°C, and 5% CO_2.

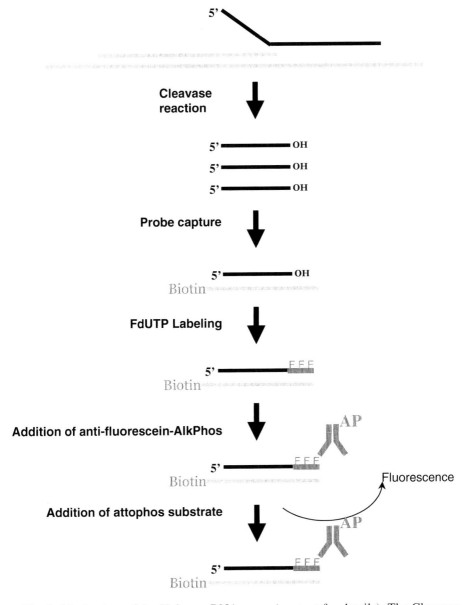

Fig. 2. Mechanism of the Xplore mRNA assay (*see* text for details). The Cleavase reaction cuts the Signal probe (black) to produce multiple Signal probe fragments (black) for each copy of target RNA. These Signal probe fragments are captured in a streptavidin-coated microwell (via biotin label on the capture probe) and tagged by labeling with fluorescein-12-dUTP and an antifluorescein antibody conjugated with alkaline phosphatase. Detection is accomplished by the reaction of the alkaline phosphatase with the substrate, which is converted to a fluorescent molecule.

3. Methods
3.1. Preparation of mRNA Standards
3.1.1. Attachment of a T7 Phage Promoter to Template DNA Using PCR

Templates for in vitro transcription were constructed by adding the phage T7 promoter sequence upstream of sequences encoding mouse TNF-α and mouse IL-6 *(5,6)*.

1. RT-PCR primer pairs and a positive control amplified fragment for each cytokine gene were obtained from Clontech (Palo Alto, CA). A new version of each 5′ primer was synthesized that contains (from 5′ to 3′) a GC clamp, a *Hin*dIII site, the 21-base T7 promoter (which includes the +1 to +4 region of the T7 transcript), and the sequence complementary to the cytokine gene **(Fig. 3)**. The *Hin*dIII site is optional, as the PCR product with the T7 promoter can be transcribed directly without subcloning.
2. A 100-μL PCR reaction was assembled containing 1X cloned *Pfu* buffer (Stratagene, La Jolla, CA), 0.2 μ*M* dNTPs, 0.4 μ*M* modified 5′ primer, 0.4 μ*M* 3′ primer, 2.5 U *PfuTurbo* DNA polymerase (Stratagene), and 80 pg of positive control amplified fragment. The DNA polymerase was added after the other reaction components had been heated at 94°C for 2 min.
3. PCR was performed using the following conditions for 35 cycles: 94°C, 1 min; 60°C, 1 min; 72°C 1 min. The reaction was heated to 72°C for 10 min after the last cycle.
4. The PCR product of each reaction was purified using the High Pure PCR Product Purification Kit from Roche Molecular Biochemicals (Indianapolis, IN). The size of each PCR product was analyzed by agarose gel electrophoresis.

3.1.2. In Vitro Synthesis of Cytokine mRNA Transcripts

Synthetic mRNA transcripts for mouse TNF-α and mouse IL-6 were produced with the T7-MEGAshortscript in vitro transcription kit for large-scale synthesis of short-transcript RNAs (Ambion, Austin, TX).

1. A 20 μL in vitro transcription reaction was assembled containing 1X transcription buffer, 75 m*M* NTPs, 300 ng T7 template DNA, and 2 μL T7 MEGAshortscript enzyme mix. The reaction was incubated at 37°C for 5 h.
2. The DNA template was removed by addition of 1 μL of RNase-free DNase I (2 U/μL) and incubation at 37°C for 20 min. The reaction was stopped by addition of 5 μL of 5 *M* ammonium acetate, 100 m*M* EDTA.

3.1.3. Purification and Quantification of Cytokine mRNA Transcripts

Synthetic mRNA transcripts for mouse TNF-α and mouse IL-6 were purified by denaturing polyacrylamide gel electrophoresis (*see* **Note 1**).

1. The products of two identical in vitro transcription reactions were pooled and combined with an equal volume of 95% formamide, 10 m*M* EDTA with crystal violet dye. RNA Century™-Plus molecular weight markers (Ambion) were mixed

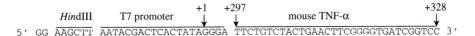

Fig. 3. 5' PCR primer for amplification of template containing T7 polymerase promoter and the mTNF-α coding sequence. +1 refers to the initiation site for T7 RNA polymerase transcription. The numbers above the mTNF-α sequence region refer to the position in the mRNA sequence.

    with an equal volume of 95% formamide, 0.5 mM EDTA, 0.025% xylene cyanol, 0.025% bromophenol blue, and 0.025% sodium dodecyl sulfate (SDS).

2. The samples were heat denatured for 3 min at 95°C and then cooled on ice.
3. The samples were loaded on a precast preparative 5% polyacrylamide gel with 1X TBE and 6 M urea (Bio-Rad). The samples were electrophoresed at 4 W until the xylene cyanol was 1.5 cm from the bottom of the gel.
4. The RNA transcript was visualized by ultraviolet (UV) shadowing.
5. The RNA band was excised, cut into small pieces, and transferred to a 1.5-mL microfuge tube containing 450 µL 0.5 M ammonium acetate, 1 mM EDTA, 0.2% SDS. The gel fragments were incubated for 15 h at 37°C with shaking.
6. The eluate was removed, combined with 2 vol of ethanol, and incubated at –20°C for at least 1 h. The RNA was pelleted by centrifuging at 15,000g for 20 min.
7. The RNA pellet was washed with 70% ethanol, centrifuged at 15,000g for 5 min, air-dried briefly, and resuspended in 60 µL RNase-free H$_2$O.
8. The concentration and purity of the transcript was determined by diluting an aliquot of the RNA in TE and measuring the OD$_{260}$ and OD$_{280}$. We routinely observe OD$_{260}$/OD$_{280}$ ratios of 1.8–2.0.
9. The integrity of the purified transcript was assessed by running a sample on a denaturing polyacrylamide gel with RNA molecular weight standards.

3.2. Xplore mRNA Assays

Mouse TNF-α and IL-6 Xplore mRNA assays were performed as follows:

1. Cleavase reactions were assembled in RNAse-free 200-µL thin walled tubes. Each 15-µL reaction consisted of 500 ng of total RNA target, 0.5 µM Invader™ oligo, 0.8 µM Signal Probe Oligo, 10 mM MOPS, pH 7.5, 100 mM KCl, 0.05% Tween-20 and Nonidet-NP40, 5 mM MgSO$_4$, 2.5 µM fluorescein-12-dUTP, 10 ng of CleavaseVII enzyme, and RNAse-free water to the final volume. All samples were assayed as duplicate samples, and standard curves for the assays were run with known amounts of IL-6 or TNF-α mRNA, which had been prepared by in vitro transcription. The mixtures were incubated in an oven at 54°C for 4 h.
2. The cleavage products (5' arms of the Signal probes) from the Cleavase reaction were labeled with fluorescein dUTP (FdUTP) using Klenow/Exo-polymerase. This is performed by transferring 15 µL of each Cleavase reaction to a streptavidin-coated microtiter plate well containing 90 µL/well of DNA polymerase reaction mix consisting of 10 nM 3' biotinylated capture/hybridization

template (complementary to the cleaved 5' arm of the Signal probe), 10 m*M* MOPS, pH 7.5, 10 m*M* MgSO$_4$, 1 U Klenow/Exo-enzyme, and RNase-free water. Solid phase hybridization and FdUTP extension was performed for 15 min at 37°C.

3. The plate was washed 3× with a TBS wash solution (25 m*M* Tris, pH 7.2, 150 m*M* NaCl , 0.1% Tween-20) to remove any unhybridized components. The fluorescein label was detected by adding 100 µL of a dilution of antifluorescein-AP(Alkaline Phosphatase)-Fab fragments to each microtiter well and incubating for 15 min at 37°C. The free antibody was washed away with TBS wash solution.

4. Bound antibody was detected by addition of 100 µL of AttoPhos™ reagent (JBL Scientific, San Louis Obispo, CA), and the plate was incubated for 30 min at 37°C. The reaction was stopped by the addition of 100 µL of 0.36 *M* K$_2$HPO$_4$. The fluorescence was measured on a Cytofluor plate reader (PE Biosystems, Framingham, MA; excitation = 450/50, emission = 580/50, gain = 45, reads/well = 10, temperature = 37°C).

3.3. Design of Probes for Detection of mIL-6 and mTNF-α mRNA

3.3.1. Target Site Selection

The target sites for probe hybridization were selected as close to a splice junction as possible to avoid detection of contaminating genomic DNA in total RNA preparations. Because mRNA secondary structure can have an effect on the accessibility of a target site to oligonucleotide hybridization, probe sets targeting different splice junctions were designed and compared directly in assays of natural samples to determine which target site produces the best assay performance. We have also used computer-generated mRNA secondary structure maps (*7*) to determine which regions of an mRNA sequence have a high probability of being base paired and therefore are expected to be poor target sites (*see* **Note 1**).

3.3.2. Design of Invader Probes

Invader probes were designed to have a T$_m$ between 76 and 84°C so that they will form a stable complex with the target sites at the reaction temperature of 54°C. The 3' terminal base of each Invader probe was designed to be mismatched with the corresponding base on the target mRNA and to "invade" the 5' terminal base pair between the Signal probe and the mRNA target. The one base invasion structure is essential for Signal probe cleavage by the Cleavase enzyme, and the presence of a base mismatch at the invasion site enhances the rate of cleavage (**Fig. 1**) (*2,3*). The Invader probes were analyzed with DNA sequence analysis software (Lasergene, DNA Star, Madison, WI) to determine whether intermolecular secondary structures exist that could have an adverse effect on the assay.

3.3.3. Design of Signal Probes

Signal probes were designed to have a 3' target specific region and a 5' arm, which is cleaved during the reaction and used for detection (**Fig. 1**) (*2–4*). The target-specific region of each Signal probe was designed to have a T_m between 42 and 44°C so that it will rapidly cycle on and off the target site at the reaction temperature of 54°C. The sequence of the 5' arm of each Signal probe (nine nucleotides) was chosen so that it does not base pair with the target or the target-specific region of the Signal probe, which could interfere with assay performance. In addition, each Signal probe sequence was designed to avoid the formation of intramolecular secondary structures with the corresponding Invader probe (*see* **Note 2**).

3.3.4. Design of Capture Probes

The Capture probe for each assay was designed to be complementary to the ten-nucleotide cleaved 5' arm of the Signal probe (**Fig. 4**) *(2–4)*. A biotin molecule was covalently attached to the 3' or penultimate 3' nucleotide of the Capture probe during synthesis to enable binding of the oligonucleotide to the streptavidin-coated plate. Each Capture probe was designed so that when it is base paired to the cleaved 5' arm of the Signal probe there is a single-stranded 5' extension of 3 dA residues, which serves as a template for incorporation of FdUTP by DNA polymerase.

3.4. Temperature Optimization of the Cleavase Reaction

The temperature optimum of each Xplore assay was determined by performing simultaneous Cleavase reactions with identical amounts of synthetic RNA target (150 amole) at 46, 50, 54, and 58°C. The optimal temperature of the reaction can be adjusted by changing the length of the signal probe. Increasing the length of the signal probe should raise the temperature optimum, and decreasing the length should decrease the temperature optimum. The temperatures of all the Xplore assays have been adjusted to 54°C using this technique. An example of the effect of Signal probe length and temperature on the Cleavase reaction rate is presented in **Fig. 5A,B**.

3.5. Optimization of Cleavase Reaction Rate by Shifting the Signal Probe Cleavage Site

Shifting the Signal probe cleavage site by a few nucleotides can have a significant effect on the rate of Signal probe cleavage. Three probe sets were designed targeting the region around splice junction 3 of mouse IL-6 mRNA (**Fig. 6A**). The cleavage site in Signal probe 2 is shifted two bases towards the 5' end of the mRNA compared with Signal probe 1, and the cleavage site in Signal probe 3 is shifted five bases toward the 5' end of the mRNA compared with Signal probe 1. The lengths of each Signal probe and the corresponding invader probe were adjusted so that the T_ms of the Signal probes were approximately the same, and the T_ms of the invader probes were approximately the same. Cleavase reactions containing identical amounts of the mouse IL-6 synthetic transcript

```
                          5 '  TGGCGTATCT 3 '
                     3 '  CTCGACACCGCATAGAAAA 5 '
                                   /
                                biotin
```

Fig. 4. Design of biotinylated Capture oligonuleotide probe. The biotinylated Capture probe is shown 3' to 5'. The corresponding Signal probe cleavage fragment is shown annealed above the Capture probe.

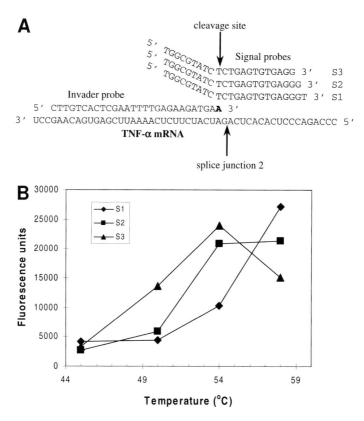

Fig. 5. Influence of mTNF-α Signal probe length on optimal cleavase reaction rate. (**A**) Signal probes for mTNF-α were prepared that varied in length of the 3' end of the probe. (**B**) The influence of reaction temperature on Cleavase reaction was determined for these probes in Xplore assays performed at 46, 50, 54, and 58°C as described in the text.

(150 amole) and each of the different probe sets were performed at 46, 50, 54, and 58°C (**Fig. 6B**). The optimal temperature for reactions with Signal probe 1 was 54°C, and the optimal temperature for reactions with signal probes 2 or 3 was between 50 and 54°C. However, the fluorescent signals generated by the

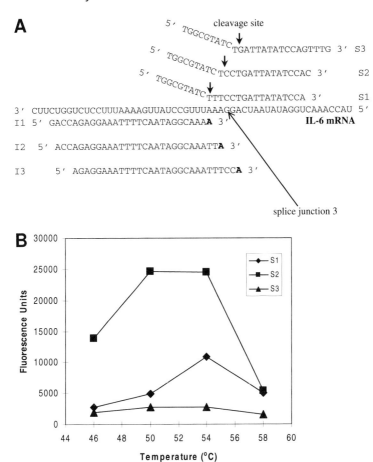

Fig. 6. Effect of cleavage site position shift on cleavase reaction rate. **(A)** Invader and Signal probes were prepared that hybridized near splice junction 3 of mIL-6 mRNA. **(B)** The effect of these two base-pair shifts of the binding sites on the Cleavase reaction rate was determined in Xplore assays performed at 46, 50, 54, and 58°C as described in the text.

three probe sets at 54°C were very different. The rate of Signal probe cleavage in reactions containing signal probe 2 was two- and ninefold higher than in reactions containing Signal probes 1 and 3, respectively **(Fig. 6B).**

3.6. Xplore Assay

3.6.1. Performance

Representative standard curves for the mTNF-α and mIL-6 assays are shown in **(Fig. 7)**. The limit of detection for these assays is typically 0.5–1 amol of target mRNA (*see* **Notes 3** and **4**).

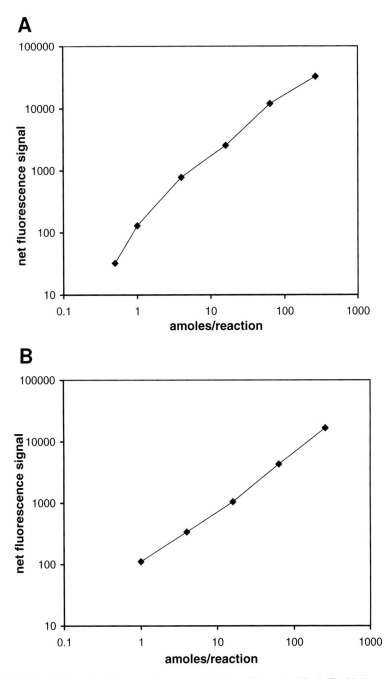

Fig. 7. Typical standard curves for mouse TNF-α (**A**) and mIL-6 (**B**) Xplore mRNA assays. Xplore assays were performed as described in the text, using dilutions of in vitro transcribed mRNA as the sample. The values shown are the average of duplicates.

3.6.2. Reproducibility

Intraassay reproducibility was evaluated by measuring IL-6 mRNA in 16 replicates of a total RNA sample. The results (**Table 1**) show that consistent concentrations were obtained for each sample; the coefficient of variation (standard deviation divided by the average value) of the assay was 6.7%.

3.6.3. Influence of RNA Concentration of Sample on Xplore Assay Performance

To investigate the influence of the amount of RNA tested in the sample on assay performance, we spiked synthetic IL-6 mRNA into 500 ng of mouse cell total RNA. Serial twofold dilutions of this sample were made in RNAse-free water and then assayed in the Xplore assay. The results show that the assay continued to measure the IL-6 mRNA accurately over a 16-fold dilution (from 500 to 31 ng) (**Table 2**) (*see* **Note 5**).

3.7. Detection of IL-6 mRNA in Stimulated J774 Cells

3.7.1. Stimulation of Mouse J774 Cells

J774 cells were plated at 4×10^6 cells/well (6-well plate) and stimulated with the addition of 5 ng/mL lipopolysaccharide (LPS; Sigma, St. Louis, MO) and 100 μM dibutyryl cyclic adenosine monophosphate (AMP; Sigma). At selected intervals the media were removed, and cells in the plate were prepared for RNA isolation by the addition 1 mL of TRIzol (Gibco LTI). The cells were then stored at $-70°$ C until further processing.

3.7.2. Total RNA Isolation

Total RNA was isolated from the frozen J774 cells using TRIzol reagent (Gibco LTI) according to the manufacturer's specifications. RNA pellets were dissolved in 20 μL of RNAse-free water, and the concentration was determined by measuring the absorbance at 260 nM (an aliquot was diluted into TE buffer for this measurement).

3.7.3. Measurement of mIL-6 mRNA

Approximately 0.5 amol of IL-6 mRNA was detected in 500 ng of total RNA from the cells processed from the time zero control cells (**Fig. 8**). The IL-6 mRNA increased to 2 amole after 1 h of induction and continued to increase steadily, reaching a peak of approx 11 amole at 5 h post-induction.

4. Notes

1. We have found that the PAGE-purified Signal probes from some sources produce a high signal in the absence of target and are not suitable for use in the assay. We believe this is due to trace contamination of the Signal probe with incomplete probe

Table 1
Intra-Assay Precision of the mIL-6 Assay

Replicate	Fluorescence signal	amol/reaction
1	3965	79.0
2	3310	65.5
3	3714	73.8
4	3834	76.3
5	4010	80.0
6	3624	72.0
7	3665	72.8
8	4005	79.9
9	3665	72.8
10	3832	76.3
11	3606	71.6
12	3422	67.8
13	3834	76.3
14	4010	80.0
15	4265	85.2
16	3965	79.0
Average value	3795.4	75.5
Standard deviation	244.9	5.1
% CV	6.5	6.7

Table 2
Effect of Total RNA Sample Size on mIL-6 Assay Performance

	Total RNA in reaction (ng)				
Nanograms of total RNA in reaction	500	250	125	62	31
IL-6 mRNA (amol/reaction)					
Observed	130	60	28	10	6
Expected		65	33	16	8

sequences that can hybridize to the Capture oligonucleotide and then be extended with FdUTP by the DNA polymerase. We have had success with all PAGE-purified Signal probes obtained from Midland Certified Reagent Company (Midland, TX).

2. We have used the mfold program (7) to identify splice junction regions of the mRNA target that are free from secondary structure. Although we have found that regions with predicted high secondary structure do not perform well, not all regions predicted to be open perform well. The optimal splice junction site for probes should be determined empirically.

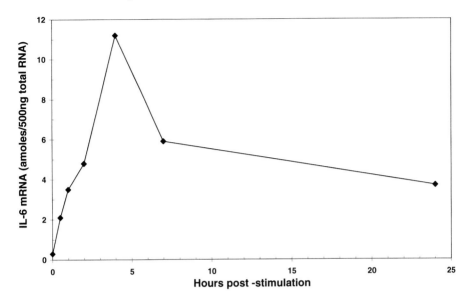

Fig. 8. Detection of mIL-6 mRNA expression in stimulated J774 cells. IL-6 mRNA was measured in 500-ng samples of total RNA isolated from J774 cells as described in the text. The values reported for each time-point are the average of duplicate analysis of the total RNA sample for that time point.

3. As is typical of fluorescence-based assays, the signal observed in the assay is dependent on the instrumentation. The filters used to control the excitation and emission wavelengths, as well as the gain setting of the photomultiplier tube, can greatly impact the signal. We have found that the Xplore assay provided consistent results even when the signal varied over an eightfold range due to variation in the gain setting.

4. The ability of the Xplore assays to detect low-abundance transcripts can be improved by using a mRNA preparation as a sample instead of total RNA. We tested the use of 500 ng mRNA prepared using the Ambion MicroPoly(A)Pure method as a sample and found that this material gave a value approx 10 times greater than than the value observed in 500 ng of total RNA. This is expected, as only 5–10% of the RNA in a cell is mRNA.

5. The use of more than 500 ng of total RNA in the assay can inhibit the signal produced. If more than 500 ng is used, we recommend checking for sample inhibition by spiking a reaction with the lowest assay standard and determining whether the signal produced reflects the added amount of target.

Acknowledgments

We wish to thank Robert Kwiatkowski, Tsetska Takova, and Bruce Neri for their generous help in developing assays using the Invader probe and Cleavase enzyme technology.

Endogen, Inc. no longer markets Xplore assays. Interest in Cleavase enzymes and Invader probe technology should be directed to Third Wave Technologies, Inc., Madison, WI.

References

1. Lyamichev, V., Brow, M. A. D., and Dahlberg, J. E. (1993) Structure-specific endo-nucleolytic cleavage by eubacterial DNA polymerases. *Science* **260,** 778–783.
2. Lyamichev, V., Mast, A. L., Hall, J. G., Prudent, J. R., Kaiser, M. W., Takova, T., et al. (1999) Polymorhism identification and quantitative detection of genomic DNA by invasive cleavage of oligonucleotide probes. *Nature Biotechnol.* **17,** 292–296.
3. Kaiser, M. W., Lyamicheva, N., Ma, W., Miller, C., Neri, B., Fors, L., and Lyamichev,V.I. (1999) A comparison of euabacterial and archaeal structure-specific 5'-exonucleases. *J. Biol. Chem.* **274,** 21,387–21,394.
4. Griffin, T. J., Hall, J. G., Prudent, J. R., and Smith, L. M. (1999) Direct genetic analysis by matrix-assisted laser desorption/ionization mass spectroscopy. *Proc. Natl. Acad. Sci. USA* **96,** 6301–6306.
5. Milligan, J. F., Groebe, D. R., Witherell, G. W., and Ulhenbeck, O. C. (1987) Oligoribonucleotide synthesis using T7 RNA polymerase and synthetic DNA templates. *Nucleic Acids Res.* **15,** 8783–8798.
6. Fahy, E., Kwoh, D. Y., and Gingeras, T. R. (1991) Self-sustained sequence replication (3SR): An isothermal transcription-based amplification system alter-native to PCR. *PCR Methods Applic.* **1,** 25–33.
7. Mathews, D. H., Sabina, J., Zucker, M., and Turner, D. H. (1999) Expanded sequence dependence of thermodynamic parameters improves prediction of RNA secondary structures. *J. Mol. Biol.* **288,** 911–940.

11

Measurement of Cytokine and Chemokine mRNA Using Nonisotopic Multiprobe RNase Protection Assay

Zheng-Ming Wang and Roman Dziarski

1. Introduction

The multiprobe ribonuclease protection assay (RPA) is a highly sensitive and specific method for simultaneous detection and quantification of several species of mRNA. Three most distinct advantages of the multiprobe RPA method are: high sensitivity and specificity, capacity to simultaneously quantify more than a dozen different mRNA transcripts in a single sample of total RNA, and the flexibility of multiple probes (cDNA, antisense RNA, oligo probe, etc.) that can be used for hybridization with mRNA (**Table 1**). This method allows one to compare relative mRNA levels of multiple genes, or to compare changes in mRNA levels among various treatments or among various tissues. For such comparisons, the results can be normalized based on the amount of mRNA for housekeeping genes.

Development of this assay was made possible by the discovery of DNA-dependent RNA polymerases from the bacteriophages T7, T3, and SP6 (*1–4*). These polymerases exhibit a high degree of fidelity for their promoters, polymerize RNA at a very high rate, efficiently transcribe long segments, and do not require high concentrations of rNTPs. Therefore, these polymerases could be applied for the synthesis of RNA probes with high specific activity from cDNA fragments subcloned into plasmids that contain bacteriophage T7, T3, or SP6 promoters.

1.1. Overview of the Assay

An overview of the multiprobe nonisotopic RPA assay *(5)* is shown in **Fig. 1**.

1. A set of up to 12 linearized plasmid cDNA templates, each of a different size and representing a unique sequence of interest, and each under the regulation of the T7 bacteriophage promoter, is constructed or purchased from Pharmingen (San Diego, CA) or Ambion (Austin, TX).

From: *Methods in Molecular Medicine, vol. 60: Interleukin Protocols*
Edited by: L. A. J. O'Neill and A. Bowie © Humana Press Inc., Totowa, NJ

Table 1
Comparison of Direct RNA Quantification Methods[a]

Method	Sensitivity/features	Advantages	Disadvantages
RPA	High. 1–100 µg RNA/lane. Bands correlate with the protected probe size and the amount of hybridized RNA, but not the size of original mRNA.	Measures expression of 10–20 genes in one RNA sample. No need to reprobe. More sensitive than Northern. Tolerates partially degraded RNA. Once the conditions are set up generates more data in less time. Templates and kits available commercially.	Technically demanding.
Northern blot	Low. 10–20 µg RNA/lane. Bands correlate with both the amount and size of of original mRNA.	Traditional gold standard method for measurement of mRNA. Serves both as a qualitative (size of transcript) and quantitative method to evaluate RNA.	Detects one gene per experiment. Needs reprobing for other genes. Signal diminished with reprobing and time. Needs more and higher quality RNA. Large variation from lab to lab.
Dot/slot blot	Intermediate. 4–10 µg RNA/dot or slot. Spots or bands correlate only with the amount but not the size of original mRNA.	One experiment can measure 100 RNA samples. Very small variation in results. Quantification of RNA more accurate than Northern. Needs less experience to run.	Needs large amount of high quality RNA. Laborious.

[a]Other (indirect) mRNA quantification methods include reverse-transcriptase polymerase chain reaction (RT-PCR) and Quantikine (R&D Systems) and Xplore (Endogen) colorimetric methods.

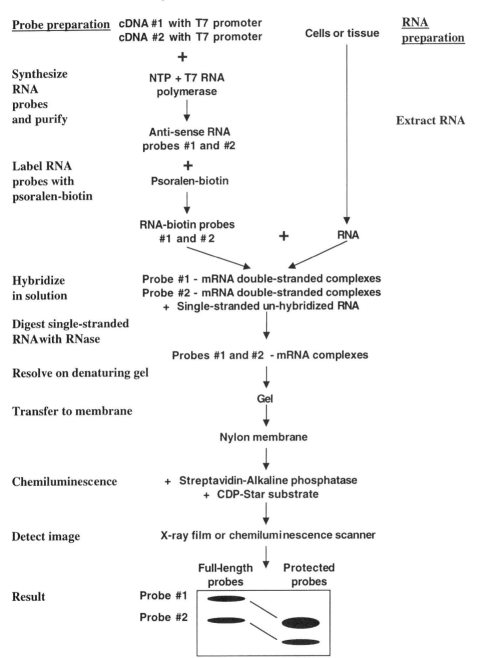

Fig. 1. Overview of the multiprobe nonisotopic RPA assay.

2. A mixture of antisense RNA probes, complementary to the cDNA templates, is synthesized using T7 polymerase, and the RNA probes are purified.
3. The probes are labeled with psoralen-biotin. Psoralens are tricyclic compounds that intercalate between bases and can be covalently attached to nucleic acids with UV irradiation. This attachment does not compromise hybridization efficiency.
4. RNA is extracted from cells.
5. An excess of biotin-labeled probes is hybridized with the RNA.
6. Labeled probes hybridize with the complementary sequences of mRNA and form double-stranded complexes.
7. The unhybridized single-stranded RNA is digested with RNases. The hybridized double-stranded probe RNA—mRNA complexes are not digested. These undigested (RNase-protected) species contain the labeled probe fragments (protected probe) that are 20–30 nucleotides shorter than the original full-length probes, because flanking sequences in the probes that are derived from the plasmid do not hybridize with target mRNA and are digested with RNase. The amounts of protected probes for each antisense RNA are proportional to the amounts of each complementary target mRNA.
8. The mixture of protected probes and target mRNA is resolved on a polyacrylamide gel and transferred to a positively-charged nylon membrane.
9. The location of the biotin-labeled protected probe fragments on the membrane is revealed by chemiluminescence, based on the binding of alkaline phosphatase-tagged streptavidin to biotin-labeled protected probes, and by emission of light from the CDP-Star substrate.
10. The chemiluminescence in full-length probe and protected probe bands is detected using X-ray film or a chemiluminescence detector (e.g., Kodak Digital Science Image Station). The amount of chemiluminescence can be measured using the above mentioned detector and is proportional to the amount of the protected probe. The amount of the protected probe is in turn proportional to the amount of complementary target mRNA. If the probes for the housekeeping gene mRNA are included in the assay, along with the inducible mRNA, the amounts of inducible mRNA can be normalized based on the amount of housekeeping gene mRNA.

This assay is highly specific and quantitative because of the exquisite RNase sensitivity of the mismatched base pairs (single-stranded RNA), but not of the hybridized base pairs (double-stranded RNA). The assay gives quantitative results that reflect the total amount of each mRNA complementary to the probes, because hybridization in solution with an excess of labeled probe saturates all of the complementary mRNA. The excess of unhybridized labeled probes is digested together with all the other noncomplementary single-stranded RNA. This RPA assay can be performed on total RNA prepared from tissues or primary or cultured cells by any of the standard RNA extraction procedures, without the need for purification of [polyA]⁺RNA. This method can even tolerate partially degraded RNA, because the labeled probes bind only to short RNA fragments, which makes this assay the most reliable for comparing the amounts of mRNA. The features of the RNase protection assay are compared in **Table 1** to two other standard methods of directly measuring mRNA.

In this chapter, we will describe the use of a nonisotopic multiprobe RPA assay for measuring the amounts of mRNA for eight chemokines and nine cytokines in human monocytes stimulated with bacterial components (*see* **Note 1**). This assay uses the chemokine and cytokine cDNA templates from Pharmingen and RPA kit and nonisotopic psoralen-biotin labeling system from Ambion. We have selected the nonisotopic labeling system because large amounts of probes need only be synthesized and labeled once, and then they can be stored frozen and used in all experiments.

2. Materials
2.1. cDNA Template Sets (Pharmingen)

1. The human chemokine template set (50 ng/µL, total 10 µL) includes 8 chemokines: Ltn, RANTES, IP-10, MIP-1β, MIP-1α, MCP-1, IL-8, and I-309, and 2 house-keeping genes, L32 and GAPDH; with the following lengths of RNA transcripts: 433, 390, 349, 314, 256, 231, 204, 191, 141, and 125 bases respectively.
2. The human cytokine template set (50 ng/µL, total 10 µL) includes 9 cytokines: IL-12p35, IL-12p40, TNF-α, IL-1α, IL-1β, IL-1Ra, G-CSF, IL-6, IFN-γ, and 2 housekeeping genes, L32 and GAPDH; with the following lengths of RNA transcripts: 389, 349, 314, 283, 257, 230, 222, 211, 173, 141 and 125 bases respectively (*see* **Notes 2** and **3**).

2.2. Other Reagents, Kits, and Equipment

Most reagents are provided in the kits listed below. Reagents made in the laboratory and glassware need to be nuclease-free (DEPC- or RNase ZAP-treated).

1. RNA Century Marker Plus template (Ambion).
2. MEGAscript In Vitro Transcription kit (Ambion).
3. MAXIscript In Vitro Transcription kit (Ambion).
4. BrightStar Psoralen-Biotin Nonisotopic Labeling kit (Ambion).
5. RPA III Ribonuclease Protection Assay kit (Ambion).
6. BrightStar BioDetect Nonisotopic Detection kit (Ambion).
7. RNase-free siliconized nonstick microcentrifuge tubes (Ambion).
8. RNase ZAP (Ambion).
9. GeneElute agarose spin column (Sigma 5-6500).
10. Gel band elution buffer: 0.5 M ammonium acetate, 1 mM EDTA, 0.1 % SDS.
11. Fluor-coated TLC plastic plate (Ambion).
12. 10X TBE: 108 g Tris, 55 g boric acid, 40 mL 0.5 M EDTA, pH 8.0. Do *not* treat with DEPC.
13. 10% (w/v) Ammonium persulfate.
14. TEMED.
15. Urea.
16. Ethanol (absolute and 70%).
17. 40% Acrylamide/*bis* acrylamide (19:1 ratio, Ambion).

18. Glycogen: 10 µg/µL.
19. Diethylpyrocarbonte (DEPC).
20. Nylon membrane, positively charged (Ambion or Amersham).
21. Spectroline mini 254 nm UV short-wave lamp (Fisher).
22. Potable 365 nm UV light (Fisher or Ambion).
23. UV crosslinker.
24. Hybridization incubator.
25. X-ray film or Kodak Digital Science Image Station.

3. Methods

The RPA assay is a very sensitive and demanding procedure that requires very careful attention to all the details.

3.1. Human Monocyte Isolation and Stimulation

Human monocytes are isolated, purified, cultured and stimulated with bacterial products (peptidoglycan and lipopolysaccharide) or bacteria (*Staphylococcus aureus*) as described in Chapter 36 on cDNA arrays.

3.2. RNA Preparation

RNA is isolated from monocytes as described in Chapter 36 on cDNA arrays by the single-step phenol-chloroform method (*6*) or using the QIAGEN RNeasy kit (Valencia, CA) (*see* **Note 4**). RNA is stored at –70°C.

3.3. In Vitro Transcription to Synthesize RNA Probes

The reaction described below synthesizes antisense RNA probes from linearized plasmid cDNA templates containing T7 bacteriophage promoter (chemokine and cytokine templates from Pharmingen) using T7 polymarase and MAXIscript kit. The amount of labeled probes actually needed for the RPA experiments is very small. However, we usually transcribe a large amount of RNA (2–10 µg) to make purification of the probes and measurement of probe concentration easier. We strongly recommend *the use of siliconized microcentrifuge tubes to perform all RPA experiments* (*see* **Note 5**).

1. Thaw and place the reagents on ice. Keep the 10X transcription buffer at room temperature (if placed on ice, spermidine will precipitate, which will result in subsequent precipitation of template DNA!).
2. Add the following amounts of the indicated reagents in the order shown to a 1.5-mL microcentrifuge tube at room temperature:

dH$_2$O (nuclease-free)	8 µL
DNA template	4 µL (200 ng)
10X transcription buffer	2 µL
10 mM ATP	1 µL
10 mM CTP	1 µL
10 mM GTP	1 µL

10 m*M* UTP	1 µL
T7 polymerase + ribonuclease inhibitor	2 µL

3. Mix contents and incubate for 6 h at 37°C to maximize yield.
4. Add 1 µL of RNase-free DNase I (2 U/µL) to the reaction and incubate at 37°C for 15 min to remove template DNA (complete digestion of DNA templates is essential).
5. Purify the transcribed RNA probes on a gel (*see* **Subheading 3.5.**) and label with psoralen-biotin (*see* **Subheading 3.6.**).

3.4. Synthesis of RNA Markers

The reaction described below synthesizes RNA molecular weight markers of 100, 200, 300, 400, 500, 750, and 1000 bases from RNA Century Marker Plus template using MEGAscript kit.

1. Thaw and place the reagents on ice. Keep the 10X transcription buffer at room temperature (if placed on ice, spermidine will precipitate, which will result in subsequent precipitation of template DNA!).
2. Add the following amounts of the indicated reagents in the order shown to a 1.5 mL microcentrifuge tube at room temperature:

dH$_2$O (nuclease-free)	6 µL
DNA template	2 µL (1 µg)
10X transcription buffer	2 µL
75 m*M* ATP	2 µL
75 m*M* CTP	2 µL
75 m*M* GTP	2 µL
75 m*M* UTP	2 µL
T7 polymerase + ribonuclease inhibitor	2 µL

3. Mix contents and incubate for 6 h at 37°C to maximize yield.
4. Add 1 µL of RNase-free DNase I (2 U/µL) to the reaction and incubate at 37°C for 15 min to remove template DNA.
5. Purify the transcribed RNA markers on a gel (*see* **Subheading 3.5.**) and label with psoralen-biotin (*see* **Subheading 3.6.**).

3.5. Gel Purification of Transcribed RNA

Gel purification of the transcribed RNA probes is required to separate full-length transcripts from prematurely terminated transcription products and from unincorporated nucleotides. Gel purification of nonradioactive probe (synthesized in **Subheading 3.3.**) will yield a single clear band. Use *siliconized glass* to run the gel (*see* **Note 5**).

1. Prepare denaturing 6% polyacrylamide 8 *M* urea gel by dissolving 11.04 g urea in 8.325 mL of dH$_2$O (nuclease-free) with 2.3 ml of 10X TBE, and 3.45 mL of 40% acrylamide/*bis* acrylamide. Then add 184 µL of 10% ammonium persulfate and 24.5 µL of TEMED, mix, and immediately cast into a 14 × 16 cm gel. We use a standard Hoefer Western blot gel apparatus with 1.0 mm thick gel and 10-well-comb.

2. Add equal volume of 2X gel loading buffer to the transcribed RNA probes (*see* **Subheading 3.3., step 4**), mix, heat at 95°C for 2 min, put on ice, and then load on the gel.

3. Run the gel with 1X TBE at 250 V until the first bromophenol blue dye reaches the bottom of the gel.

4. Turn off the current and remove the glass plates with the gel. Remove one glass plate, cover the gel with plastic wrap, and remove the second glass plate. Place the gel (gel side up) on a plastic TLC plate, and in a darkened room visualize the RNA with a hand-held 254 nm UV light (300 nm light will not work). RNA transcripts will appear as purple bands.

5. Cut out the RNA bands from the gel, and put each band into a tube. In a template set of several probes, you can extract each probe (band) individually, or you can put all the bands together in one tube, if they will always be used together. Add 150–350 µL of RNase-free water (e.g., DEPC-treated) or elution buffer. The elution buffer should be sufficient to completely cover the gel slices. You can use a pipet tip to smash the gel into small pieces. Incubate the tube on a shaker at room temperature for 2 h or at 4°C overnight to elute RNA from the gel.

6. Add 100 µL of TE to each of the GeneElute agarose spin columns, place each column in a 1.5-mL microcentrifuge tube, and spin for 5 s at maximum speed (14,000 rpm, 16,000g) in a microcentrifuge at room temperature. Discard the TE collected in the tube. Transfer all the contents of each RNA elution tube from **step 5** (both gel and solution) into the washed GeneElute agarose spin column, put the columns in 1.5 microcentrifuge tubes, and spin at maximum speed in a microcentrifuge for 10 min at room temperature.

7. Discard the column, add 1/10 vol of the 5 *M* ammonium acetate to the eluted RNA, 1 µL of glycogen, and 3 vol of ethanol to precipitate the RNA transcripts. Put at –20°C for 30 min.

8. Centrifuge at 4°C in a microcentrifuge at maximum speed (14,000 rpm, 16,000g) for 15 min, then discard the supernatant, wash the precipitated RNA with 200 µL 70% ethanol, centrifuge again for 10 min, thoroughly drain the supernatant, and air-dry the RNA pellet at room temperature.

9. Dissolve the RNA pellet in 10–50 µL of nuclease-free dH$_2$O (about 0.5–1 µg/µL), and measure the RNA concentration in a spectrophotometer. Immediately proceed to **Subheading 3.6.** or store RNA at –70°C.

3.6. Psoralen-Biotin Labeling of RNA

The reaction described below labels purified RNA probes and molecular weight RNA markers with psoralen-biotin complex using BrightStar Psoralen-Biotin Nonisotopic Labeling kit (Ambion). Biotin-labeled psoralens intercalate between RNA bases and are then covalently attached to RNA with UV irradiation. This attachment does not compromise RNA's hybridization efficiency. Biotin is then detected with streptavidin-alkaline phosphatase and a chemiluminescent substrate.

The advantages of the psoralen labeling include the ability to label either RNA, DNA, or oligonucleotides, high efficiency of labeling (almost three times higher than radioactive labeling), ability to store the labeled probes at –70°C for more than a year and, therefore the ability to perform all experiments with the same probe (the conditions of the assay have to be optimized only once), and convenience of not having to handle radioisotopes (*see* **Note 6**).

Use noncoated (untreated) 96-well microtiter plates. Treat the plate with RNase ZAP (or soak for 30 min in 0.1 N NaOH), rinse in DEPC-dH$_2$O, and dry. For the labeling, RNA does not need to be denatured (in contrast to DNA, which must be denatured by boiling for 10 min and chilling). Note that *Psoralen-Biotin reagent is light-sensitive* and must be stored in the dark (wrapped in aluminum foil) at –20°C, and should be handled in dim light. Also, nucleic acids cannot be quantified by absorbance at 260 nm after psoralen-biotin labeling, because psoralen absorbs light at 260 nm.

1. Centrifuge the stock lyophilized psoralen-biotin tube at 10,000 rpm (8000g) for 15 s, then add 33 µL of dimethylformamide (provided in the kit), mix to dissolve, and place at 4°C in the dark.
2. Place the 96-well plate on ice. Add a total of 10 µL of dH$_2$O with 0.5 µg of the purified RNA probe or RNA markers (*see* **Subheading 3.5.**, **step 9**) per well. Add 1 µL psoralen-biotin per 10 µL of RNA solution and mix. The concentration of RNA should be 50 ng/µL or less, the pH should be between 2.5 and 10, and the salt concentration should be less than 20 nM.
3. Keep the plate on ice and place a 365 nm UV light source 2 cm or less directly over the samples in the plate and irradiate for 45 min.
4. Dilute the sample to 100 µL by adding 89 µL of 1X TE, mix, and transfer into a 1.5-mL microcentrifuge tube.
5. Add 200 µL of dH$_2$O-saturated n-butanol (shake well before use), vortex, and centrifuge at 10,000 rpm (8000g) for 1 min. Discard the *top n-butanol* layer. Repeat the n-butanol extraction of the bottom layer and discard the top n-butanol layer.
6. Aliquot the labeled probe or markers in 10–50 µL vol and store in 0.5-mL tubes at –20°C for short-term storage (few days) or at –80°C for up to a year. The probe concentration is approx 5 ng/µL, but the accurate concentration of the probe must be determined by the dot blot procedure described below (*see* **Subheading 3.7.**) by comparison with a DNA standard.

3.7. Measurement of Probe Concentration by a Dot Blot Assay

1. Prepare groups of seven microcentrifuge tubes and make serial 10 times dilutions of standard psoralen-biotin-labeled DNA (1 ng/µL) and of your labeled probes. Place 3 µL of the standard DNA (1 ng/µL) in the first tube of the first group, put 9 µL of dH$_2$O in the six remaining tubes, and make serial dilutions of the DNA by transferring 1 µL of DNA from the first tube to the second, then from the second to the third, etc. The DNA concentrations in the seven tubes should be: 1 ng/µL, 100 pg/µL, 10 pg/µL, 1 pg/µL, 100 fg/µL, 10 fg/µL, and 1 fg/µL.
2. Prepare similar serial dilutions of the labeled probes, by mixing 1 µL of the probe with 4 µL of dH$_2$O in the first tube, and then making six 10 times dilutions (1 µL

+ 9 µL dH$_2$O) in the remaining tubes. If the stock concentration of the probe is 5 ng/µL, the concentrations of the diluted probe in the seven tubes should be the same as the concentrations of the DNA standard.

3. Spot 1 µL from each tube onto a positively charged nylon membrane (mark the membrane with a pencil). Let the membrane air-dry for 1–2 h at room temperature. Develop the dot blot using the BrightStar chemiluminescence detection procedure (described in **Subheading 3.9.**). Obtaining reliable results in this dot blot assay does not require UV crosslinking of DNA and RNA to the membrane (air-drying is sufficient). After chemiluminescent detection of the labeled spots and standards, a concentration curve can be constructed based on the chemiluminescence of the DNA standard, and concentrations of the RNA probes can be determined based on this curve.

4. Sensitivity: This method can detect 10–100 fg-labeled DNA or RNA per spot.

3.8. Ribonuclease Protection Assay (RPA)

The assay described below measures the amounts of mRNA for eight chemokines and nine cytokines in human monocytes stimulated with bacterial products, using the psoralen-biotin labeled RNA probes synthesized using Pharmingen chemokine and cytokine cDNA templates and Ambion RPA III Ribonuclease Protection Assay kit.

First, a pilot experiment should be performed to determine the optimal conditions for RNase digestion, because this step is the most critical for the performance of the assay. However, the conditions for the RNase digestion vary depending on the source of mRNA, the types of probes, hybridization conditions, etc. Once the optimal conditions are established, they should always work for the given set of probes and mRNA preparations.

1. Prepare 0.5 mL microcentrifuge tubes as outlined in **Table 2**. Calculate the concentrations of RNA in the samples to be assayed. The amount of total cellular RNA to be used in the experiment depends on the level of expression of your target mRNA in the sample. For human monocytes, 5 µg of total RNA gives us a very strong signal, but for the monocytic THP-1 cell line, 10 µg of RNA has to be used. For poly(A)$^+$RNA use 10 times less. Then add yeast RNA to bring the final amount of total RNA in all tubes to 50 µg.

2. Add 1 ng of each labeled probe to each tube (for a set of probes, use 1 ng of *each* probe, e.g., for a set of 10 probes, use a total of 10 ng of the probes).

3. Add 1/10 vol of 5 *M* ammonium acetate to each tube, and 2.5 vol of ethanol, mix, and put at –20°C or –80°C for at least 15 min to precipitate RNA (*see* **Note 7**).

4. Pellet RNA by centrifuging at maximum speed (14,000 rpm, 16,000*g*) in a microcentrifuge for 15 min at 4°C. Discard the supernatants (be careful not to dislodge the small RNA pellets) and wash the pellets with 70% ethanol (but do not resuspend the pellets), centrifuge for 10 min, discard the supernatants, and air-dry the pellets at room temperature.

5. Add 10 µL of hybridization buffer to each tube, vortex for at least 15 s until the pellets dissolve.

Table 2
Pilot Experimental Plan for RNase Digestion

Tube no.	Target RNA (µg)	Yeast RNA (µg)	Each probe (ng)	RNase A/T1 dilution[a]	RNase T1 dilution[b]
1	1.25	48.75	1	1:100	
2	2.5	47.5	1	1:100	
3	5	45	1	1:100	
4	10	40	1	1:100	
5	10	40	1	1:50	
6	10	40	1	1:250	
7	10	40	1	1:500	
8	10	40	1	1:1000	
9	10	40	1		1:10
10	10	40	1		1:50
11	10	40	1		1:100
12		50	1	1:100	
13		50	1		
14		50	1[c]	1:100	

[a]From stock 250 U/ml RNase A and 10,000 U/mL RNase T1.
[b]From stock 5000 U/ml RNase T1.
[c]Labeled DNA probe (provided with the kit).

6. Heat all the tubes at 95°C for 4 min, then incubate at 56°C for 16 h (see **Note 8**). For best hybridization results, we put the 0.5 mL tubes in roller hybridization bottles in a preheated (56°C) hybridization incubator and rotate at 3–5 rpm/min. The long hybridization time allows the hybridization to go to completion, which is required for obtaining quantitative results.

7. Turn the hybridization incubator to room temperature, do not open the incubator and do not stop the rotation. Let the temperature of the hybridization tubes to go down gradually; after 1 h stop the rotation, take out the tubes, and spin for 1 min in a microcentrifuge at 5000 rpm (2,040g) at room temperature.

8. Prepare 1 mm thick 6% acrylamide 8 M urea denaturing gel with a 20-well comb. We use a standard 14 × 16 cm Hoefer Western blot gel apparatus (the same as in **Subheading 3.5.**), but other gels (mini gels, precast gels, etc.) can also be used.

9. Make dilutions of RNase T1 and RNase A in the RPA III digestion buffer (provided with the Ambion RPA III Ribonuclease Protection Assay kit) to obtain the final concentrations indicated in **Table 2** (use 150 µL/sample as total volume of the reaction mix to calculate dilutions). *Do not put on ice.*

10. Add 150 µL per tube of the above diluted RNases, mix well, and incubate the tubes at 37°C for 30 min to 1 h, vortex the tubes every 15 min. Note that each series of tubes contains three control tubes (#12, #13, and #14) that contain 50 µg of irrelevant (yeast) RNA only (see **Note 9**). RNases are added to tubes #12 and #14. Tube #12 will serve as a positive control for the function of RNases and will

also show if the probes are being protected in the absence of homologous RNA. There should be no signal at all on the gel in lanes with reaction mix from tube #12. Tube #14 contains control DNA probe (provided with the kit). Tube #13 receives RNase digestion buffer only without the RNases and serves as a control for probe integrity. Tubes #13 and #14 should yield only bands migrating at the positions of the full-length probes. Once the optimal concentrations of RNases and RNA are established in a pilot experiment, these conditions are used to run all the samples by following the same protocol (*see* **Note 10** for optimal conditions in our assay).

11. Spin the tubes for 1 min in a microcentrifuge at 5000 rpm (2040g) at room temperature to pull down the solutions, add 2 µL (10 µg) of yeast RNA, 1 µL of glycoblue dye, and 225 µL of RPAIII inactivation/precipitation buffer to each tube. Then add 150 µL of ethanol to each tube and put at −20°C for at least 15 min to precipitate RNA (*see* **Note 11**).

12. Pellet RNA by centrifuging at maximum speed (14,000 rpm, 16,000g) in a microcentrifuge for 15 min at 4°C. Discard the supernatant completely, add 150 µL of 70% ethanol to wash the blue pellets, centrifuge again for 10 min, discard the supernatant completely, and air-dry the pellets at room temperature.

13. Dissolve the blue pellets in 10 µL of denaturing gel loading buffer. Heat the tubes at 90–95°C for 4 min to denature RNA and then immediately place the tubes on ice.

14. Wash the wells of the gel with 1X TBE buffer, fill the wells with 1X TBE, and load the samples on the gel. Note that the signal of the non-RNase digested samples and RNA markers are very strong, and, therefore, load only 1/10 or less compared to the digested samples, to prevent later overexposure. Load the RNA markers and undigested probe sample in the first or last lanes. Run the gel in 1X TBE buffer at 250 V for several hours, until the first bromophenol blue dye reaches the bottom of the gel or just runs off the gel.

15. Turn off the current, remove the gel, and transfer the RNA fragments onto a positively-charged membrane using a standard Western blotting apparatus with 0.5X TBE buffer at 1 amp for 2 h. We usually trim off the portions of the gel that do not contain the samples to decrease the size of the membrane. This allows the use of smaller amounts of reagents in the subsequent steps.

16. Use a pencil to mark the sample side of the membrane (*see* **Note 12**). Crosslink RNA to the membrane by UV (in a UV-crosslinker, keep the membrane wet during the crosslinking) and dry the membrane with the sample side up.

3.9. Detection of RNA by Chemiluminescence

The assay described below detects the biotin-labeled full length and protected probes generated in the RPA assay and blotted onto a nylon membrane using the Ambion BrightStar BioDetect kit. The procedure is based on high affinity binding of alkaline phosphatase-conjugated streptavidin to biotin-labeled RNA, and detection of complexes by chemiluminescence using the CDP-Star substrate. The amount of biotin-labeled RNA can be quantified, because the amount of chemiluminescence is proportional to the amount of biotin contained in the RNA blotted onto the membrane.

1. Measure the surface area of your membrane to determine the amounts of the washing and assay buffers needed. Dissolve the precipitate in the 5X washing buffer at 37–65°C. Dilute the 5X washing buffer and 10X assay buffer to 1X working buffers before the experiment, prepare enough for one experiment only (discard the unused diluted buffer after each experiment). For example, for a 10×10 cm membrane (100 cm^2), 100 mL of washing buffer and 30 mL of assay buffer are needed (the volumes below are given for a 100 cm^2 membrane). Place the RPA membrane (*see* **Subheading 3.8., step 16**) *sample side up* in a plastic box, which is approximately the size of the membrane. *Do not allow the membrane to dry* throughout the entire procedure. The procedure is performed at room temperature on a rocking shaker at medium speed (10–20 rockings/min).
2. Wash the membrane 2 times, 5 min each, in 20 mL 1X washing buffer.
3. Wash the membrane 2 times, 5 min each, in 10 mL 1X blocking buffer.
4. Wash the membrane once for 30 min in 20 mL 1X blocking buffer.
5. Incubate the membrane for 30 min in 10 mL of the conjugate solution (10 mL blocking buffer plus 1 µL of streptavidin-alkaline phosphatase conjugate).
6. Wash the membrane once for 15 min in 20 mL 1X blocking buffer.
7. Wash the membrane 3 times, 15 min each, in 20 mL 1X washing buffer.
8. Wash the membrane 2 times, 2 min each, in 15 mL 1X assay buffer.
9. Incubate the membrane in 5 mL CDP-star solution for 5 min. Make sure that the solution evenly covers the entire membrane (we rotate the box by hand).
10. Take out the membrane with forceps. Let the excess of CDP-star solution drip off, place the membrane in a transparent plastic bag, remove all the air, and heat-seal the bag.
11. Expose the membrane to an X-ray film at room temperature. Usually 1 min to 2 h exposure is sufficient (*see* **Note 13**). The CDP-star reaches peak light emission in 2–4 h, and the light emission persists at the high level for several days. The image can also be obtained and quantified using Kodak Digital Science Image Station (*see* **Subheading 3.10.**).

3.10. Analysis of Results

1. The lane with free probes should yield distinct bands of similar intensity corresponding in size and number to the size and number of the full-length probes used (**Fig. 2**). Hybridization of cellular RNA with specific RNA probes protects labeled RNA probes from RNase digestion and yields protected probe fragments, which are 20–30 nt shorter than the unprotected probes (*see* **Note 14**). Therefore, the RPA lanes should yield bands of protected probes for the housekeeping genes and for the genes whose mRNA is present in the cells (e.g., chemokine and cytokine mRNA induced in human monocytes by bacterial stimulants, *see* **Fig. 2**) and they should be 20–30 nt smaller than the full-length probes.
2. The results can be compared visually (**Fig. 2**) and the bands can be identified based on their size (by comparing with the size markers). We usually expose our membranes to both to an X-ray film (which is somewhat more sensitive and can give a sharper image) and to a Kodak Digital Science Image Station 440CF

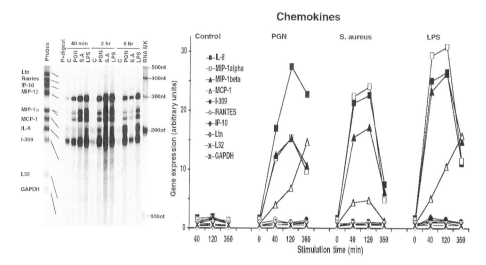

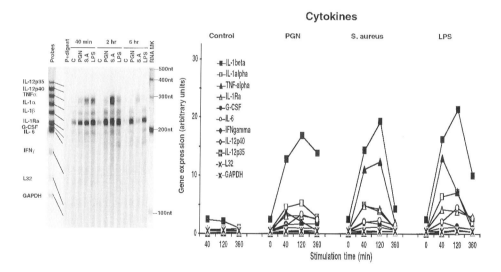

Fig. 2. Kinetics of expression of chemokine and cytokine mRNA in human monocytes stimulated with bacterial peptidoglycan (PGN), lipopolysaccharide (LPS), or *S. aureus* cells, quantified by RPA. Human monocytes were unstimulated (control) or stimulated with PGN, LPS, or *S. aureus* for the indicated lengths of time, and mRNA for the indicated chemokines, cytokines, and housekeeping genes was detected and quantified by RPA. Representative blots are shown on the left (in lane P+digest, the probe alone was digested with RNase). The graphs show means from three experiments on three different donors, normalized for each membrane based on expression of two housekeeping genes. The SE were less than 10% and are not shown. Reproduced with permission from **ref. 5**.

(which is somewhat less sensitive, but gives a digital image that can be used for publication or presentation, and also allows accurate quantification of the intensity of chemiluminescence).

3. The amount of chemiluminescence in each band can be quantified using Kodak Digital Science Image Station 440CF and the Image Analysis Software 3.0. The results can be normalized based on the amount of chemiluminescence of housekeeping genes, whose expression does not significantly change upon stimulation (L32 and GAPDH in the sets used here). The amount of chemiluminescence is proportional to the amount of mRNA present in the sample that hybridized with the labeled probe (because an excess of the labeled probe is used for hybridization). This procedure allows direct comparison of the results from different membranes and donors. The quantitative results can be expressed as a graph (**Fig. 2**).

4. The RPA assay described here proved to be useful, sensitive, and reliable for detection and quantification of chemokine and cytokine mRNA in human monocytes stimulated with bacterial products (*5*). The results revealed induction of high levels of chemokine mRNA and also high, but somewhat lower levels of cytokine mRNA (**Fig. 2**) (*5*). These results were consistent with detection of high levels of chemokine and cytokine mRNA using cDNA arrays (*5*) and also with high levels of chemokine and cytokine secretion revealed by the ELISA assays and bioassays (*5*). The RPA assay also showed very high specificity, as evidenced by high induction of mRNA for chemokines and cytokines typically produced by monocytes, and no induction of mRNA for chemokines and cytokines typically produced by lymphocytes and other cells (**Fig. 2**) (*5*). The RPA assay has been successfully used in other laboratories for simultaneous measurement of mRNA for several cytokines, cytokine receptors, and other genes both in humans and experimental animals (*7–16*).

This RPA method is convenient to use and does not require any special equipment, so it can be performed in any laboratory equipped to perform basic molecular biology experiments. The RPA method is also more sensitive (and, therefore, requires much less RNA) than the traditional Northern blot and dot/slot blot methods (**Table 1**), which is a great advantage if small amounts of cells (e.g., from normal donors or patients) are available. There is little variation from experiment to experiment when using the same probes and the same RNA or even different RNA batches obtained from the same donor. However, different donors show some variation in the level of expression of the same genes and in their ability to respond to the same stimulants. Therefore, we recommend averaging the results from at least three donors. The main disadvantage of the RPA method is its relative complexity and the time that has to be spent in optimizing the conditions of the assay. However, once the optimal conditions are established, the method is very reliable and can generate large amount of information in a single experiment.

4. Notes

1. The method described here can be used (with only minor modifications in the procedure for obtaining and treating the cells) for analysis and comparison of chemokine and cytokine mRNA levels in various other primary cells, in cells from patients with different diseases, or in vitro cultured cell lines exposed to various treatments. We have obtained very similar results using the same RPA assay for the analysis of chemokine and cytokine mRNA levels in human THP-1 monocytic cell line activated with the same bacterial stimulants *(5)*. Application of this method to measure chemokine and cytokine mRNA levels in other cells may only require slight modifications in the amounts of RNA used for the assay, because levels of chemokine and cytokine mRNA in various cells may be different (lower expression in other cells may require more RNA). This method can also be used for the analysis and comparison of mRNA levels for other genes in various cells, but the steps for synthesizing the probes and for hybridization and RNase digestion most likely will have to be optimized. Numerous commercial ready-made sets or custom sets of templates are now available from Pharmingen, Ambion, and other sources, and can be easily used in this assay. Templates, probe synthesis kits, and RPA assay kits do not have to be from the same company. We have found that Pharmingen templates work very well with Ambion probe synthesis and RPA assay kits.
2. Careful selection of the templates is important. To start, it may be wise to try commercial preassembled sets of templates, because they are much less expensive than the custom-made templates. The templates and the RPA kit or reagents do not have to be from the same company. We usually use templates from Pharmingen and the probe synthesis and RPA kits from Ambion. Select the template with housekeeping genes that are expressed in the cells of interest and whose expression does not substantially change with the treatments that are to be used.
3. If you design your own template set, the probes must be about 100–1000 bp long (optimum size is 200–500 bp), have unique sequences for each cDNA, and must be preferably 20–30 bp (at least 10–20 bp) different in size from each other (smaller differences will be very difficult to resolve on the gel).
4. Although this procedure can tolerate RNA of somewhat lower quality, the best and most consistent results will be obtained with high quality RNA. For tips on high quality RNA, *see* Chapter 36 on cDNA arrays. If the RNA is partially degraded and the breaks are within the segments complementary to the probes, the degraded RNA will not be detected or will give bands of protected probe of the wrong size. When comparing different RNA samples (different treatments of the same cells, different donors, different cell types, etc.), all RNA samples should be obtained by the same method and the quality of RNA in all the samples should be similar.
5. Using siliconized microcentrifuge tubes and siliconized nonstick glass plates to run the gel will yield much better results.
6. Another version of the RPA assay (in addition to the nonisotopic RPA presented in this chapter) is the isotopic RPA *(18)*. The advantages of the nonisotopic method are described above and in **Subheading 1.** In the isotopic method, the

RNA probes are synthesized in the presence of ^{32}P-UTP, which yields ^{32}P-labeled probes. The probes are purified by ethanol precipitation (gel purification is difficult and not necessary) and can then be used directly for hybridization, without the need for psoralen-biotin labeling. The hybridization, RNase digestion, and resolving the RPA products on a gel are the same in both procedures. In the isotopic method, the gel is then dried and the radioactive bands corresponding to the full-length and protected probes are detected by autoradiography. The quantification of the radioactivity in the bands can be done using a phosphorimager. The isotopic assay, therefore, has fewer steps than the nonisotopic assay, because there is no need for the labeling of probes with psoralen-biotin, and no need to blot the final gel onto a membrane and detect the bands by chemiluminescence. The main disadvantage of the isotopic assay, however, is that new probes have to be synthesized and purified, and their use optimized every 2 wk, because of the short half-life and high energy of ^{32}P, which quickly causes radiation lysis of the labeled probes. Moreover, the use of ^{32}P requires additional precautions, generates radioactive waste, and repetitive probe labeling is more expensive. In the nonisotopic assay, the probes can be synthesized once, their use can be optimized, and they can be stored and reused for more than a year.

7. Coprecipitation of the probes plus RNA mix before hybridization, dissolving the precipitated RNA in a small volume of hybridization buffer, and then denaturing RNA increases hybridization efficiency.

8. The optimal hybridization temperature and time may vary from 42°C for 10–48 h (recommended by Ambion for RPA III kit) to 68°C for 3 h (for Ambion Hybspeed RPA kit) and needs to be optimized for each system. For multiprobe protocols, higher stringency at higher temperature reduces nonspecific cross-hybridization without affecting probe:target mRNA hybridization. Longer hybridization times allow for binding of all complementary mRNA to the probe, which is important for quantifying the amount of mRNA. In our system, the optimal conditions were 56°C for 16 h.

9. The use of the positive and negative control (described in **Subheading 3.8., step 10**) is critical to check the function of RNases and to check if the probes are being protected in the absence of homologous RNA (positive control for digestion, no bands in this lane) and to check if the probes are not "spontaneously" digested in the absence of RNases (negative control for digestion, full-length probe bands in this lane, no bands corresponding to protected probes).

10. The concentrations of the RNases are crucial for the outcome of the RPA assay. Several different concentrations of RNases need to be tested, often outside the range given for the first pilot experiment **(Table 2)**. In the pilot experiments, vary the concentrations of the sample RNA and the RNases and keep the concentration of the probes constant (because the assay uses a relatively large excess of the labeled probes). If the double-stranded probe:mRNA hybrid is A-U rich, local denaturation ("breathing") may occur, which may lead to cleavage of the double stranded regions by RNase A, which cleaves 3' to C and U residues. If this problem is suspected, use RNase T1 alone (which cleaves 3' to G residue only) or substantially decrease the amount of RNase A. For our experimental conditions, 500 U/mL (1:10 dilution) of RNase T1 and 0.25 U/mL (1:40,000 dilution) of RNase A gave the best results.

11. **Subheading 3.8., step 11**, that inactivates RNases after RNase digestion, also precipitates the RNA fragments. The RNase inactivation/precipitation III solution in the Ambion kit may not efficiently precipitate all small RNA fragments (especially <150 bases). Therefore, the precipitation is improved by adding 150 µL of ethanol. The precipitated RNA fragments, if desired, can be stored frozen for extended periods of time in the nonisotopic assay, but extended storage of ^{32}P-labeled RNA fragments in the isotopic assay is not recommended, because, in addition to the loss of total radioactive signal, it will also result in radiolysis of the probe, causing high background on the autoradiograph.

12. Always mark the sample side of the nylon membrane. This side has to face up during the chemiluminescence detection step, and then it needs to face the X-ray film or the screen of the imaging apparatus.

13. Several concentrations of undigested full-length probes and RNA may have to be tried to get the right exposure that matches the exposure of RPA results (use approx 10–20 times less RNA than the amount of the labeled probe in the RPA assay).

14. Occasionally, some probes may yield two bands of the protected probe, most likely due to incomplete hybridization and/or alternative digestion of the protected probe by the RNases. This, or other spurious bands that may sometimes appear, may complicate identification of the bands corresponding to each protected probe in a multiprobe assay. If the identity of some bands in the protected probes lane is in doubt and cannot be determined based on their size, the experiment may have to be repeated either with the probes in question individually omitted from the set or with single probes used individually. Using a given probe individually will positively identify which protected probe band (or bands) corresponds to this probe. These bands should be differentiated from other spurious bands that result from contamination of the probe (e.g., if template DNA is not completely removed from the probe, it will hybridize with the probe and generate additional bands in all lanes) or from underdigestion or overdigestion with the RNases. Underdigestion will usually yield a ladder of bands in between the full-length probe and the protected probe fragment, and will also leave leftover full-length probe in the no target RNA plus RNase control lane. Overdigestion will usually yield a ladder or smear of bands below the expected size of the protected fragment. This means that the conditions of digestion are not optimal. The instruction manual provided with the Ambion RPA kit has an excellent section on optimization and troubleshooting for the RPA assay and should be consulted if problems persist.

References

1. Melton, D. A., Krieg, P. A., Rebagliati, M. R., Maniatis, T., Zinn, K., and Green, M. R. (1984) Efficient in vitro synthesis of biologically active RNA and RNA hybridization probes from plasmids containing a becteriophage SP6 promoter. *Nucl. Acids Res.* **12,** 7035–7056.

2. Schenborn, E. T. and Mierendorf, R. C. (1985) A novel transcription property of SP6 and T7 RNA polymerases: dependence on template structure. *Nucl. Acids Res.* **13,** 6223–6236.

3. Milligan, J. F., Groebe, D. R., Witherell, G. W., and Uhlenbeck, O. C. (1987) Oligonucleotide synthesis using T7 RNA polymerase and synthetic DNA template. *Nucl. Acids Res.* **15,** 8783–8798.

4. Calzone, F. J., Britten, R. S., and Davison, E. H. (1987) Mapping of gene transcripts by nuclease protection assays and cDNA primer extension. *Meth. Enzymol.* **152,** 611–632.

5. Wang, Z.-M., Liu, C., and Dziarski, R. (2000) Chemokines are the main proinflammatory mediators in human monocytes activated by *Staphylococcus aureus*, peptidoglycan, and endotoxin. *J. Biol. Chem.* **275,** 20,260–20,267.

6. Chomczynski, P. and Sacchi, N. (1987) Single-step method of RNA isolation by acid guanidinium thiocyanate-phenol-chloroform extraction. *Anal. Biochem.* **162,** 156–159.

7. Stalder, A. K. and Campbell, I. L. (1994) Simultaneous analysis of multiple cytokine receptor mRNAs by RNase protection assay in LPS-induced endotoxemia. *Lymphokine Cytokine Res.* **13,** 107–112.

8. Tang, W. W., Feng, L., Mathison, J. C., and Wilson, C. B. (1994) Cytokine expression, upregulation of intercellular adhesion molecule-1, and leukocyte infiltration in experimental nephritis. *Lab. Invest.* **70,** 631–638.

9. Banner, L. R. and Patterson, P. H. (1994) Major changes in the expression of the mRNA for cholinergic differentiation factor/leukemia inhibitory factor and its receptor after injury to adult peripheral nerves and ganglia. *Proc. Natl. Acad. Sci. USA* **91,** 7109–7113.

10. Pearce, B. D., Hobbs, M. V., McGraw, T. S., and Buchmeier, M. J. (1994) Cytokine induction during T-cell-mediated clearance of mouse hepatitis from neurons in vivo. *J. Virol.* **68,** 5483–5495.

11. Panja, A., Siden, E., and Mayer, L. (1995) Synthesis and regulation of accessory/proinflammatory cytokines by intestinal epithelial cells. *Clin. Exp. Immunol.* **100,** 298–305.

12. Lemay, S. Mao, C., and Singh, A. K. (1996) Cytokine gene expression in MRL/lpr model of lupus nephritis. *Kidney Internation* **50,** 85–93.

13. Chowers, Y., Marsh, M. N., De Grandpre, L., Nyberg, A., Theofilopoulos, A. N., and Kagnoff, M. F. (1997) Increased proinflammatory cytokine gene expression in the colonic mucosa of coeliac disease patients in the early period after gluten challenge. *Clin. Exp. Immunol.* **107,** 141–147.

14. Kernacki, K. A., Goebel, D. J., Poosch, M. S., and Hazlett, L. D. (1998) Early cytokine and chemokine gene expression during *Pseudomonas aeruginosa* corneal infection in mice. *Infect. Immun.* **66,** 376–379.

15. Hill, J. K., Gunion-Rinker, L., Kulhanek, D., Lessov, N., Kim, S., Clark, W. M., et al. (1999) Temporal modulation of cytokine expression following focal cerebral ischemia in mice. *Brain Res.* **820,** 45–54.

16. Ho, J. W., Liang, R. H., and Srivastava, G. (1999) Differential cytokine expression in EBV positive peripheral T cell lymphomas. *Molec. Pathol.* **52,** 269–274.

17. Gilman, M. (1993) Ribonuclease protection assay, in *Current Protocols in Molecular Biology* (Ausubel, F. M., et al., eds.), John Wiley & Sons, Philadelphia, PA, pp. 4.7.1–4.7.8.

12

Isolation of Total and Bioactive Interleukins by Immunoaffinity-Receptor Affinity Chromatography

Terry M. Phillips and Benjamin F. Dickens

1. Introduction

The isolation of total and bioactive cytokines can be achieved by a combination of immunoaffinity and immobilized receptor chromatography. The former procedure isolates the total amount of a specific cytokine, and the latter procedure isolates the bioactive fraction of the immunoaffinity-purified material. Recombinant receptors are becoming available for a number of different biologic materials and are available in forms suitable for affinity chromatography.

Immunoaffinity-receptor chromatography is based on the principle that an immobilized antibody, bound to a suitable chromatographic packing matrix, can effectively react with and bind its specific antigen. Once this binding has taken place, the antibody will retain the antigen while nonreactive materials are washed through the column, thus leaving only the specific materials bound to the antibody. Recovery of the bound ligand is achieved by introducing a dissociation agent capable of disrupting the bonds formed between the immobilized antibody and its antigen, thus releasing the latter into the running buffer. The effluent is passed through an in-line dialyzer to remove the dissociation agent and then onto the receptor affinity column. The free antigen now interacts with the immobilized receptor, which in turn repeats the process—isolating the bioactive fraction while allowing the remainder to flow through the column and be collected. Recovery of the bioactive fraction is achieved by introducing a second dissociation phase and collecting the liberated material. To utilize this procedure, suitable immunoaffinity and receptor-coated matrices have to be constructed and packed into a series of chromatography columns. When this system is used in conjunction with a high-performance liquid chromatography (HPLC) system, the process can be easily controlled and is relatively quick to perform.

From: *Methods in Molecular Medicine, vol. 60: Interleukin Protocols*
Edited by: L. A. J. O'Neill and A. Bowie © Humana Press Inc., Totowa, NJ

2. Materials
2.1. Activation of Glass Beads

1. Solid glass beads (150–220 μm diameter; Sigma).
2. 3-Aminopropyltriethoxysilane (*caution:* skin irritant).
3. 1,1'-Carbonyldiimidazole (CDI).
4. Simple reflux apparatus and heating mantle.
5. Jewellery sonicator.
6. 10% Sucrose solution (w/v) in distilled water.
7. 0.01 *M* Sodium dihydrogen phosphate buffer, pH 7.4.
8. 1 *N* Hydrochloric acid (analytical grade).
9. 1 *N* Nitric acid (analytical grade).
10. Toluene (analytical grade).
11. Methanol (analytical grade).
12. Dioxane (analytical grade).

2.2. Immunoaffinity Column Construction

1. CDI-activated glass beads.
2. Streptavidin (Pierce).
3. Long-chain hydrazine biotin (Pierce).
4. 1500 mw ethylene glycol.
6. Monoclonal antibody to recombinant human interleukin-2 (IL-2; R & D Systems).
7. Poly-ether-ether-ketone (PEEK)-biocompatible chromatography columns (*see* **Note 1**).
8. PEEK column fittings (*see* **Note 1**).
9. PEEK tubing.

2.3. Receptor Column Construction

1. CDI-activated glass beads.
2. Recombinant human soluble IL-2g receptor (*see* **Note 2**).
3. Recombinant human IL-2 (R & D Systems).
4. PEEK columns and tubing.

2.4. Sample Preparation and Isolation

1. Fluorescein isothiocyanate (FITC).
2. 50 m*M* Sodium carbonate, pH 9.0.
3. 2.0 *M* Sodium thiocyanate (w/v) in 0.01 *M* phosphate buffer, pH 7.4.

2.5. Affinity Chromatography Instrumentation

1. HPLC system.
2. Injection port equipped with a 25-μL sample loop.
3. Gradient elution pump and mixing system.
4. In-line dialyzer (Technicon IMS, Warren, MI).
5. Two four-way switching valves (Hamilton or Rheodyn).

6. Fluorescence detector, set at 495 nm$_{excitation}$, 525 nm$_{emission}$.
7. Recording integrator.
8. Fraction collector.

3. Methods
3.1. Making CDI-Activated Glass Beads

1. Fill a 100-mL glass cylinder with a 10% sucrose solution. Gently add 10 g of glass beads to the top of the sucrose and allow them to sediment by gravity (*see* **Note 3**).
2. Gently pour off the sucrose and fill the cylinder with distilled water. Cover with Parafilm and gently shake to wash the beads. Repeat this procedure three times, adding fresh distilled water each time.
3. Following the final wash and removal of the distilled water, recover the beads (*see* **Note 4**), dry the beads on clean filter paper (*see* **Note 5**), and place them in a glass beaker containing 10 mL of 1 *N* hydrochloric acid.
4. Place the beaker in a small jewellery sonicator and sonicate for 5 min.
5. Wash the beads twice in 100 mL 1 *N* hydrochloric acid or until the supernatant is clear (*see* **Note 6**). Place the damp beads in a 50-mL round-bottomed flask.
6. Assemble a simple reflux apparatus (**Fig. 1**). Attach the round-bottomed flask to the condenser and reflux the beads in 25 mL 1 *N* nitric acid for 30 min on a slow boil (*see* **Note 7**). Allow cold tap water to circulate through the condenser jacket throughout the procedure.
7. Allow the flask to cool (approx 5–10 min—do not cool by placing in an ice bath, as this will cause the flask to crack or break). Recover the beads by carefully decanting the acid, blot the beads dry on filter paper, and replace them in the round-bottomed flask.
8. Add 10 mL of a 10% solution of 3-aminopropyltriethoxysilane dissolved in toluene and reattach the flask to the reflux apparatus. Reflux for 16 h on slow boil.
9. Allow the flask to cool and carefully decant the supernatant. Add 25 mL of 95% methanol and wash the beads by rapidly hand-swirling the flask. Decant and repeat this wash procedure five times.
10. Following the last wash, add 25 mL of fresh 95% methanol, reattach the flask to the reflux apparatus, and reflux for 10 min at a slow boil. Repeat this step twice (*see* **Note 8**).
11. Finally, add 25 mL of distilled water and wash the beads three times using a rapid hand-swirling motion to ensure that the entire bead surface is washed. Recover the beads and blot them dry on filter paper prior to placing them in a 15-mL glass screw-capped tube (*see* **Note 9**).
12. Add 10 mL of dioxane to the beads and swirl to mix. Add 100 mg of CDI to the tube and swirl to mix. Place on an overhead mixer and mix for 8 h at room temperature.
13. Recover the beads and place them in a 100-mL glass cylinder filled with dioxane. Cover with Parafilm and wash by inversion and sedimentation 10 times. Change the dioxane between washes.
14. After the final wash, recover the beads and dry them on filter paper.

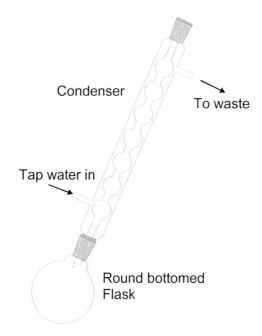

Fig. 1. Simple reflux apparatus for preparing glass beads. The reflux column condenser is clamped to a laboratory stand via a standard clamp. The angle of the condenser is set at approx 45°. The round-bottomed flask containing the glass beads plus the solution in which they are to refluxed is attached to the lower end of the condenser. Vacuum grease should be applied to the ground glass joints prior to connecting them. The assembled apparatus is placed in a fume hood with the round-bottomed flask surrounded by a heating mantle. The water jacket of the condenser should be connected to a water supply and tap water run constantly through the jacket during the reflux procedure.

3.2. Making the Immunoaffinity Support

1. To 1 g of CDI-activated glass beads add 1 mL of 50 mM sodium carbonate, pH 9.5, containing 1 mg of streptavidin (*see* **Note 10**) in a capped glass tube.
2. Place the tube on an overhead mixer and incubate for 12 h at 4°C.
3. Recover the beads and wash them five times in 0.01 M sodium phosphate buffer, pH 7.4 (*see* **Note 11**).
4. Suspend 100 µg of anti-IL-2 antibody in 250 µL of 0.1 M sodium acetate buffer, pH 5.0, and cool to 4°C (*see* **Note 12**).
5. Add 250 µL of ice-cold 10 mM sodium metaperiodate, mix well, and incubate for 20 min at 4°C, in the dark (*see* **Note 13**).
6. Stop the reaction by adding 2 mL of a 5% solution of 1500 mw ethylene glycol and dialyse the solution for 5 h against 0.01 M phosphate buffer, pH 7.0, at 4°C, in the dark (*see* **Note 13**).
7. Remove the antibody solution and place in a 15-mL capped glass tube.

8. Add 1 mL of 0.01 *M* phosphate buffer, containing 1 mg of sodium cyanoborate and 1 mg of hydrazine biotin.
9. Mix well and incubate for 1 h at room temperature.
10. Stop the reaction by dialysis against 0.01 *M* phosphate buffer overnight at 4°C.
11. Add the 0.01 *M* phosphate buffer containing the biotinylated antibody to 1 g of avidin-coated beads in a capped tube.
12. Mix for 1 h at 4°C in an overhead mixer.
13. Recover the beads and wash three times in 0.01 *M* phosphate buffer, pH 7.4.
14. Block the free biotin receptors by incubating the beads for 1 h in 5 mL 0.01 *M* phosphate buffer, pH 7.4, containing 1 mg/mL biotin, at 4°C (*see* **Note 14**).
15. Wash the beads five times in 0.01 *M* phosphate buffer, pH 7.4.

3.3. Making the Receptor Support

1. Add 2 µg of recombinant IL-2 receptor to 6 µg of recombinant IL-2 and incubate in an overhead mixer at room 37°C for 30 min (*see* **Note 15**).
2. Sediment the recombinant receptor by centrifugation of 100,000*g* for 20 min at 4°C, and resuspend the pellet in 1 mL of 50 m*M* sodium carbonate, pH 9.5.
3. Add 1 g of CDI-activated glass beads (*see* **Note 10**) to 1 mL of recombinant IL-2 receptor/IL-2 complex. Place in a capped glass tube.
4. Place the tube on an overhead mixer and incubate for 12 h at 4°C.
5. Recover the beads and wash them three times in 2.0 *M* thiocyanate, followed by 10 washes in 0.01 *M* sodium phosphate buffer, pH 7.4 (*see* **Note 11**).

3.4. Packing the Immunoaffinity and Receptor Columns (see Note 16)

1. Assemble the lower half of the PEEK column by attaching the end fitting onto the column barrel **(Fig. 2)**. Place a packing matrix retaining frit in the end fitting prior to assembly. Hand-tighten the end fitting until no further movement can be achieved.
2. Clamp the column either in a small vise or to a laboratory stand. Make sure that the column is vertical.
3. Place 250 µL of 0.01 *M* phosphate buffer in the column tube and slowly add the antibody-coated beads (*see* **Note 17**). Occasionally, cover the top of the column tube with Parafilm and bang the assembly on the bench top to eliminate air bubbles and to ensure that the beads pack properly.
4. Continue adding beads until the column tube is completely packed.
5. Using a blade spatula, smooth the packed bead surface so that it is level with the top of the column tube.
6. Carefully attach the top end fitting and hand-tighten.
7. Repeat the procedure for the receptor-coated beads using a new column assembly.

3.5. Assembly of the Immunoaffinity-Receptor System

1. Attach the inlet of the immunoaffinity column to the outlet of the injection port on the HPLC.
2. Attach the outlet of the immunoaffinity column to the inlet of the first switching valve **(Fig. 3)**.

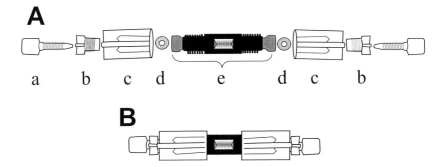

Fig. 2. Commercially available OmegaChrom PEEK columns used for immunoaffinity-receptor affinity chromatography. (**A**) Column assembly is performed by inserting the ferrule connector (b) into the column end-fitting (c) and tightened by finger pressure. The "finger-tight" connector (a) is then inserted into (b) and also tightened by finger pressure. A frit (d) is placed in the assembled column end-fitting (a–c), making sure that the frit lies flat in the fitting. The main body of the column (e) is carefully inserted into the assembled end-fitting and tightened by finger pressure. Only one end of the column is assembled. Using the star wrench and a suitable adjustable wrench, the main body of the column is securely tightened into the end-fitting until it no longer turns—do not use excessive force. Using the small end of the star wrench, the connector (b) is also securely tightened. The column is now ready to pack. After packing the column, the top end-fitting is assembled as described above and connected to the main body of the column. (**B**) The fully assembled column.

3. Attach the inlet of the on-line dialyzer (*see* **Note 18**) to the switching valve (**Fig. 3**).
4. Attach the outlet of the on-line dialyzer to the inlet of the second switching valve.
5. Attach the receptor column to the inlet on the second switching valve.
6. Connect a short length of PEEK tubing between inlet on the first switching valve and inlet on the second switching valve (*see* **Note 19**).
7. Attach the outlet of the receptor column to the flow-cell of the HPLC system (*see* **Note 20**).

3.6. Fluorochrome Labeling of Samples

1. Place 50 µL of the sample in a microcentrifuge tube.
2. Add 50 µL of a 1 mg/mL solution FITC dissolved in 50 m*M* sodium carbonate buffer, pH 9.0 (*see* **Note 21**).
3. Place on an overhead mixer for 15 min at room temperature.
4. Clarify the mixture by centrifugation for 2 min in a microcentrifuge.
5. Carefully remove the supernatant (*see* **Note 22**).

3.7. Isolation of Total and Bioactive IL-2

1. Set the first switching valve so that the effluent from the immunoaffinity column is directed to waste (*see* **Note 23**). This takes the dialyzer and receptor column off-line.

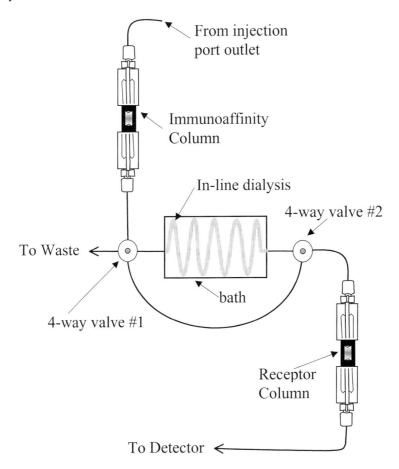

Fig. 3. The immunoaffinity-receptor system. The immunoaffinity column is attached via a short length of PEEK tubing to the outlet of the HPLC's injection port. The outlet of the immunoaffinity column is connected via a 3-cm length of PEEK tubing to the top port of the first four-way valve. The left port of this valve is connected to a length of tubing going to waste. The right port is connected via a 3-cm length of PEEK tubing to the inlet port of the "in-line" dialyzer unit. The bottom port of the valve is connected via a 10-cm length of PEEK tubing to the bottom port of another four-way valve. This forms a bypass for the dialyzer used during the elution phase of the receptor column. The left port of the second valve is attached via a 3-cm length of PEEK tubing to the inlet of the receptor column. The outlet of the receptor column is attached to the flow cell of the HPLC's detector. Switching of the first valve controls the output from the immunoaffinity column, directing it either to waste or through the dialyzer. Additionally, this valve can divert the flow past the dialyzer and directly to the receptor column. Likewise, the second valve places the dialyzer either on- or off-line depending on the stage of the process. The use of these valves is essential for the elution phase of the receptor column.

2. Using a Hamilton gas-tight syringe (100- or 50-μL vol) inject 25 μL of the sample into the injection port of the HPLC.

3. Run 0.01 M phosphate buffer, pH 7.4, through the system for 5 min at a flow rate of 0.5 mL/min (*see* **Note 24**).

4. Change the first and second switching valves to bring the dialyzer and receptor column on-line (*see* **Note 25**).

5. Initiate the immunoaffinity elution phase by generating a 0–2.0 M sodium thiocyanate gradient over 5 min (*see* **Note 26**).

6. Return the running buffer to 0.01 M phosphate buffer, pH 7.4, and run for a further 5 min.

7. Set the switching valves so that the dialyzer is off-line but the receptor column remains on-line.

8. Initiate the receptor elution phase by generating another 0–2.0 M sodium thiocyanate gradient over 5 min.

9. Throughout the procedure, constantly monitor the column outflow with the fluorescence detector, record the developing chromatogram, and collect the resulting peaks (*see* **Note 27**).

4. Notes

1. Short PEEK columns (5 cm long × 2.5 mm id; OmegaChrom columns) are available from Upchurch Scientific (Oak Harbor, WA). These columns are short lengths of thick-walled PEEK tubing encased in an aluminum outer tube to which PEEK end fittings can be attached. The fittings are made especially for these columns, which makes assembly very easy. When buying these columns it is important to also buy the "star" wrench offered by the company. This tool is required to fully hand-tighten the column assembly. A short length (20 cm) of PEEK tubing (0.010 inch id) is attached to the end fitting via a "fingertight" retaining fitting. This tubing provides points of attachment to either the on-line dialyzer or the HPLC system. The components of these columns are illustrated in **Fig. 2**.

2. The procedure described in this chapter refers to the use of the IL-2 receptor, which has been described in procedures for isolating IL-2 (*1–3*). However, several other soluble cytokine receptors are available from R & D Systems, and at present, this company supplies soluble forms of human IL-2α, -β, and -γ; IL-3α; Il-4; Il-5α; IL-6; IL-9; and IL-10. The procedure described is applicable for use with any of these soluble receptors.

3. Allowing the glass beads to cascade down through the sugar solution removes the fine shards of glass that are present in most commercially available sources of solid glass beads. The sucrose procedure is a quick and convenient way to remove these contaminants.

4. Beads can be recovered by using a clean spoon-shaped spatula. However, care must be taken to ensure that the beads do not roll off the spatula—this is a common cause of bead loss, especially among novices.

5. Whatman No. 1 filter paper is ideal for this procedure. Three or four sheets of filter paper are placed in a plastic tray and the beads simply placed on the filter paper and rolled until they are dry.

6. The safest approach to washing glass beads in acid is to place Parafilm over the mouth of the cylinder and wash the beads by inversion and sedimentation. Repeat this process three times per wash cycle and wear gloves to protect your hands from accidental leaks. It is also wise to perform this procedure over a sink.

7. The most convenient way to maintain a slow boiling action during the reflux stage is to place the round-bottomed flask in a heater unit. A slow boil is defined as a bubble being produced approximately every 30–45 s depending on the type of heater unit.

8. The purpose of the methanol washes with interspersed refluxes is required in order to remove the excess silane completely.

9. Glass tissue culture tubes are excellent for this stage of the protocol. Usually these tubes are sealed with a solvent-resistant cap equipped with an inert liner. These tubes are easily sealed with Parafilm, providing the perfect container for placing in an overhead mixer.

10. Once the CDI attachment groups have been synthesized onto the glass surface, the group quickly loses activity, especially when exposed to air. Dried beads can be kept for considerable lengths of time sealed under nitrogen, but for most practical purposes, the beads should be coated with protein within 12–24 h. This ensures that the activities of the coupling groups are maximized.

11. Allowing them to sediment through 100 mL of distilled water can easily wash glass beads. If this procedure is performed in a measuring cylinder, then covering the top with Parafilm and rolling the beads back and forth through the water effectively washes the beads. Change the distilled water twice during each wash.

12. Prior to attachment to streptavidin-coated glass beads, antibodies have to be biotinylated. The use of long chain (LC) hydrazine biotin ensures that the biotin will be derivatized into the Fc or tail portion of the antibody molecule. This portion contains the sugar molecules that are the target of the biotinylation process. However, these sugars have to be oxidized prior to attachment of the biotin *(4,5)*. This procedure is described in **Subheading 3.2., steps 4–10**. A potential problem with this form of biotinylation is that some monoclonal antibodies lack sugar in their Fc portions. It is a wise precaution to check that the antibodies contain sugar before attempting hydrazine biotinylation. Nonglycosylated antibodies can be biotinylated using succinimide ester biotin. In this latter case, the biotin is simply attached by incubating it with the target immunoglobulin at pH 9.0 in 50 mM sodium carbonate buffer.

13. It is extremely important to keep the reaction mixture in the dark as fluorescent lighting can seriously inhibit the reaction. To overcome this effect, the tube can simply be wrapped in aluminum foil. Reaction can then take place either on the bench or in a drawer.

14. Usually the biotinylated antibody utilizes the majority of the biotin receptors present on the streptavidin. However, it is good practice to make sure that all available biotin receptors are blocked to reduce nonspecific binding during the isolation process. This is simply achieved by incubating the beads with free biotin.

15. The receptor is incubated with its substrate prior to immobilization to ensure protection of the receptor binding site. Receptors bound to the packing matrix via the ligand are simply removed during the washing phase, as is the substrate bound to immobilized receptors.

16. The packing procedure is identical for both antibody- and receptor-coated beads. Care should be taken not to use excessive force, as this could shear the protein coat off the bead surface.

17. Wet beads can be introduced into the column tube by making a small funnel using a large (1000-μL) pipet tip. Place the tip into the column tube and mark where it fits tightly into the tube. Remove the tip and cut it approx 2 mm below the mark. Use either a scalpel or a razor blade to remove the lower end of the tip. The final product should just fit into the column tube yet also provide a funnel for guiding the wet beads into the column.

18. Commercial on-line dialyzer units are available from Technicon (Warren, MI).

19. The purpose of this tubing is to take the dialyzer off-line during the second elution phase. This ensures that the elution buffer will pass directly into the receptor column and release the bound bioactive cytokine.

20. Attachment of the packed column to the HPLC system involves connection of the antibody column inlet tubing to the outlet of the injection port. This ensures that the sample is immediately injected into the column. The outlet tubing of the column should be connected to the inlet of the switching valve. This valve is used to (a) direct the nonreactive materials to waste, and (b) direct the eluted cytokine into the on-line dialyzer. The on-line dialyzer is used to remove the chaotropic ion prior to introduction of the sample into the receptor column. The outlet of the dialyzer is connected to the inlet of the receptor column, the outlet of which is then coupled to the flow-cell inlet **(Fig. 3)**. Ideally, the tubing connecting the columns to the switching valve, dialyzer, and HPLC system should be as short as possible. However, the length of the tubing required to attach the columns to the HPLC will vary with different HPLC systems.

21. Only FITC isomer I should be used as this is the purest form of this fluorochrome. FITC is poorly soluble in aqueous buffers and must be dissolved in a acetone (10 μL) prior to addition to the aqueous conjugation buffer.

22. An advantage of the immunoaffinity step is that one does not need to remove free fluorochrome. The immobilized antibody will select only labeled cytokine, the free fluorochrome passing through the column along with the other nonreactive materials.

23. The switching valve is used to isolate the receptor column during the initial phase of the separation. This ensures that only immunoaffinity-purified cytokine enters the on-line dialyzer and then the receptor column. In this way, the incidence of nonspecific binding when isolating cytokines from complex biologic fluids can be overcome.

24. During this phase, the total cytokine binds to the immobilized antibody while nonreactive materials are washed through the column and discarded.

25. The materials eluted from the immunoaffinity column must pass through an on-line dialyzer prior to entry into the receptor column. This ensures that the elution or dissociation agent is adequately removed from the isolated cytokine prior to interaction with the immobilized receptor. Without this step, the binding of the cytokine to the immobilized receptor would be minimal or nonexistent.

26. The thiocyanate gradient is run through the immunoaffinity column to recover the bound cytokine. Sodium thiocyanate effectively dissociates the binding of antigen to the immobilized antibody, thus releasing the bound cytokine into the on-line dialyzer.

27. A typical chromatogram will produce two peaks; the first is the nonactive cytokine and the second is the bioactive cytokine. Total cytokine is calculated by adding the concentrations of the materials in peaks 1 and 2, whereas the bioactive is the material contained in peak 2. To improve the working life of the receptor column, it should be at 4°C by either encasing the column in a water jacket connected to a circulating water bath or by keeping the system in a controlled temperature chromatography cabinet.

References

1. Bailon, P. and Weber, D. V. (1988) Receptor-affinity chromatography. *Nature* **335,** 839–840.
2. Nachman, M., Azad, A. R., and Bailon, P. (1992) Membrane-based receptor affinity chromatography. *J. Chromatogr.* **597,** 155–166.
3. Phillips, T. M. (1997) Measurement of total and bioactive interleukin-2 in tissue samples by immunoaffinity-receptor affinity chromatography. *Biomed. Chromatogr.* **11,** 200–204.
4. O'Shannessy, D. J. and Quarles, R. H. (1987) Labeling of the oligosaccharide moieties of immunoglobulins. *J. Immunol. Methods* **99,** 153–161.
5. Phillips, T. M. (1992) *Analytical Techniques in Immunochemistry.* Marcel Dekker, NY.

13

Detection of Cytokines by Immunohistochemistry

Mahmoud Huleihel

1. Introduction

Cytokines belong to a family of immunoregulatory peptide growth factors that are produced mainly by immune cells after immune challenge. Various cells of nonimmune cell origin such as epithelial and muscle cells are also capable of producing cytokines, as well as many tumor cells *(1,2)*. We have recently demonstrated that sperm cells are capable of producing interleukin-1 (IL-1) *(3)*. The autocrine and paracrine effects excerted by cytokines may therefore play an important role, not only in physiologic processes but also in pathophysiologic situations. The cytokine family includes interleukins (IL-1–IL-18), colony-stimulating factors (macrophage-colony-stimulating factor [M-CSF], granulocyte-CSF [G-CSF], granulocyte macrophage-CSF [GM-CSF]), tumor necrosis factors (TNF-α and -β), interferons (IFN-α, -β, and -γ), transforming growth factor families (TGF-α and -β), activin, inhibin, chemotactic factors, and epidermal, fibroblast, insulin-like, nerve, and platelet-derived growth factors.

Cytokines do not act in an isolated manner but form part of a cascade of local events in which the surrounding cells function. The amplitude of an immune response may be mediated by cytokines, through feedback inhibition of proinflammatory cytokines and through downregulator cytokines such as IL-4, IL-10, IL-12, and/or cytokine-soluble receptors and the IL-1 receptor antagonist. Since cytokines, like hormones, also have systemic effects, the term homeokines has been suggested. Cytokines are involved in tumor transformation, in angiogenesis, and in the regulation of tissue remodeling *(1,2)*. Cytokines are expressed by almost all tissues and cells and also in plasma and various other body fluids of humans and animals *(1,2)*. Various methods are used to determine the levels of expression of cytokines, such as bioassays, immunoassays, Northern blot analysis to assess RNA levels, *in situ* hybridization (ISH), and

From: *Methods in Molecular Medicine, vol. 60: Interleukin Protocols*
Edited by: L. A. J. O'Neill and A. Bowie © Humana Press Inc., Totowa, NJ

immunohistochemical staining (IHC). The IHC and ISH methods permit the localization of cytokines within producing cells and within distinct compartments without the need to change the original microenvironment of the tissue.

This chapter deals with immunohistochemical staining, a sensitive method for determining the cellular compartment in which a substance is localized. This determination gives additional information to that achieved by qualitative and quantitative assessment.

2. Materials

1. Antigen retrieval (AR) agents: trypsin, proteanase L, urea, or citrate buffer.
2. 3% (v/v) H_2O_2 in 80% (v/v) methanol.
3. Phosphate-buffered saline (PBS), pH 7.4: Dissolve 80 g NaCl, 2.0 g KCl, 11.5 g Na_2HPO_4, and 2.0 g KH_2PO_4 in 900 mL distilled water. Adjust pH to 7.4 with 1 M NaOH if necessary. Make volume up to 1 L with distilled water. Store at room temperature. Dilute 1 in 10 with distilled water for use.
4. PBS containing 0.05% (w/v) casein.
5. Anticytokine antibodies.
6. Biotinylated secondary antibody and matched normal serum.
7. Diaminobenzidine tetrahydrochloride (DAB).
8. Eukitt for mounting.
9. Mayer's hematoxylin for counterstaining.
10. Acetone.
11. Alternative reagents for background staining: Tris-HCl buffer, or Triton X-100.
12. Paraffin wax.
13. B5 solution fixative, Bouin's solution fixative, or formalin.
14. Xylol.

3. Methods

Prior to immunohistochemical staining, tissues and cells need to be processed or fixed. Cytokines, like other antigens, can be detected after various forms of fixation. Formalin- or acetone-fixed tissues and cell imprints may be used for staining most of cytokines, using anticytokine antibodies (polyclonal or monoclonal) by direct or indirect immunohistochemical methods. When applying the indirect staining method, the secondary antibody is biotinylated. This approach is inexpensive compared with the direct method, using labeled anticytokine antibodies. AR is sometimes required to unmask the effect some fixatives have on antigens (*4,5*).

3.1. Basic Protocol for Immunohistochemical Staining of Tissues

1. Immunohistochemistry for most antigens does not require fresh tissue samples but can be performed on formalin-fixed, paraffin-embedded tissues (*4,5*). Tissue processing, embedding, and fixation are described in **Subheadings 3.2., 3.3.,** and **3.4.,** respectively. Saline-coated slides are preferred to ensure attachment of sections to the slide on which sections are mounted (*see* **Note 1**). The mounted sections are usually dried at 37°C or 60°C (*see* **Note 2**).

2. It is important to choose an optimal procedure for AR *(6–9)*. To determine the most suitable AR agent for a particular antigen, the sections are exposed to one of the following most commonly used AR agents: trypsin, proteanase L, urea, or citrate buffer *(6,9)*. For urea and citrate buffer, microwave or pressure cooking are the most commonly used methods. To bring the AR agent to boiling point, the sections are exposed to an increased temperature for 5, 10, or 15 min, depending on the agent. It is essential to leave the sections in the AR agent for a 20-min cooling—off period to ensure optimum results.
3. To block endogenous peroxidase, the specimen is treated with 3% H_2O_2 in 80% methanol for 15–20 min. Subsequently, nonspecific background is blocked with PBS containing 0.05% casein according to Tacha and McKinney *(10)* or PBS containing normal serum from the animal species in which the secondary antibody was prepared (*see* **Note 3**).
4. The primary antibody (for optimal concentrations, *see* **Note 4**) is then added (*11,12*; *see* **Notes 5–8**).
5. The biotinylated antibody is applied. Development of the stain is achieved by 0.06% DAB + H_2O_2. Mayer's hematoxylin is used for counterstaining *(13)*. Eukitt is used for mounting the sections.

3.2. Tissue Processing

Basically, processing means embedding the tissue to be examined in a firm, solid medium, which will allow thin, soft sections to be cut *(14)*. Paraffin wax is the most widely used material for this purpose. It is of course of utmost importance that the liquid wax thoroughly permeate the tissue in its fluid form and that it does as little damage as possible to the tissue upon solidification. Tissues should not be processed before it has been unequivocally determined that the fixation process has been completed. Rapid fixation can be achieved by heat. If buffered formalin at 60°C is used, one need not wait longer than 60 min to fix 5-mm slices for most tissues. The size of the tissue blocks in relation to the container used for processing is also important. They must be small enough to move freely within the container and to be exposed to the processing material solution from all sides. Otherwise, poor processing results can be expected.

3.3. Embedding

Higher temperatures of the wax will cause denaturation of the antigens during embedding. Therefore, one should choose a paraffin wax with a melting temperature of not more than 56°C. The tissue blocks should be prepared at a maximal thickness of 5 mm.

If slides are precoated with poly-L-lysine or other adhesives like rubber solutions or egg albumin the detachment of sections from the slides may be prevented.

3.4. Fixation

The purpose of fixing the sample is literally to "fixate" it, e.g., to retain a given situation of the morphology of cells and tissues and to stabilize the proteins in these cells and tissues *(15)*. The fixation process aims to fixate the cytokines to be measured in their *in situ* conditions. In choosing an appropriate fixative it has to be taken into account that the type of fixative may directly affect a variety of tissue and cell features.

A fixative may interfere with the immunoreactivity of the antigen and with cell morphology. It may also adversely affect various reaction, like extraction, diffusion, and displacement of the antigen during the steps of fixation. Finally, effects during fixation may interfere with subsequent antigen-antibody reactions employed in the localization of the antigen.

Recommended fixatives are B5, acetone, Bouin's solution, and formalin, the latter being most commonly used at a concentration of 10% (v/v). It is advisable to use formalin diluted in PBS. The time of fixation should not be longer than required for optimal preservation of the morphology. Prolonged fixation times may reduce the immunoreactivity of many antigens. Prolonged fixation with formalin may also cause shrinkage and hardening of the tissue.

The penetration of fixatives into tissues/cells is an important step in IHC. To allow penetration of the fixative (which is usually slow) into tissues/cells, the blocks prepared should be thin and small (4 μm).

Some cell surface antigens and antigens of cell membranes or nuclear receptors cannot be detected in conventionally fixed tissues. For determination of these antigens, sections of unfixed frozen material should be used and the mounted sections air-dried and fixed in cold acetone for 10 min.

3.5. Preparing and Storing Smears and Imprints for IHC Staining

Smears are air-dried, fixed in cold acetone, and then stored at –20°C or below. Before storage, sections are wrapped in foil. Before staining, care should be taken not to unwrap the slides before they have again reached room temperature. The slides are then air-dried and immersed in PBS.

3.6. Immunohistochemical Staining of Cells in Tissue Culture Suspension

To obtain a suitable cell concentration, the suspension is centrifuged at 300*g* for 10 min. The sediment is washed with PBS, and cells are resuspended in a saline/PBS solution. Then 100 μL of this suspension is mounted on saline-coated slides and dried at room temperature. The slides are fixed with acetone for 10 min, air-dried, wrapped in foil, and stored at –20°C until stained. Prior to the staining procedure, slides should be incubated for 15 min in Xylol.

4. Notes

1. During the whole staining procedure, the slides should always be kept in a moist atmosphere.
2. It should be noted that some antigens are lost if stored more than 4 wk at room temperature (RT). It is advisable to store sections that are not stained within a few days wrapped in foil, at –20° C to minimize antigen loss.
3. Background staining: Immunohistochemistry may produce uniform staining of the specimen, which will affect the sensitivity for identifying the cytokine (antigen) examined. This background staining is usually due to nonimmunologic binding of the specific antibodies to certain molecules or sites within the tissue. To achieve meaningful results, it is necessary to block these molecules and sites, thereby reducing this background stain. One method used for this purpose is preincubation of the sections with an immunoglobulin that does not interfere with the primary specific antibody, as in **Subheading 3.1.** Other methods involve the use of Tris-HCl buffer, high dilutions of the primary antibodies, or the addition of detergents such as Triton X-100. Pretreatment with enzymatic digestion is recommended *(4,5)*.
4. It is important to use optimal dilutions for each anticytokine antibody used to avoid false-negative results or increased background staining. Signal amplification is dependent on the avidity of the binding between the primary and the secondary antibody. This in turn, is dependent not only on the concentration of the secondary antibody but also on the concentration of immobilized primary antibody in the tissue.
5. Negative controls are important for each specimen using PBS/normal casein instead of the primary antibodies, or diluted normal serum from the animal source of the primary antibody instead of the primary antibody. Preabsorption of the primary antibodies with the relevant recombinant cytokine will show significant decrease in positive staining. As positive controls for the antibody-cytokine interaction, known positive tissues for the respective cytokines should be included whenever possible.
6. Unresponsiveness to the complete cytokine protein may be due to species homology in cytokine sequences. This problem may be overcome by analysis of putative antigenic sites in the amino acid chain and subsequent induction of anticytokine antibodies using coresponding synthetic peptides. Numerous monoclonal and polyclonal antibodies against human cytokines are available for IHC staining. Monoclonal antibodies are better suited for cytokine staining, since they produce less background than polyclonal antisera. IHC staining is not an off-the-shelf procedure whereby a set of given antibodies are used. One of the important prerequisites is to choose the optimal antibody out of a spectrum of different antibodies, which have to be screened.
7. Between antibody incubation periods, the sections should be thoroughly washed using PBS (3×5 min between reagents).
8. For decalcification, EDTA is preferred since greater retention of immunoreactivity can be achieved than with acid decalcification. The latter will also reduce the antigenicity of cell components, including immunoglobulins.

Acknowledgments

The author expresses his gratitude to Drs. M. Glezerman and I. Prinsloo for helpful suggestions and comments.

References

1. Abbas, A. K., Lichtman, A. H., and Pober, J. S. (1997) *Cellular and Molecular Immunology,* 3rd ed., W. S. Saunders, London, pp. 249–296.
2. Dinarello, C. A. (1996) Biological basis for interleukin-1 in disease. *Blood* **87,** 2095–2147.
3. Huleihel, M., Levy, A., Lunenfeld, E., Horowitz, S., Potashnik, G., and Glezerman, M. (1997) Distinct expression of cytokines and mitogenic inhibitory factors in semen of fertile and infertile men. *Am. J. Reprod. Immunol.* **37,** 304–309.
4. Robinson, G., Ellis, I. A., and MacLennan, K. A. (1990) Immunohistochemistry, in *Theory and Practice of Histological Techniques,* 3rd ed. (Bancroft, J. D., Stevens, A., and Turner, D. R., eds.), Churchill Livingstone, NY, pp. 413–436.
5. Hoefakker, S., Boersma, W. A., and Claassen, E. (1995) Detection of human cytokines in situ using antibody and probe based methods. *J. Immunol. Methods* **185,** 149–175.
6. Pileri, S. A., Roncador, G., Ceccarelli, C., Piccioli, M., Briskomatis, A., Sabattini, E., et al. (1997) Antigen retrieval techniques in immunohistochemistry: comparison of different methods. *J. Pathol.* **183,** 116–123.
7. Shi, S.-R., Cote, R. J., and Chaiwun, B. (1998) Standardization of immunohistochemistry based on antigen retrieval technique for routine formalin-fixed tissue sections. *Appl. Immunohistochem.* **6,** 89–96.
8. Cattoretti, G. and Suurmeijer, A. J. H. (1995) Antigen unmasking on formalin-fixed paraffin-embedded tissues using microwaves. *Adv. Anat. Pathol.* **2,** 2–9.
9. Taylor, C. R., Shi, S.-R., and Cote, R. J. (1996) Antigen retrieval for immunohistochemistery status and need for greater standardization. *Appl. Immunohistochem.* **4,** 144–166.
10. Tacha, D. E. and Mckinney, L. (1992) Casein reduced non-specific background staining in immunolabelling techniques. *J. Histotechnol.* **15,** 127–134.
11. Huleihel, M., Maymon, E., Piura, B., Isebrand, P., Benharroch, D., Yanai-Inbar, I., et al. (1997) Distinct patterns of expression of interleukin-1a and b by normal and cancerous human ovarian tissues. *Eur. Cytokine Net.* **8,** 179–187.
12. Glezerman, M., Mazor, M., Maymon, E., Piura, B., Isebrand, P., Benharroch, D., et al. (1998) TNF-alpha and IL-6 are differently expressed by fresh human cancerous ovarian tissues and primary cell lines. *Eur. Cytokine Net.* **9,** 171–179.
13. Stevens, A. (1990) The hematoxylins, in *Theory and Practice of Histological Techniques,* 3rd ed. (Bancroft, J. D., Stevens, A., and Turner, D. R., eds.), Churchill Livingstone, NY, pp. 107–118.
14. Gordon, K. C. (1990) Tissue processing, in *Theory and Practice of Histological Techniques,* 3rd ed. (Bancroft, J. D., Stevens, A., and Turner, D. R., eds.), Churchill Livingstone, NY, pp. 43–59.
15. Hopwood, D. (1990) Fixations and fixatives, in *Theory and Practice of Histological Techniques,* 3rd ed. (Bancroft, J. D., Stevens, A., and Turner, D. R., eds.), Churchill Livingstone, NY, pp. 21–43.

14

Whole Blood Assays and the Influence of Circadian Rhythmicity on Human Cytokine Measurement

Nikolai Petrovsky

1. Introduction
1.1. Relevance of Circadian Rhythms to Immune Assays

Circadian rhythmicity is a prominent feature of many important biologic functions. Failure to take such variation into account when performing assays may lead to increased assay variation or, most importantly, an erroneous result. Circadian rhythms of immunologic relevance include variation in the number of circulating T cells *(1)*, the autologous mixed lymphocyte reaction *(2)*, the phagocytic index *(3)*, and urinary neopterin secretion *(4)*.

1.2. Whole Blood Cytokine Assays

The investigation of cellular immunity and T-cell function in humans is increasingly turning away from a reductionist approach and instead focusing on the study of natural mixed cell populations, e.g., whole blood *(5)*. Isolation of cells into artificial medium usually containing fetal calf serum has profound modifying effects on T-cell function. For example, serum, which contains transforming growth factor-β (TGF-β) and other cytokine/growth factor products from platelets, modifies the T-cell cytokine response profile in vitro *(6)*. Changes in the function of antigen-presenting cells (APC), e.g., dendritic cells, removed from their physiologic environment *(7)* are also likely to affect T-cell responses adversely. When peripheral blood mononuclear cell (PBMC) cultures are compared with whole blood, interleukin-1 (IL-1) and IL-2 production are higher whereas tumor necrosis factor-α (TNF-α) and interferon-γ (IFN-γ) production are lower *(8)*. Simply adding autologous red blood cells to human PBMC cultures enhances production of IL-2, IL-6, IFN-γ, and TNF-α and increases IL-2 receptor expression and T-cell proliferation *(9)*.

From: *Methods in Molecular Medicine, vol. 60: Interleukin Protocols*
Edited by: L. A. J. O'Neill and A. Bowie © Humana Press Inc., Totowa, NJ

1.3. Cytokine Assays for Assessment of T-Cell Function

Cytokine-based assays offer important advantages and are steadily replacing traditional T-cell proliferation assays as the index of T-cell activation. Cytokine assays are often more sensitive and specific for T-cell responses to both mitogens and antigens *(10)*. Furthermore, the pattern of cytokine production may assist in determining functional significance; IFN-γ and IL-2 are produced by Th1 cells that mediate delayed type hypersensitivity (DTH) reactions whereas IL-4, -5, -6, and -10 are produced by Th2 cells that mediate humoral immunity and allergy *(11)*. Cytokines are readily measurable in the plasma above whole blood cultures, and antigen-specific whole blood cytokine production has been documented as a diagnostic test for tuberculosis in cattle *(12)* and for immunity to *Francisella tularensis (13)*, leprosy *(14)*, and cutaneous leishmaniasis *(15)* in humans. The advantage of unmanipulated whole blood for cytokine assays is that it most closely approximates the state of circulating cells in vivo and contains physiologic concentrations of factors that influence T-cell function *(16)*.

1.4. Evidence of Circadian Variation of Cytokine Production

Until recently little was known about circadian influences on cytokine production. Such variation would have important implications for the timing and interpretation of serum, plasma, or whole blood cytokine measurements. Early evidence that human cytokine production was under circadian influence came from findings that IL-1 and IL-6 were detectable in the serum of healthy subjects only between midnight and 3 am *(17)*. With more sensitive cytokine assays, serum IL-6 values have been shown to peak around 1 am and reach a nadir at 10 am *(18,19)*. Serum granulocyte macrophage colony-stimulating factor (GM-CSF) *(20)*, IL-2 *(21)*, soluble p75 TNF receptor *(22)*, and plasma-soluble IL-2 receptor *(23,24)* levels also exhibit circadian rhythmicity.

With currently available assays, however, many cytokines are not easily detectable in human plasma or serum. This makes it difficult to know whether all cytokines are subject to circadian rhythmicity. To address this question, we tested for circadian rhythmicity of cytokine production in whole blood stimulated ex vivo *(25)*. These experiments confirmed that whole blood IL-1 production demonstrated a circadian rhythm identical to the previously described rhythm of plasma IL-1 levels *(17)* with peak IL-1 production in blood taken around 3 am *(16)*. Similarly whole blood IFN-γ production in response to mitogens or tetanus exhibited circadian rhythmicity ($p < 0.001$ by Cosinor analysis) with a peak at approx 1 am and a nadir at 8 am *(25)* (*see* **Note 1**). In individual subjects, the time of peak IFN-γ production can range from 8:30 pm to 4 am and the time of the nadir from 7 am to 1:30 pm with peak IFN-γ production up to 40-fold higher than nadir levels. The mean IFN-γ peak-to-nadir interval is 9 h. IL-12 production exhibits a circadian rhythm (peak around 11 pm) almost synchronous with that of IFN-γ and demonstrating a similar amplitude. Whole blood IL-1, IL-10, and TNF-α production also exhibits significant 24-h rhythmicity in the majority of subjects *(16,26)*. The rhythms of IL-1, IL-10, and TNF-α are closely synchronous with peaks in blood taken at approx 9 pm or 3 h earlier than peak IFN-γ production and nadirs around 9 am.

Other studies have reported the absence of circadian cytokine rhythms of serum IL-10 and IL-12 *(21)* and mitogen-stimulated IL-2 production *(2)*. These negative results could be explained on the basis of methodologic problems, namely, the dilution of whole blood with culture medium or the culture of purified PBMCs in other than 100% autologous plasma. What these manipulations have in common is that they markedly reduce the concentration of important plasma hormones that are responsible for regulating cytokine production, in vivo.

1.5. Sex Differences in Circadian Cytokine Production

Analyzed on the basis of gender, there was no significant difference found among the phases or amplitudes of the circadian cytokine rhythms of IL-1, 6, 10, 12, IFN-γ, or TNF-α.

1.6. Relationship Between Circadian Cytokine Rhythms and White Cell Subsets

Cytokine circadian rhythms could reflect underlying changes in the number of circulating cytokine-producing blood cells. Both the peripheral blood white cell count (WBC) and the lymphocyte count demonstrate circadian rhythmicity, peaking around 11 pm and reaching a nadir at 9 am. Although there was a strong correlation between whole blood IFN-γ, IL-12, TNF-α, and IL-10 production and either the WBC or lymphocyte count, this does not prove a causal relationship as each of the above cytokines, and also both the WBC and lymphocyte count were all strongly negatively correlated with plasma cortisol, which could therefore be the common factor entraining both the WBC count and the cytokine production. The only exception to the above pattern was plasma macrophage inhibitory factor (MIF) levels, which were positively correlated with plasma cortisol.

In subjects given oral cortisone acetate 25 mg at 9 pm there was a reduced or absent correlation between each of the above cytokines and the WBC or lymphocyte count, suggesting the absence of a causal relationship between the circadian rhythms of lymphocyte numbers and cytokine production.

1.7. Circadian Entrainment of Cytokine Production by Plasma Hormones

Following oral administration of cortisone acetate, whole blood production of IFN-γ, IL-12, IL-1, and TNF-α exhibited a sharp fall (*see* **Note 2**). One hour after cortisone ingestion, IFN-γ, IL-12, TNF-α, and IL-1 production was suppressed by 84, 90, 95, and 62%, respectively. IL-10 production was reduced in only a minority of subjects 1 h after cortisone administration. In all cases, cytokine production recovered over 6–8 h concomitant with the decay in plasma cortisol levels consistent with an inverse causal relationship between plasma cortisol and IFN-γ, IL-12, TNF-α, and IL-1 production. One hour after cortisone administration, at a time when cytokine production was maximally suppressed, there was no significant reduction in the total WBC count, lymphocyte count, or numbers of CD3+, CD4+, CD8+, and CD56+ cells (see **Note 3**). The lymphocyte fraction decrease by 30–40%, but with a lag of 2–3 h after the plasma cortisol peak, whereas the nonlymphocyte fraction (principally monocytes and polymorphonuclear cells) increased by 15–20%.

The rhythm in plasma melatonin was in reverse phase to that of cortisol; melatonin peaked at approx 4 am and was low or unmeasurable during the daytime, whereas cortisol peaked during the late morning (9 am) and reached a nadir at 4 am. The peak in the IFN-γ coincided temporally with the peak in plasma melatonin, and this relationship held true even when the normal nighttime fall in plasma cortisol was prevented by oral cortisone acetate given at 9 pm. There was a significant positive correlation between plasma melatonin and whole blood IFN-γ and IL-12 but not TNF-α, IL-1, or IL-10 production. Furthermore, oral administration of melatonin 3 mg at 9 pm accentuated the nighttime peak of IFN-γ production while at the same time reducing nighttime IL-10 production and having no measurable effect on the circadian rhythms of IL-12 or TNF-α. Overall, cortisol, 17-hydroxyprogesterone, prolactin, and androstenedione were negatively and melatonin and growth hormone were positively, correlated with cytokine production (**Table 1**).

1.8. Circadian rhythmicity of Th1/Th2 Balance

To determine whether there is circadian variation in Th1/Th2 balance, the IFN-γ/IL-10 ratio was calculated for each study time point. As a result of the peak of IL-10 preceding that of IFN-γ production, and the subsequent steeper fall in IL-10, the IFN-γ/IL-10 ratio exhibited considerable 24-h variation, peaking around 4 am and reaching a nadir at 3 pm (*26*). The peak in the IFN-γ/IL-10 ratio coincided almost exactly with the time of the cortisol nadir. Furthermore, the IFN-γ/IL-10 ratio was reduced by 73% after oral administration of cortisone acetate 25 mg at 9 pm. The Th1 cytokines, IFN-γ and TNF-α, were inhibited to a much greater degree than the Th2 cytokines, IL-6 and IL-10, 1 h after oral cortisone (see **Note 4**). There was a close temporal relationship between the time of the IFN-γ/IL-10 and plasma melatonin peak. Following melatonin administration, the peak of the IFN-γ/IL-10 ratio was phase advanced by 3 h, peaking at 1:30 am rather than 4:30 am. This reflected the dual effect of melatonin in accelerating and accentuating the nighttime peak of IFN-γ production while reducing

Table 1
Correlation Matrix of Circadian Cytokine Production Against Plasma Hormone Levels[a]

	IFN–γ	IL–1	IL–10	IL–12	TNF–α
Melatonin	0.69	0.0	0.14	0.28	0.1
	(<0.001)	ns	ns	(<0.002)	ns
Androstenedione	–0.42	–0.37	–0.5	–0.38	–0.52
	(<0.001)	(<0.001)	(<0.001)	(<0.001)	(<0.001)
DHEAS	–0.47	–0.18	0.0	–0.17	0.0
	(<0.001)	ns	ns	ns	ns
Hydroxyprogesterone	–0.57	–0.56	–0.64	–0.73	–0.69
	(<0.001)	(<0.001)	(<0.001)	(<0.001)	(<0.001)
Growth hormone	0.4	0.0	0.2	0.2	0.28
	(<0.001)	ns	(<0.05)	(<0.05)	(<0.005)
Prolactin	–0.26	–0.28	–0.42	–0.5	–0.47
	(<0.005)	(<0.005)	(<0.001)	(<0.001)	(<0.001)
Cortisol	–0.87	–0.26	–0.6	–0.65	–0.6
	(<0.001)	(<0.005)	(<0.001)	(<0.001)	(<0.001)

[a]Correlation coefficients *(r)* are presented as a matrix table of cytokines (*x*-axis) against 24-h plasma hormone levels (*y*-axis). Subjects (*n* = 5) had blood taken hourly for 24 h for measurement of LPS-stimulated whole blood IFN-*g*, IL-1, IL-10, IL-12, and TNF-α production. Cytokine data were correlated with representative 24-h plasma melatonin, androstenedione, DHEAS, 17-hydroxy progesterone, growth hormone, prolactin, and cortisol levels. ns, not significant. The *p* values are in parenthesis.

nighttime IL-10 production. There was a positive correlation between the IFN-γ/IL-10 ratio and plasma melatonin that remained even in subjects receiving cortisone acetate 25 mg at 9 pm (N. Petrovsky, manuscript in preparation). The IFN-γ/IL-10 ratio was negatively correlated with plasma dihydroepiandrostenedione (DHEAS) and cortisol (**Table 2**).

2. Materials

1. Venesection: Vacutainer blood collection system (Becton-Dickinson).
2. Mitogen/antigen: *E. coli* lipopolysaccharide (LPS) serotype 0127:B8 (Gibco), preservative-free tetanus toxoid (CSL, Australia).
3. Mitogen/antigen buffer: Human tonicity (HT)-RPMI.
4. Blood culture: Eight-channel multipipet (Titertek), V-bottomed plastic trough, round-bottomed 96-well tissue culture plates (Falcon).
5. Cytokine measurement: Cytokines were assayed by enzyme-linked immunosorbent assay (ELISA) as follows; IFN-γ (CSL, Australia), IL-1 and IL-6 (Biosource International), and TNF-α, IL-10, and IL-12 (PharMingen antibody pairs).
6. Circadian analysis software: Chronolab (Dr. Fernida, Bioengineering and Chronobiology Lab., ETSI Telecommunie, University of Vigo, Spain).

Table 2
Correlation Matrix of Circadian Plasma Hormone Levels Against the IFN–γ/IL–10 Ratio[a]

	IFN–γ/IL–10 ratio		
	Normal	After melatonin	After cortisone
Androstenedione	0.29	–0.55	–0.1
	(<0.002)	(<0.001)	ns
DHEAS	–0.57	–0.35	–0.5
	(<0.001)	(<0.001)	(<0.001)
Hydroxyprogesterone	0.0	–0.64	–0.3
	ns	(<0.001)	(<0.001)
Growth hormone	0.0	0.5	0.0
	ns	(<0.001)	ns
Prolactin	0.32	–0.33	0.1
	(<0.001)	(<0.001)	ns
Melatonin	0.68	na	0.51
	(<0.001)		(<0.001)
Cortisol	–0.57	–0.68	–0.56
	(<0.001)	(<0.001)	(<0.005)

[a]Correlation coefficients *(r)* are presented as a matrix of the IFN-γ/IL-10 ratio *(x–axis)* under normal conditions (first column) or after oral melatonin (second column) or cortisone (third column) against plasma hormone levels *(y–axis)*. Subjects *(n* = 5) had blood taken hourly for 24 h for measurement of the ratio of IFN-γ to IL-10 in LPS-stimulated whole blood. These experiments were repeated on two further occasions when the subjects either received 3 mg melatonin or 25 mg cortisone acetate at 9 pm. Cytokine data were correlated with representative 24-h plasma androstenedione, DHEAS, 17–hydroxy progesterone, growth hormone, prolactin, and cortisol levels. na, not assessed; ns, not significant. The *p* values are in parenthesis.

3. Methods

3.1. Measurement of Circadian Cytokine Variation

Venous blood is drawn at regular time intervals, e.g., each hour for 24 h, from human volunteers. Circulating levels of serum or plasma cytokines can then be directly measured by ELISA. For cytokines such as IFN-γ, which are normally undetectable in plasma, a system of short-term ex vivo whole blood cultures is used to stimulate measurable cytokine production. This reflects the capacity of blood taken at a particular time of day to produce particular cytokines. Whole blood cytokine production can be elicited using either a mitogen, e.g., *lipopolysaccharide* LPS, phytohemaglutinin, (PHA) or concavalin A (Con A), or a recall-antigen, e.g., tetanus toxoid (*see* **Note 5**). Blood samples are taken hourly via an indwelling venous cannula inserted in a forearm cubital fossa vein. During the study period the subjects should be encouraged to maintain their normal sleep/wake cycle and activity patterns (*see* **Note 6**). During the day the intravenous cannula (IVC) can be capped and kept patent with a saline flush. During the night the IVC can be kept patent by connecting it to a normal saline infusion (500 mL over 12 h), thereby allowing venous blood samples to be taken during the night without disturbing or waking the subject. To avoid blood dilution with saline, the first 10 mL of blood withdrawn is discarded prior to collection of the actual study sample. Plasma can also be collected at each study time point for measurement of potentially relevant hormones such as cortisol, growth hormone, melatonin, prolactin, DHEAS, 17-hydroxyprogesterone, or androstenedione (*see* **Note 7**). At each time point blood can also be taken in EDTA for determination of blood counts and circulating lymphocyte subsets.

3.2. Whole Blood Assay to Assess T-Cell Function

Forearm venous blood is collected into sterile, heparinized 10-mL tubes (Vacutainer, Becton-Dickinson) as previously described *(5)* (*see* **Notes 8** and **9**). After thorough mixing by repeated inversion of the tube, 280-μL aliquots of blood are pipetted into 96-well tissue culture plate wells preloaded with 20 μL of antigen in HT-RPMI or 20 μL of HT-RPMI alone. The 96-well tissue culture plates are incubated at 37°C in a 5% CO_2 atmosphere for 48 h after which the plasma supernatants are aspirated, pooled, and stored at –20°C until assayed for cytokines by ELISA.

3.3. Analysis of Circadian Rhythmicity

For group analysis, cytokine measurements are best first expressed as a percentage of the 24-h individual mean. Circadian rhythmicity is analyzed by Chronolab, a software package for chronobiologic time series analysis *(27)* available from Dr. Fernida, Bioengineering and Chronobiology Lab., ETSI Telecommunie, University of Vigo, Spain.

3.4. Plasma Cytokine Measurement

Cytokine levels in plasma supernatants are most conveniently measured by ELISA. To avoid the expense of preprepared coated ELISA plate kits, it is now possible to obtain reliable antibody pairs, e.g., from Pharmigen, which can be used to prepare ELISAs according to the following sample protocol. The capture monoclonal antibody (MAb) was coated overnight at 4 μg/mL onto Nunc Maxisorb plates at a concentration of 5 μg/mL. The plates were then washed and blocked with 10% bovine serum albumin for 1 h at room temperature (RT). Samples (50 μL) were added to wells and incubated for 2 h at RT followed by washing and incubation with a secondary biotin-conjugated detection MAb at 1 μg/mL for 1 h. After washing, this was followed by incubation with 100 μL streptavidin-peroxidase (1:500) for 1 h. Color was developed with 100 μL tetramethylbenzidine (TMB) peroxidase substrate.

4. Notes

1. IFN-γ has an important role in natural killer (NK) cell activation, and increased nighttime IFN-γ production could, therefore, explain the increased NK cell function seen in human blood samples taken at night *(28)*.

2. Of the human cytokines we have studied to date, IFN-γ, IL-12, and TNF-α are the most sensitive, with IL-1 being intermediate and IL-6 and IL-10 least sensitive to inhibition by physiologic levels of cortisol *(16)*. Plasma MIF levels are increased by physiologic levels of cortisol (N. Petrovsky, manuscipt in preparation). The ranking of human cytokines on the basis of sensitivity to cortisol differs a little from that of mice, in which IFN-γ, IL-1, IL-4, and IL-10 are the most sensitive and TNF-α, GM-CSF, IL-2, and IL-3 the most resistant to suppression by supraphysiologic doses of dexamethasone *(29)*. Human cytokine sensitivity to inhibition by cortisol closely matches sensitivity to inhibition by IL-10, with IFN-γ being most sensitive and IL-6 most resistant to IL-10 inhibition *(30)*.

3. Cortisol downregulates cytokine gene expression by binding to and activating negative regulatory elements in the promoters of cytokine genes *(31–33)*. Consequently, it seems likely that cortisol reduces whole blood cytokine production by directly downregulating cytokine gene transcription. IL-10 has anti-inflammatory actions *(34)*, which may explain why it is relatively resistant to cortisol suppression.

4. The bias toward Th1 cytokine production during the night and early morning when the IFN-γ/IL-10 ratio is high may explain why symptoms of chronic inflammatory disorders, e.g., rheumatoid arthritis, are most severe during the night and early morning *(35)*. Patients with rheumatoid arthritis have significant circadian variation in plasma IL-6 with peak values in the morning and low values in the afternoon and evening *(36,37)*. In asthma, bronchoalveolar lavage fluid concentrations of IL-1β are significantly greater at 4 am than at 4 pm in patients with nocturnal airflow obstruction. *(38)*.

5. Whether a mitogen or recall antigen is used for whole blood stimulation does not appear to affect the phase of circadian cytokine rhythms *(25)*.

6. In shift workers, cytokine rhythms may be phase advanced or retarded in accordance with these individuals' altered sleep/wake cycle *(25)*.

7. Cortisol and melatonin are unlikely to be the only neuroendocrine hormones that entrain cytokine rhythms; other potential candidates that exhibit both circadian rhythmicity and immunomodulatory actions include 17-hydroxy progesterone, DHEAS, prolactin, growth hormone, and triiodothyronine. Plasma levels of melatonin and androstenedione peak at approx 3 am, whereas levels of growth hormone (GH) and prolactin peak soon after the onset of sleep. Levels of 17-hydroxyprogesterone and cortisol both peak at approx 9 am. Melatonin stimulates IL-1 *(39)* and IFN-γ *(40)* production by human macrophages and mouse splenocytes, respectively, and counteracts the immunosuppressive effects of glucocorticoids on antiviral resistance and thymic weight in mice *(41)*. Similarly, DHEAS biases toward type 1 cytokine production *(6,42)*. GH activates human macrophages and primes them for enhanced H_2O_2 release *(43)* and when given to hypopituitary animals augments antibody synthesis and skin graft

rejection *(44,45)*. Melatonin therapy in patients with solid tumors induced a significant decline in plasma TNF-α *(46)* consistent with a role of melatonin in regulating cytokine production. Interestingly, another pineal indole, 5-methoxytryptophol, which reaches its highest levels during the light phase of the day, significantly increases serum concentrations of IL-2 while decreasing IL-6 *(47)*. A strong negative correlation has been reported between the circadian rhythm of β-endorphin and plasma IL-1β levels *(48)*.

8. In view of the circadian nature of cytokine production, interassay variation in whole blood cytokine responses will be minimized if blood is drawn at a fixed time of day. Ideally, for maximal responsiveness of proinflammatory cytokines, blood would need to be drawn in the late evening or early morning hours. Alternatively, for maximal responsiveness of plasma MIF blood would need to be taken in the late morning. Purification of PBMCs from blood prior to culture or dilution of whole blood 1:10 with culture medium will reduce plasma hormone levels and will thereby significantly dampen any circadian influence on cytokine production. However, the resultant cytokine production is less likely to reflect the situation in vivo.

9. In view of the causal relationship between high plasma cortisol and low proinflammatory cytokine production, the effect on cytokine production of an acute increase in plasma cortisol induced, for example, by anxiety in anticipation of venesection may need to be considered.

References

1. Miyawaki, T., Taga, K., Nagaoki, T., Seki, H., Suzuki, Y., and Taniguchi, N. (1984) Circadian changes of T lymphocyte subsets in human peripheral blood. *Clin. Exp. Immunol.* **55,** 618–622.
2. Indiveri, F., Pierri, I., Rogna, S., Poggi, A., Montaldo, P., Romano, R., et al. (1985) Circadian variations of autologous mixed lymphocyte reactions and endogenous cortisol. *J. Immunol. Methods* **82,** 17–24.
3. Melchart, D., Martin, P., Hallek, M., Holzmann, M., Jurcic, X., and Wagner, H. (1992) Circadian variation of the phagocytic activity of polymorphonuclear leukocytes and of various other parameters in 13 healthy male adults. *Chronobiol. Int.* **9,** 35–45.
4. Auzeby, A., Bogdan, A., Krosi, Z., and Touitou, Y. (1988) Time-dependence of urinary neopterin, a marker of cellular immune activity. *Clin. Chem.* **34,** 1866–1867.
5. Petrovsky, N. and Harrison, L. C. (1995) Cytokine-based human whole blood assay for the detection of antigen-reactive T cells. *J. Immunol. Methods* **186,** 37–46.
6. Daynes, R. A. and Araneo, B. A. (1992) Natural regulators of T-cell lymphokine production in vivo. *J. Immunother.* **12,** 174–179.
7. Romani, L., Puccetti, P., Mencacci, A., Cenci, E., Spaccapelo, R., Tonnetti, L., et al. (1994) Neutralization of IL-10 up-regulates nitric oxide production and protects susceptible mice from challenge with *Candida albicans*. *J. Immunol.* **152,** 3514–3521.
8. De Groote, D., Zangerle, P. F., Gevaert, Y., Fassotte, M. F., Beguin, Y., Noizat-Pirenne, F., et al. (1992) Direct stimulation of cytokines (IL-1 beta, TNF-alpha, IL-6, IL-2, IFN-gamma and GM-CSF) in whole blood. I. Comparison with isolated PBMC stimulation. *Cytokine* **4,** 239–248.

9. Kalechman, Y., Herman, S., Gafter, U., and Sredni, B. (1993) Enhancing effects of autologous erythrocytes on human or mouse cytokine secretion and IL-2R expression. *Cell. Immunol.* **148,** 114–129.

10. Hao, X. S., Le, J. M., Vilcek, J., and Chang, T. W. (1986) Determination of human T cell activity in response to allogeneic cells and mitogens. An immunochemical assay for gamma-interferon is more sensitive and specific than a proliferation assay. *J. Immunol. Methods* **92,** 59–63.

11. Mosmann, T. R. and Coffman, R. L. (1989) TH1 and TH2 cells: different patterns of lymphokine secretion lead to different functional properties. *Annu. Rev. Immunol.* **7,** 145–173.

12. Rothel, J. S., Jones, S. L., Corner, L. A., Cox, J. C., and Wood, P. R. (1992) The gamma-interferon assay for diagnosis of bovine tuberculosis in cattle: conditions affecting the production of gamma-interferon in whole blood culture. *Aust. Vet. J.* **69,** 1–4.

13. Karttunen, R., Ilonen, J., and Herva, E. (1985) Interleukin 2 production in whole blood culture: a rapid test of immunity to *Francisella tularensis. J. Clin. Microbiol.* **22,** 318–319.

14. Weir, R. E., Morgan, A. R., Britton, W. J., Butlin, C. R., and Dockrell, H. M. (1994) Development of a whole blood assay to measure T cell responses to leprosy: a new tool for immuno-epidemiological field studies of leprosy immunity. *J. Immunol. Methods* **176,** 93–101.

15. Frankenburg, S. (1988) A simplified microtechnique for measuring human lymphocyte proliferation after stimulation with mitogen and specific antigen. *J. Immunol. Methods* **112,** 177–182.

16. Petrovsky, N., McNair, P., and Harrison, L. C. (1998) Diurnal rhythms of pro-inflammatory cytokines: regulation by plasma cortisol and therapeutic implications. *Cytokine* **10,** 307–312.

17. Gudewill, S., Pollmacher, T., Vedder, H., Schreiber, W., Fassbender, K., and Holsboer, F. (1992) Nocturnal plasma levels of cytokines in healthy men. *Eur. Arch. Psychiatry Clin. Neurosci.* **242,** 53–56.

18. Sothern, R. B., Roitman-Johnson, B., Kanabrocki, E. L., Yager, J. G., Fuerstenberg, R. K., Weatherbee, J. A., et al. (1995) Circadian characteristics of interleukin-6 in blood and urine of clinically healthy men. *In Vivo* **9,** 331–339.

19. Sothern, R. B., Roitman-Johnson, B., Kanabrocki, E. L., Yager, J. G., Roodell, M. M., Weatherbee, J. A., et al. (1995) Circadian characteristics of circulating interleukin-6 in men. *J. Allergy Clin. Immunol.* **95,** 1029–1035.

20. Akbulut, H., Icli, F., Buyukcelik, A., Akbulut, K., and Demirci, S. (1999) The role of granulocyte-macrophage-colony stimulating factor, cortisol, and melatonin in the regulation of the circadian rhythms of peripheral blood cells in healthy volunteers and patients with breast cancer. *J. Pineal Res.* **26,** 1.

21. Lissoni, P., Rovelli, F., Brivio, F., and Fumagalli, L. (1998) Circadian secretions of IL-2, IL-12, IL-6 and IL-10 in relation to the light/dark rhythm of the pineal hormone melatonin in healthy humans. *Nat. Immun.* **16,** 1.

22. Liebmann, P., Reibnegger, G., Lehofer, M., Moser, M., Purstner, P., Mangge, H., et al. (1998) Circadian rhythm of the soluble p75 tumour necrosis factor (sTNF-R75) receptor in humans—a possible explanation for the circadian kinetics of TNF-alpha effects. *Int. Immunol.* **10,** 1393.
23. Lemmer, B., Schwulera, U., Thrun, A., and Lissner, R. (1992) Circadian rhythm of soluble interleukin-2 receptor in healthy individuals. *Eur. Cytokine Netw.* **3,** 335–336.
24. Jones, A. C., Besley, C. R., Warner, J. A., and Warner, J. O. (1994) Variations in serum soluble IL-2 receptor concentration. *Pediatr. Allergy Immunol.* **5,** 230–234.
25. Petrovsky, N., McNair, P., and Harrison, L. C. (1994) Circadian rhythmicity of interferon-gamma production in antigen-stimulated whole blood. *Chronobiologia* **21,** 293–300.
26. Petrovsky, N. and Harrison, L. C. (1997) Diurnal rhythmicity of human cytokine production: a dynamic disequilibrium in T helper cell type 1/T helper cell type 2 balance? *J. Immunol.* **158,** 5163–5168.
27. Mojon, A., Fernandez, J. R., and Hermida, R. C. (1992) Chronolab: an interactive software package for chronobiologic time series analysis written for the Macintosh computer. *Chronobiol. Int.* **9,** 403–412.
28. Angeli, A., Gatti, G., Sartori, M. L., and Masera, R. G. (1992) Chronobiological aspects of the neuroendocrine-immune network. Regulation of human natural killer (NK) cell activity as a model. *Chronobiologia* **19,** 93–110.
29. Kunicka, J. E., Talle, M. A., Denhardt, G. H., Brown, M., Prince, L. A., and Goldstein, G. (1993) Immunosuppression by glucocorticoids: inhibition of production of multiple lymphokines by in vivo administration of dexamethasone. *Cell. Immunol.* **149,** 39–49.
30. Bejarano, M. T., de Waal Malefyt, R., Abrams, J. S., Bigler, M., Bacchetta, R., de Vries, J. E., et al. (1992) Interleukin 10 inhibits allogeneic proliferative and cytotoxic T cell responses generated in primary mixed lymphocyte cultures. *Int. Immunol.* **4,** 1389–1397.
31. Kelso, A. and Munck, A. (1984) Glucocorticoid inhibition of lymphokine secretion by alloreactive T lymphocyte clones. *J. Immunol.* **133,** 784–791.
32. Mukaida, N., Gussella, G. L., Kasahara, T., Ko, Y., Zachariae, C. O., Kawai, T., et al. (1992) Molecular analysis of the inhibition of interleukin-8 production by dexamethasone in a human fibrosarcoma cell line. *Immunology* **75,** 674–679.
33. Ray, A., LaForge, K. S., and Sehgal, P. B. (1990) On the mechanism for efficient repression of the interleukin-6 promoter by glucocorticoids: enhancer, TATA box, and RNA start site (Inr motif) occlusion. *Mol. Cell. Biol.* **10,** 5736–5746.
34. Li, L., Elliott, J. F., and Mosmann, T. R. (1994) IL-10 inhibits cytokine production, vascular leakage, and swelling during T helper 1 cell-induced delayed-type hypersensitivity. *J. Immunol.* **153,** 3967–3978.
35. Harkness, J. A., Richter, M. B., Panayi, G. S., Van de Pette, K., Unger, A., Pownall, R., et al. (1982) Circadian variation in disease activity in rheumatoid arthritis. *Br. Med. J. Clin. Res.* **284,** 551–554.
36. Arvidson, N. G., Gudbjornsson, B., Elfman, L., Ryden, A. C., Totterman, T. H., and Hallgren, R. (1994) Circadian rhythm of serum interleukin-6 in rheumatoid arthritis. *Ann. Rheum. Dis.* **53,** 521–524.

37. Crofford, L. J., Kalogeras, K. T., Mastorakos, G., Magiakou, M. A., Wells, J., Kanik, K. S., et al. (1997) Circadian relationships between interleukin (IL)-6 and hypothalamic-pituitary-adrenal axis hormones: failure of IL-6 to cause sustained hypercortisolism in patients with early untreated rheumatoid arthritis. *J. Clin. Endocrinol. Metab.* **82,** 1279–1283.

38. Jarjour, N. N. and Busse, W. W. (1995) Cytokines in bronchoalveolar lavage fluid of patients with nocturnal asthma. *Am. J. Respir. Crit. Care Med.* **152,** 1474–1477.

39. Morrey, K. M., McLachlan, J. A., Serkin, C. D., and Bakouche, O. (1994) Activation of human monocytes by the pineal hormone melatonin. *J. Immunol.* **153,** 2671–2680.

40. Colombo, L. L., Chen, G. J., Lopez, M. C., and Watson, R. R. (1992) Melatonin induced increase in gamma-interferon production by murine splenocytes. *Immunol. Lett.* **33,** 123–126.

41. Maestroni, G. J., Conti, A., and Pierpaoli, W. (1986) Role of the pineal gland in immunity. Circadian synthesis and release of melatonin modulates the antibody response and antagonizes the immunosuppressive effect of corticosterone *J. Neuroimmunol.* **13,** 19–30.

42. Rook, G. A., Hernandez-Pando, R., and Lightman, S. L. (1994) Hormones, peripherally activated prohormones and regulation of the Th1/Th2 balance. *Immunol. Today* **15,** 301–303.

43. Warwick-Davies, J., Lowrie, D. B., and Cole, P. J. (1995) Growth hormone is a human macrophage activating factor. Priming of human monocytes for enhanced release of H2O2. *J. Immunol.* **154,** 1909–1918.

44. Comsa, J., Leonhardt, H., and Schwarz, J. A. (1975) Influence of the thymus-corticotropin-growth hormone interaction on the rejection of skin allografts in the rat. *Ann. NY Acad. Sci.* **249,** 387–401.

45. Nagy, E., Berczi, I., and Friesen, H. G. (1983) Regulation of immunity in rats by lactogenic and growth hormones. *Acta Endocrinol.* **102,** 351–357.

46. Lissoni, P., Barni, S., Tancini, G., Brivio, F., Tisi, E., Zubelewicz, B., et al. (1994) Role of the pineal gland in the control of macrophage functions and its possible implication in cancer: a study of interactions between tumor necrosis factor-alpha and the pineal hormone melatonin. *J. Biol. Regul. Homeostatic Agents* **8,** 126–129.

47. Lissoni, P., Pittalis, S., Rovelli, F., Zecchini, S., Casati, M., Tremolada, M., et al. (1996) Immunomodulatory properties of a pineal indole hormone other than melatonin, the 5-methoxytryptophol. *J. Biolog. Regul. Homeostatic Agents* **10,** 27–30.

48. Covelli, V., Massari, F., Fallacara, C., Munno, I., Jirillo, E., Savastano, S., et al. (1992) Interleukin-1 beta and beta-endorphin circadian rhythms are inversely related in normal and stress-altered sleep. *Int. J. Neurosci.* **63,** 299–305.

II

ILLUSTRATION OF METHODOLOGIES USING INDIVIDUAL INTERLEUKINS

15

Assaying Interleukin-8

Paul N. Moynagh

1. Introduction

Interleukin-8 (IL-8) is a member of the rapidly expanding chemokine family, which consists of a large number of small (8–10 kDa) secreted proteins with the capacity to act as leukocyte chemoattractants *(1)*. Chemokines are crucial mediators of inflammation as they are able to enhance migration selectively of specific types of leukocytes from blood vessels into damaged and/or infected tissue, where the leukocytes will effect elimination of the infectious agent and healing of any tissue damage. However, inappropriate or chronic triggering of the inflammatory response can lead to excessive infiltration of normal tissue by various types of leukocytes, ultimately culminating in inflammation-based pathologic states *(2,3)*.

Since chemokines are crucial players in regulating leukocyte migration into tissues, there has been much recent research in the area of dysregulated expression of chemokines, in terms of both correlating chemokine levels with onset, progression, and outcome of disease *(4,5)* and resolving the mechansims underlying their expression. IL-8 has been especially subjected to such close scrutiny because of its effectiveness in facilitating migration of neutrophils to inflammatory sites *(6)*. Thus, the assaying of IL-8 has been performed in tissue, plasma, and serum samples from various disease states *(7)* and also in cell culture supernatants from experiments probing the signal transduction pathways utilized by proinflammatory cytokines (e.g., IL-1 and tumor necrosis factor [TNF]) in inducing IL-8 *(8–12)*. The assaying of IL-8 can be performed at a number of levels. It may be measured at the mRNA stages or protein or at the functional level *(13)*. The latter necessitates a bioassay system whereby the sample is measured for its ability to influence the migration of leukocytes in an in vitro cell culture system. However, the major disadvantage of this approach is the difficulty in distinguishing between the different members of the chemokine family.

From: *Methods in Molecular Medicine, vol. 60: Interleukin Protocols*
Edited by: L. A. J. O'Neill and A. Bowie © Humana Press Inc., Totowa, NJ

The recent explosion in identification of new members of the chemokine family has highlighted a redundancy phenomenon, which has been evident in the cytokine family as a whole. The redundant nature of cytokine action is especially true in the chemokine family: Here a number of different chemokines can act as chemoattractants for the same population of leukocytes *(14)*. A number of chemokines share with IL-8 the ability to act as a neutrophil chemoattractant, and thus the bioassay approach does not provide a specific measure of IL-8 in a sample of unknown content. Indeed, it is rare in biologic samples to detect elevation of chemokines restricted to a single member. It is more common to detect increased levels of cocktails of chemokines, since the expression of different chemokines is frequently controlled by common mechanisms *(4)*. The bioassay system may be used in conjunction with blocking anti-IL-8 antibodies to define IL-8 activity in the sample, but this adds considerable expense, especially in high-throughput screening of samples. There is thus a need for more specific assay systems for IL-8. This chapter describes a protocol that achieves specific measurement of IL-8 by measuring IL-8 at the protein level using a sandwich enzyme-linked immunosorbent assay (ELISA) approach (**Fig. 1**).

The use of a sandwich ELISA system to quantitate levels of IL-8 offers the major advantage of specificity but also lends itself to high-throughput screening of samples for IL-8. The system described measures human IL-8 and is based on use of an anti-IL-8 antibody to capture standard IL-8 or IL-8 from serum, plasma, or cell supernatant samples onto 96-well microtiter plates. A detection anti-IL-8 antibody, which has been biotinylated, is added to the captured IL-8. The capture antibody is generally monoclonal in nature, whereas the detection antibody is usually polyclonal, to allow simultaneous recognition of the IL-8 by both antibodies. The amount of detection antibody adsorbed by the captured IL-8 is proportional to the quantity of the latter in the original sample or standard. The amount of detected antibody is in turn measured by addition of steptavidin-conjugated horseradish peroxidase and subsequently a peroxidase substrate. The latter is acted on by peroxidase and converted into a colored product that can be measured spectrophotometrically. The optical density is thus a measure of the original concentration of IL-8. A standard curve is constructed relating standard IL-8 concentration to optical density; this can be used to compute levels of IL-8 in unknown samples.

The IL-8 standard is a recombinant form, which minimizes expense. The capture and detection antibodies have become available from many commercial companies in recent years as matched antibody pairs. Previously, companies offered only ELISA kits, with all necessary components included, for measuring IL-8. Indeed, such kits are still available today, but the cost may be an order of magnitude higher than that incurred with the purchase of matched antibody pairs and the development of ones own ELISA system.

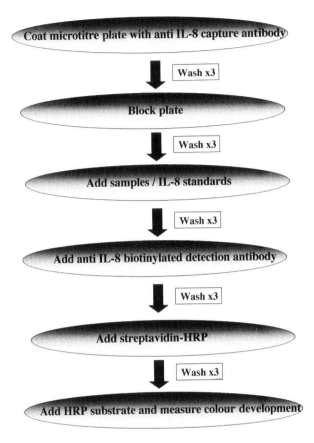

Fig. 1. Flowchart summary of sandwich ELISA for IL-8.

2. Materials

1. DuoSet^R ELISA Development System (human IL-8; R&D Systems Europe, Oxon, UK). This system contains mouse anti-human IL-8 (capture antibody), biotinylated goat anti-human IL-8 (detection antibody), standard recombinant human IL-8, and streptavidin conjugated to horseradish peroxidase.
2. Phosphate-buffered saline (PBS), pH 7.4: Dissolve 80 g NaCl, 2.0 g KCl, 11.5 g Na_2HPO_4, and 2.0 g KH_2PO_4 in 900 mL distilled water. Adjust pH to 7.4 with 1 *M* NaOH if necessary. Make volume up to 1 L with distilled water. Store at room temperature. Dilute 1 in 10 with distilled water for use.
3. PBS, pH 7.4, containing 0.05% (v/v) Tween-20 (wash buffer).
4. PBS, pH 7.4, containing 1% (w/v) bovine serum albumin (BSA) and 5% (w/v) sucrose (block buffer).
5. Dulbecco's modified Eagle's medium (DMEM; *see* **Note 1**).
6. 0.11 *M* Sodium acetate buffer, pH 5.5.

7. Tetramethylbenzidine (TMB; 6 mg/mL in DMSO; *see* **Note 2**; Sigma, Poole, UK).
8. 3% (v/v) Hydrogen peroxide (Sigma).
9. 2 *N* H_2SO_4.
10. ELISA grade microtiter plates (Maxisorp, Nunc, Life Technologies).

3. Methods

The method described here is based predominantly on the suggested protocol that accompanies the DuoSet ELISA Development System. Some differences in detail are included, and the notes also include potential problems and advice on useful modifications to the overall protocol. The protocol described below is used routinely in the author's laboratory to measure production of IL-8 by various primary human cells and cell lines **(Fig. 2)**, which are generally grown in DMEM containing 10% fetal calf serum (FCS).

1. Coat the 96-well microtiter plate with 100 µL of mouse anti-human IL-8 (4 µg/mL in PBS, pH 7.4; *see* **Note 3**), and incubate overnight at room temperature.
2. Aspirate each well and wash three times with 300 µL of wash buffer using a multichannel pipettor (*see* **Note 4**). After the addition of each round of wash buffer ensure that all contents are removed from the wells by forcibly inverting the plate onto clean paper toweling.
3. Add 300 µL of block buffer to each well and incubate at room temperature for 2 h.
4. Decant the block buffer and wash as described in **step 2**.
5. Add 100 µL of cell culture supernatants, diluted in DMEM (*see* **Notes 1** and **5**) or standard recombinant human IL-8 (0–2000 pg/mL; *see* **Note 6**) to wells and incubate for 1 h at room temperature.
6. Decant the samples or standards and wash as described in **step 2**.
7. Add 100 µL of biotinylated goat anti-human IL-8 (20 ng/mL in DMEM), and incubate for 1 h at room temperature.
8. Decant the detection antibody and wash as described in **step 2**.
9. Add 100 µL of working dilution (specified on vial) of streptavidin conjugated to horseradish-peroxidase in DMEM, and incubate for 20 min in the dark at room temperature.
10. Decant the contents of the wells and wash as described in **step 2**.
11. Add 100 µL of freshly prepared substrate solution to each well (For each 96-well microtiter plate, substrate solution is prepared by mixing 10 mL 0.11 *M* sodium acetate buffer, pH 5.5, 167 µL TMB [6 mg/mL in DMSO] and 10 µL of 3% [v/v] hydrogen peroxide). Incubate with substrate solution for 20 min in the dark at room temperature.
12. Add 50 µL of 2 *N* H_2SO_4 to each well to terminate reaction.
13. Read the optical density of each well on a spectophotometric microtiter plate reader set to 450 nm, with a reference wavelength of 570 nm to correct for optical imperfections in the plate. Use the average readings of the zero standard to blank the plate reader.
14. Average the replicate readings for each standard, plot the mean absorbance for the standards on the *y*-axis against the mean concentration of the standards on

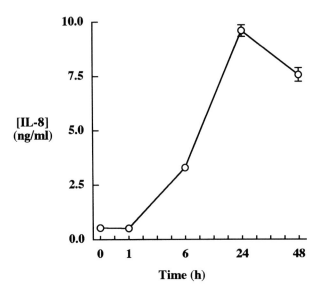

Fig. 2. Time-dependent induction of IL-8 in 1321N1 astrocytoma by IL-1β (10 ng/mL) as determined by IL-8 sandwich ELISA.

the *x*-axis, and construct the best-fit line curve through the points. The data can be linearized by using log-log paper and subjecting the log transformation to regression analysis.

15. Locate the absorbance reading of each sample on the *y*-axis, and extend a horizontal line to intersect the standard curve. Drop a perpendicular line from the point of intersection to the *x*-axis to define the corresponding concentration of IL-8. Multiply the concentration by any dilution factor applied in **step 5**.

4. Notes

1. In the present protocol, cell culture supernatants are diluted in DMEM because the supernatants are derived from cells that had been cultured in this medium. In the case of serum samples, dilutions may be performed using control serum. However, this may give rise to high background readings since human serum may contain endogenous levels of IL-8. An alternative diluent in the latter case is DMEM or 20 m*M* Tris, pH 7.3, containing 150 m*M* NaCl, 0.1% (w/v) BSA, and 0.05% (v/v) Tween-20 (recommended by the manufacturers of the DuoSet ELISA Development System).
2. The solution of TMB (in DMSO) should be stored for no longer than 2 wk. From experience the use of TMB beyond this storage period results in a dramatic decrease in the sensitivity of the assay.
3. The working concentrations of the capture and detection antibodies may be decreased, thus minimizing considerably the expense of the assay. This results in an assay of reduced sensitivity. However, the latter is not a problem if samples

contain sufficiently high concentrations of IL-8 to necessitate initial dilution. The reduced sensitivity can be compensated for by decreasing the dilution factor of the samples. The author has found that in routine cell culture experiments, the working concentrations of the capture and detection antibodies can be reduced fivefold and still form the basis of an assay of sufficient sensitivity.

4. The washing of wells in the present protocol is performed by a multichannel pipettor, but a squirt bottle or autoplate washer may also be used. Irrespective of the method employed, it is recommended to avoid cross-well contamination during washing especially in the wash step immediately after addition of samples and standards.

5. The standard curve will plateau at the higher concentrations of standard. Always dilute samples to achieve absorbance readings in the linear region of the standard graph.

6. In constructing a standard curve, use a range of concentrations of standards to encompass the absorbance range 0–0.8. This ensures that microtiter plate readers are working within their linear range. However, most of the recent generation of readers guarantee linearity considerably beyond this range.

References

1. Horuk, R. (1994) Molecular properties of the chemokine receptor family. *Trends Pharmacol. Sci.* **15**, 159–165.
2. Strieter, R. M., Standiford, T. J., Huffnagle, G. B., Colletti, L. M., Lukacs, N. W., and Kunkel, S. L. (1996) "The good, the bad, and the ugly." The role of chemokines in models of human disease. *J. Immunol.* **156**, 3583–3586.
3. Wenzel, U. O. and Stahl, R. A. (1999) Chemokines, renal disease, and HIV infection. *Nephron* **81**, 5–16.
4. Ranshoff, R. M. (1997) Chemokines in neurological disease models: correlation between chemokine expression patterns and inflammatory pathology. *J. Leukoc. Biol.* **62**, 645–652.
5. Yokoyama, H., Wada, T., Furuichi, K., Segawa, C., Shimizu, M., Kobayashi, K., et al. (1998) Urinary levels of chemokines (MCAF/MCP-1, IL-8) reflect distinct disease activities and phases of human IgA nephropathy. *J. Leukoc. Biol.* **63**, 493–499.
6. Mukaida, N., Harada, A., and Matsushima, K. (1998) Interleukin-8 (IL-8) and monocyte chemotactic and activating factor (MCAF/MCP-1), chemokines essentially involved in inflammatory and immune reactions. *Cytokine Growth Factor Rev.* **9**, 9–23.
7. Mitsuyama, K., Toyonaga, A., Sasaki, E., Watanabe, K., Tateishi, H., Nishiyama, T., et al. (1994) IL-8 as an important chemoattractant for neutrophils in ulcerative colitis and Crohn's disease. *Clin. Exp. Immunol.* **96**, 432–436.
8. Kasahara, T., Mukaida, N., Yamashita, K., Yagisawa, H., Akahoshi, T., and Matsushima, K. (1991) IL-1 and TNF-alpha induction of IL-8 and monocyte chemotactic and activating factor (MCAF) mRNA expression in a human astrocytoma cell line. *Immunology* **74**, 60–67.

9. Duque, N., Gomez-Guerrero, C., and Egido, J. (1997) Interactions of IgA with Fc alpha receptors of human mesangial cells activates transcription factor nuclear factor-kappa B and induces expression and synthesis of monocyte chemoattractant protein-1, IL-8, and IFN-inducible protein 10. *J. Immunol.* **159,** 3474–3482.

10. Pang, L. and Knox, A. J. (1998) Bradykinin stimulates IL-8 production in cultured human airway smooth muscle cells: role of cyclooxygenase products. *J. Immunol.* **161,** 2509–2515.

11. Krause, A., Holtmann, H., Eickemeier, S., Winzen, R., Szamel, M., Resch, K., et al. (1998) Stress-activated protein kinase/Jun N-terminal kinase is required for interleukin (IL)-1-induced IL-6 and IL-8 gene expression in the human epidermal carcinoma cell line KB. *J. Biol. Chem.* **273,** 23,681–23,689.

12. Bourke, E. and Moynagh, P. N. (1999) Anti-inflammatory effects of glucocorticoids in brain cells, Independent of NFκB. *J. Immunol.* **163,** 2113–2119.

13. Aloisi, F., Care, A., Borsellino, G., Gallo, P., Rosa, S., Bassani, A., et al. (1992) Production of hemolymphopoietic cytokines (IL-6, IL-8, colony-stimulating factors) by normal human astrocytes in response to IL-1 beta and tumor necrosis factor-alpha. *J. Immunol.* **149,** 2358–2366.

14. Power, C. A. and Wells, T. N. C. (1996) Cloning and characterization of human chemokine receptors. *Trends Pharmacol. Sci.* **17,** 209–213.

16

Measurement of Interleukin-2 by Bioassay

Lyanne Weston

1. Introduction

Bioassays are used to determine the presence and concentration of biologically active cytokines by exploiting the different activities they induce, such as cellular proliferation, chemotaxis, or cytotoxicity. These assays often use established cell lines that depend for their continued growth and survival on the presence of particular cytokine(s). The detection of the cytokine may be made directly using the cell line of choice or via a second cell line that is directly dependent on the activities or properties of the first cell line. These assays are called conversion assays. Bioassays remain a simple and relatively inexpensive method for cytokine quantification; they require no specialized equipment, and, in comparison with enzyme-linked immunosorbent assay (ELISA) methods, they are relatively easy to set up in a cell culture laboratory.

Interleukin 2 (IL-2), first described in 1976 by Morgan et al. (1) is, produced mainly by CD4 T cells following activation by mitogens or alloantigens. It is a growth factor for all subpopulations of T-lymphocytes and, in the presence of other growth factors, promotes the proliferation of activated B cells (2). A number of conditions have been associated with aberrant IL-2 expression including Hodgkin's disease, numerous autoimmune diseases, graft-vs-host disease, and the rejection of solid organ grafts after transplantation. Vie and Miller (3) estimated that after 3 d in culture, the IL-2 produced by one effector cell ranged from 0.54 to 2.42 pg (approx 3 IU). To achieve a high degree of sensitivity, a bioassay using the IL-2-dependent murine cell line (CTLL-2) is commonly used. A tumor-specific cytotoxic T-cell line, it was originally derived from C57/Bl/6 inbred mice and is capable of long-term growth in medium conditioned with the supernatant from Concanavalin-A-activated splenocyte cultures (4). IL-2 was later identified as the factor responsible for the growth of CTLL-2.

From: *Methods in Molecular Medicine, vol. 60: Interleukin Protocols*
Edited by: L. A. J. O'Neill and A. Bowie © Humana Press Inc., Totowa, NJ

The presence of IL-2 is usually assessed by measuring the incorporation of tritiated thymidine into the DNA of proliferating CTLL-2 cells *(5)*. Proliferation may also be determined using the quantitative 3-(4,5-dimethylthiazol-2-yl)-2,5-diphenyltetrazolium bromide (MTT) colorimetric assay *(6)*. The yellow tetrazolium salt is metabolized by the mitochondrial succinic dehydrogenase activity of proliferating cells to produce a purple reaction product, formazan. This assay measures the number and activity of living cells, whereas the former reflects the incorporation of radioactivity into cellular DNA. The disadvantages associated with each assay are the aqueous insolubility of the formazan end product for the MTT assay on the one hand, and the disposal of radioactive waste for the tritiated thymidine incorporation assay on the other.

2. Materials
2.1. CTLL-2 Cell Line

1. This IL-2-dependent murine cell line is responsive to both murine and human IL-2 and murine IL-4. Highly sensitive, with exacting growth requirements, it is available from the major cell line repositories of Europe (ECACC) and the United States (ATCC) (*see* **Notes 1** and **2**).

2.2. Culture Medium

1. RPMI-1640 buffered with sodium hydrogen carbonate and HEPES. This medium can be stored at 4°C for 2 mo.
2. Immediately prior to use, the medium is supplemented with 20 IU/mL penicillin, 20 µg/mL streptomycin, 20 mM L-glutamine, and 10^{-5} M 2-mercaptoethanol. Supplemented media may be stored at 4°C for 2 wk (*see* **Note 3**).
3. When setting up an assay, the culture medium should be at room temperature.

2.2.1. Culture Medium for CTLL-2

1. For the maintenance of the CTLL-2 cell line, the culture medium must be additionally supplemented with 10 IU human recombinant IL-2 (rhIL-2) per mL and 15% heat-inactivated fetal calf serum (FCS) (*see* **Note 4**).
2. Assessment of cell line performance can be made using a dose-response assay (*see* **Fig. 1** and **Subheading 3.2.**).

2.2.2. Culture Medium for Human IL-2 Assay

1. The basic medium (*see* **Subheading 2.2.**) is supplemented with 20 IU/mL penicillin, 20 µg/mL streptomycin, 20 mM L-glutamine, and 10^{-5} M 2-mercaptoethanol. To this, 7.5% heat-inactivated pooled human serum is added (*see* **Notes 5** and **6**).

3. Methods
3.1. Culturing CTLL-2

1. CTLL-2, cultured in 75-cm^2 flasks, are subcultured every 3 d with fresh culture medium containing rIL-2. CTLL-2 cell numbers must never exceed 1×10^5 cells/mL. Prior to use in a bioassay, CTLL-2 are deprived of IL-2 for 3 d.

2. Cells are spun at 200g for 10 min, the supernatant is discarded, the pellet resuspended, and the tube is topped up with the culture media (described in **Subheading 2.2.**).
3. Cells are spun again at 200g for 10 min.
4. Cells are counted, adjusted to a concentration of 1×10^5 cells/mL in culture medium, and must be used immediately.

3.1.1. Cryopreservation of CTLL-2 Cells

1. CTLL-2 cells must be cryopreserved on the morning of the third day after subculturing (*see* **Note 7**).
2. A comparison of the effects of freezing on the performance of the CTLL-2 cells can be seen in **Fig. 2**.
3. CTLL-2 cells are pooled and spun as per **Subheading 3.1.**, **steps 2** and **3**.
4. The supernatant is discarded and the pellet resuspended in the culture medium described in **Subheading 2.2.**, supplemented with 15% FCS.
5. Cells are adjusted to a volume appropriate for freezing. The number of CTLL-2 cells required for assay purposes will dictate this volume. In general, 5×10^6 cells would be adequate for most assay needs.
6. Freezing medium (15% FCS supplemented with 20% DMSO) is prepared and cooled to 4°C. CTLL-2 cells, in the desired volume, are cooled to 4°C. Cryoamps are labeled and cooled. In an ice bath, freezing medium is added dropwise to the cell suspension in a 1:1 ratio with constant mixing. A 1-mL vol is dispensed into the cooled amps. The amps are frozen in a controlled rate freezer and stored in liquid nitrogen until required for assay use (*see* **Note 8**).
7. Cryopreserved cells are assessed in dose-response assays before and after freezing. Batches capable of detecting 0.01 IU of IL-2 are retained for future use (*see* **Note 9**).

3.1.2. Thawing of CTLL-2 Cells

1. CTLL-2 cells are thawed at 42°C, and 20% FCS in culture medium (*see* **Subheading 2.2.**) without IL-2 must be added dropwise for the initial 10 mL and then topped up to 50 mL and centrifuged at 200g for 10 min.
2. The supernatant is discarded, the pellet is resuspended, and the tube is topped up with culture medium (without serum or IL-2 supplements). The cells are spun again as above.
3. After this final spin, cells are resuspended in culture medium, counted, adjusted to a concentration of 1×10^5 cells/mL, and used immediately.

3.2. Dose-Response Assay

1. In a 96-well U-bottomed sterile microtiter tray, 100 µL of culture medium (*see* **Subheading 2.2.**) is dispensed into each well. Ten serial twofold dilutions of culture medium containing IL-2 are made, the resulting concentration ranging from 10 to 0.009 IU/mL of IL-2, using 12 replicates for each dilution.
2. To calculate the cutoff for the assay, 12 replicates of 100 µL of background media (culture media without IL-2) are used.

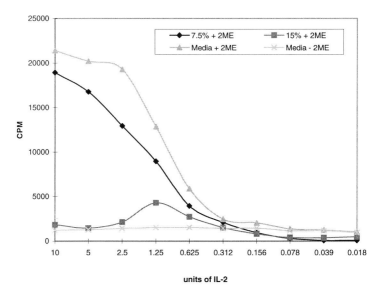

Fig. 1. Dose response curves in different media. Tritiated thymidine incorporation (CPM), plotted on the *y*-axis, against doubling dilutions of recombinant human IL-2 plotted on the *x*-axis. CTLL-2 cells were cultured in four different media. For an assay requiring the culturing of human cells, culture medium supplemented with 2ME and 7.5% heat-inactivated pooled human serum (♦) is the optimal choice compared with culture medium supplemented with 15% pooled human serum and 2ME (■), which is toxic for CTLL-2 cells. Optimal CTLL-2 growth is in culture medium supplemented with 15% heat-inactivated FCS and 2ME (▲). This dose response demonstrates the necessity of 2ME since culture medium supplemented with 15% heat-inactivated FCS without 2ME (✕) gave no response. The use of 7.5% heat-inactivated pooled human serum satisfies all assay cell growth requirements.

3. The CTLL-2 cells are thawed (as per **Subheading 3.1.2.**), and 10 μL is added to each well.
4. Trays are incubated for 4 h. At the end of this time each well is labeled with 1 μCi of tritiated thymidine and incubated for a further 16 h. Proliferation of the CTLL-2 cells is measured by the incorporation of tritiated thymidine and represented on the graphs as counts per minute (cpm).
5. The mean cpm plus 3 standard deviations of the 12 replicates of background media (**step 2**) is used to calculate the cutoff for the assay. Any counts above this point are considered positive for IL-2 detection.

3.3. Limiting Dilution Analysis

To assess the IL-2 produced by human effector T cells, the IL-2 bioassay can be used in combination with a limiting dilution analysis (LDA). Effector cell IL-2 production may be in response to mitogenic or specific allogenic stimulation.

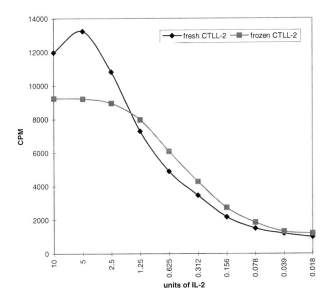

Fig. 2. Dose-response using fresh or frozen CTLL-2. Dose-response curves plotting tritiated thymidine incorporation (CPM) against recombinant human IL-2 concentration. The graph compares CTLL-2 cells that have been cultured, washed, and prepared prior to cryopreservation (◆) with CTLL2 cells after cryopreservation (■).

1. Prepared peripheral blood mononuclear cells (PBMCs) are washed, counted, and diluted in culture medium supplemented with 7.5% heat-inactivated human serum, to a concentration of 1×10^6 cells/mL.
2. Seven serial twofold dilutions are made with 24 replicates at each dilution. PBMCs (50 µL) are added to each well of a 96-well U-bottomed plate (*see* **Note 10**). The highest concentration of effector cells in the first row being 50,000 cells/well, by the eighth row this concentration is approx 390 responding cells/well.
3. The stimulators, kept at one concentration, are dispensed into each well. In the case of cells responding to alloantigen, the stimulating cells are irradiated to prevent them from contributing to the IL-2 produced by the effector cells (*see* **Note 11**). Allostimulators are γ-irradiated (25 grays), and 50 µL (50,000 cells) is added to all wells.
4. To establish the cutoff point for each assay, 24 wells containing background medium and 50 µL of allostimulators from **step 3** are used.
5. Trays are incubated at 37°C in a humidified 5% CO_2 atmosphere for 72 h.
6. All trays are γ-irradiated to prevent further production or consumption of IL-2, and CTLL-2 cells are added as per **Subheading 3.2.**, **steps 3** and **4**. (*see* **Note 12**).
7. A well is scored positive if the cpm are greater than the mean plus 3 standard deviations of the control (**step 4**), and the frequency of donor IL-2-producing effector cells is determined using maximum likelihood estimation (*see* **Note 13**).

4. Notes

1. Regular monitoring to avoid overcrowding and thus depletion of nutrients is necessary; otherwise this cell line can inexplicably lose sensitivity or die. Normally grown in continuous culture, the cells are denied IL-2 for 3 d prior to their use in an assay. Overcrowding of CTLL-2 cells in culture is a major obstacle, which can be avoided by daily monitoring of the cells. If the cells appear to be confluent, then additional media without IL-2 may be added to each flask. When farming large quantities of CTLL-2 cells, careful adherence to asceptic technique is essential. An infected cell line can introduce an additional variable and has a questionable ability to detect IL-2. When CTLL-2 cells are inspected macroscopically using phase contrast microscopy, viable cells should have an intact membrane and appear to be surrounded by a halo of light.

2. In our experience, a major drawback to this bioassay is the variable sensitivity of the indicator cell line. To minimize the day-to-day variability seen with what is normally a continuously cultured cell line, large batches of CTLL-2 are prepared and then frozen. Only batches that satisfy a set criterion of sensitivity are used in subsequent assays.

3. The inclusion of 2-mercaptoethanol (2ME) is fundamental to the growth and survival of CTLL2. **Figure 1** demonstrates the effect on the dose-response of CTLL-2 cells when 2ME is not included in the culture medium.

4. A suitable batch of FCS should be chosen, not only on the basis of response of the CTLL-2 in dose-response assays but also for each batch's ability to satisfy the growth requirements of the cell line while in culture. Some batches of FCS are more suited to CTLL-2 growth than others, and suppliers will provide small sample quantities for batch assessment. Having selected a suitable batch, FCS can be stored for long periods at –80°C. When required, a 500-mL vol is thawed, and aliquots are heat inactivated at 56°C for 30 min. Heat-inactivated FCS can be stored at –20°C for up to 6 mo.

5. Human serum, to supplement culture medium for assay use, is pooled from nontransfused male donors that have been tested for the absence of HLA antibodies and for ability to support cell growth. An additional screening process is to assess the performance of CTLL-2 cells in a dose-response assay in culture medium supplemented with various batches of human serum. Additionally, the concentration of human serum must be considered, as it must be capable of supporting human cell growth and proliferation.

6. The most suitable dilution of human serum can be determined by performing assays such as an LDA or mixed lymphocyte reaction (MLR) (7). Evaluation of the most appropriate concentration of serum must take into account the needs of both the CTLL-2 cells and the human cells.

7. Our experience working with continuously cultured CTLL-2 has shown that variable sensitivity of the indicator cell line is a drawback of this assay (**Fig. 3**). Even with regular monitoring to avoid overcrowding, which leads to the depletion of nutrients, this cell line can inexplicably lose sensitivity. To minimize the day-to-day variability, large batches of CTLL-2 were prepared and then cryopreserved.

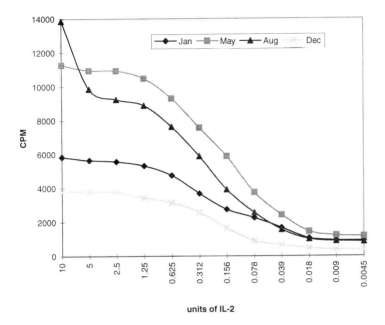

Fig. 3. Dose-response of continuously cultured CTLL-2. A dose-response assay is a useful means of assessing the sensitivity and monitoring the growth of the continuously cultured CTLL-2 cell line. This figure demonstrates the variance seen over an 8-mo period.

8. When there is a plentiful supply of frozen CTLL-2 cells capable of detecting low levels of IL-2, then seed aliquots of the cell line should be frozen and stored for later reactivation. These seed aliquots should be frozen as described; however, IL-2 should be included in the media.

9. The reproducibility of cryopreserved CTLL-2 cells is very important for use in a routine assay as it minimizes interassay variation. The four dose-response curves in **Fig. 4** were determined on different occasions over a 4-mo period using the same batch of frozen CTLL-2 cells. These results demonstrate that there is a remarkable similarity in the performance and sensitivity of these cryopreserved indicator cells.

10. Effector cells used for IL-2 determination may be PBMCs, sorted T cells, or a cell line of interest. The example used here was developed for PBMCs responding to alloantigen.

11. Stimulation may be induced by alloantigen, antigen, mitogen, viral peptides, tetramers, or any agent suspected of inducing the production of IL-2 in the effector cells.

12. The plentiful supply of sensitive indicator cells represents a significant advance in the reliability of this bioassay.

13. The work presented here demonstrates the basic requirements for an IL-2 bioassay. The procedure followed could be applied satisfactorily to other bioassay systems.

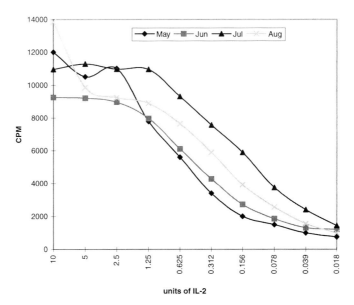

Fig. 4. Reproducibility of cryopreserved CTLL-2 cells. To minimize day-to-day variability, large batches of CTLL-2 are prepared and then cryopreserved. The four dose-response curves represented here were performed using samples of CTLL-2 cryopreserved from the same large batch. There is a remarkable similarity in the performance of these cryopreserved indicator cells. The plentiful supply of indicator cells of a known sensitivity represents a significant advance in the reliability of this bioassay.

References

1. Morgan, D. A., Rucsetti, F. W., and Gallo, R. C. (1976) Selective *in vitro* growth of T lymphocytes from normal human bone marrow. *Science* **193,** 1007–1008.
2. Gillis, S., Mochizuki, D. Y., Conlon, P. J., Hefeneider, S. H., Ramthun, C. A., Gillis, A. E., et al. (1982) Molecular characterization of interleukin 2 *Immunol. Rev.* **63,** 167–209.
3. Vie, H. and Miller, R. A. (1986) Estimation by limiting dilution analysis of human IL 2-secreting T cells: detection of IL 2 produced by single lymphokine-secreting T cells *J. Immunol.* **136,** 3292–3297.
4. Gillis, S. and Smith, K. (1977) Long term culture of tumor-specific cytotoxic T cell lines. *Nature* **268,** 154–156.
5. Weston, L., Geczy, A., and Farrell, C. (1998) A convenient and reliable IL-2 bioassay using frozen CTLL-2 to improve the detection of helper T lymphocyte precursors. *Immunol. Cell Biol.* **76,** 190–192.
6. Mosmann, T. (1983) Rapid colorimetric assay for cellular growth and survival: application to proliferation and cytotoxicity assays. *J. Immunol. Methods* **65,** 55–63.
7. Sprent, J. (1992) Mixed lymphocyte reaction, in *Encyclopedia of Immunology* (Roitt, I. M. and Delves, P. J., eds.), Academic, NY, pp. 1079–1082.

17

Assaying Interleukin-15

Amos Douvdevani, Michal Weiler, and Eli Lewis

1. Introduction

Interleukin 15 (IL-15) has been described as a cytokine with biologic functions similar to those of IL-2. IL-2 and IL-15 utilize a receptor composed of three subunits: IL-2 receptor β-chain, the γ- chain (γc) shared by IL-15, IL-2, IL-4, IL-7, and IL-9 receptors, and a unique α-chain. The α-chain of the IL-15 receptor (IL-15Rα) and IL-2Rα share a fragmentary sequence homology and structural similarities, and both proteins contain a conserved "sushi domain" binding motif. IL-15 is a potent T-cell activator that induces the effector function of cytotoxic T cells and lymphokine-activated killer cells. IL-15, like IL-2, stimulates the proliferation of activated CD4, CD8, B cells, and natural killer (NK) cells (1).

IL-15 mRNA has been demonstrated to be present in placenta, skeletal muscle, kidney, lung, heart, keratinocytes, macrophages, Langerhans cells, dendritic cells, astrocytes, microglia cells, endothelial cells, and intestinal epithelial cells. In contrast to IL-2, IL-15 is not produced by T-lymphocytes (2,3).

Although IL-15 mRNA is abundant in many tissues, it is not obvious that cells expressing IL-15 mRNA are also expressing the protein. This is because of the tight posttranscriptional regulation of IL-15 expression. IL-15 mRNA is not efficiently translated because of abundant AUG codons in the 5' UTR of IL-15 mRNA that attenuate translation. Transcripts that do get translated to protein are not efficiently secreted because of an unusually long leader peptide (4). Thus, IL-15 seems to exist in mRNA inactive pools and in intracellular protein stores.

Because of its complex regulation we suggest that IL-15 expression be analyzed at both mRNA and protein levels, and we also propose to demonstrate its biologic activity. In this chapter we describe three methods that we currently use for assaying IL-15: reverse transcriptase polymerase chain reaction (RT-PCR) for mRNA levels, enzyme-linked immunoabsorbent assay (ELISA) for IL-15 protein, and a bioassay based on the proliferation of a T-cell line (CTLD) (5).

From: *Methods in Molecular Medicine, vol. 60: Interleukin Protocols*
Edited by: L. A. J. O'Neill and A. Bowie © Humana Press Inc., Totowa, NJ

1.1. Human IL-15 mRNA Analysis by RT-PCR

We found RT-PCR to be a good method for analysis of IL-15 mRNA levels. We used this method on various types of cells and tissues with satisfactory results. The major advantages are the requirement of low amounts of RNA, the simplicity of the procedure, and its rapidity. However, one should take into account that this method is only partially quantitative, and only notable changes in RNA levels (about twofold) could be detected by the basic protocol we describe.

In this procedure, RNA is extracted from cells and then reverse transcribed to complimentary DNA (cDNA). The cDNA is a "mirror" replicate of the mRNA from which it was produced; the number of a specific transcript, such as IL-15, is kept in cDNA form and can serve as a template for PCR amplification. PCR amplification specifically increases the levels of a specific DNA sequence and allows, in most cases, its detection by simple DNA staining, without the need for radioactive material.

Under optimal conditions the level of RT-PCR products from one sample can be compared with other samples and thus can give an indication of the relative levels of a specific mRNA. β-actin mRNA levels are usually highly expressed and are less affected by various treatments than other mRNA species. β-actin is therefore commonly used as an internal standard for the amount and quality of mRNA samples.

The sensitivity of RT-PCR enables the analysis of small samples, such as primary cultures of 1×10^5 kidney tubular epithelial cells. For this assay we usually grow our cells and perform the experiments in 24-well plates. RNA analysis for each treatment should be performed in triplicate. If experiments are performed on primary cultures, experiments should be repeated on cells prepared from different donors.

Basically, the RT-PCR procedure can be divided into four steps: (a) RNA extraction, (b) reverse transcription, (c) PCR amplification, and (d) analysis of PCR products (*see* **Note 1**).

1.2. ELISA of Human IL-15 Protein

This assay employs the quantitative sandwich enzyme immunoassay technique. First, 96-well plates are coated with a monoclonal antibody specific for IL-15. Standards and samples are pipetted into the wells, and the immobilized antibody binds any IL-15 present. After washing away any unbound substances, a second biotinylated antibody specific for IL-15 is added to the wells; then streptavidin conjugated to horseradish peroxidase (HRP) is added and binds to the biotinylated antibody. A chromogenic HRP substrate solution is added to give color with intensity that correlates to the amount of IL-15 bound in the first step. The reaction is stopped by administration of acid, and the intensity of the color is measured by an ELISA reader. The assay can detect IL-15 levels as low as 10 pg/mL (*see* **Note 2**).

1.3. Assessment of Human IL-15 Biologic Activity

Of the multiple biologic activities that IL-15 exhibits, the activity that is being assessed in this chapter is the proliferative response of an IL-2-dependent murine T-cell line, namely, CTLD *(5)*. The proliferative effect attributed to IL-15 may be examined in a variety of samples, such as an accumulated cell culture supernatant or cell culture lysate, purified protein, and various body fluids such as serum (*see* **Note 3**). The assay employs a 96-well plate in which CTLDs are evenly applied over the tested samples and over a standard solution of increasing concentrations of recombinant human IL-15 (rhIL-15). The proliferative response occurs for a period of 48–72 h. The cell population is then quantified by XTT, a tetrazolium salt, which is modified by a mitochondrial reaction to a soluble red salt *(6)*. Using this nonradioactive bioassay it is possible to detect as low as 30 pg/mL of rhIL-15. Since the tested biologic fluid may contain factors other than IL-15, it is essential to determine the specific contribution of IL-15 to the proliferative response by blocking its activity with a specific antibody.

2. Materials
2.1. RT-PCR for IL-15 mRNA
2.1.1. Total RNA Extraction

1. RNeasy Mini Kit (cat. no. 74104; Qiagen, Hilden, Germany). This kit contains affinity columns and reagents for 50 RNA preparations (*see* **Note 4**). The kit includes RLT, RW1, and RPE buffers, RNase-free water, minicolumns, and 1.5- and 2-mL collecting tubes.
2. β-Mercaptoethanol (β-ME, Sigma). For safety, open in fume hood.
3. Ethanol (analytic grade).

2.1.2. cDNA Preparation

1. Moloney murine leukemia virus-reverse transcriptase (MMLV-RT, 200 U/μL; Gibco BRL, Gaithersburg, MD).
2. 5X Reverse transcriptase buffer (supplied with the MMLV-RT enzyme).
3. Dithiothreitol (DTT, 0.1 *M*; Gibco BRL, supplied with the MMLV-RT enzyme).
4. RNase-free water (Sigma).
5. RNase inhibitor (40 U/μL, Roche, Molecular Biochemicals).
6. Oligo-d(T) 15-mer (8 nmol; Roche). Reconstitute the lyophilized content of the vial with 200 μL of RNase-free water to obtain a solution of 40 pmol/μL.
7. dNTP mix (10 m*M* of each nucleotide; Sigma).

All reagents except water should be stored at –20°C.

2.1.3. PCR

1. β-actin primers (expected product size 237 bp):
   Sense primer   5'-GGGTCAGAAGGATTCCTATG-3'.
   Antisense primer   5'-GGTCTCAAACATGATCTGGG-3'.

2. IL-15 primers (expected product size 290 bp):
   Sense primer   5'-CCATAGCCAGCTCTTCTTC -3'.
   Antisense primer 5'-GGTGAACATCACTTTCCG-3'.
   The primers should be reconstituted in water and stored in small aliquots.
3. dNTP mix (10 mM of each nucleotide; Sigma).
4. *Taq* DNA polymerase (5 U/µL, available from Sigma or other sources).
5. 10X reaction buffer (usually supplied with the *Taq* polymerase).
   All reagents listed above should be stored at –20°C.
6. 0.6-mL PCR microtubes.
7. Light mineral oil (needed only if the thermal cycler is not equipped with a heated cover).
8. DNA programmable thermal cycler.
9. DNA horizontal mini-gel electrophoresis apparatus.
10. Standard reagents and apparatus for DNA gel electrophoresis (agarose, buffer TBE, ethidium bromide, loading buffer, 100-bp ladder, horizontal mini-gel system, and power supply).
11. Video imaging system and densitometry software.

2.2. ELISA for IL-15 Protein

1. 96-well polystyrene microtiter plate (MA #25920; Corning Costar, Cambridge, MA).
2. Tween-20 (ICN, Costa Mesa, CA).
3. NP-40 (Calbiochem, La Jolla, CA).
4. Bovine serum albumin (BSA).
5. Sodium azide (NaN$_3$; Sigma). **Caution:** Sodium azide is a dangerous poison.
6. Sucrose (Sigma).
7. Phosphate-buffered saline (PBS).
8. Trizma base (Sigma).
9. NaCl (Sigma).
10. Coating antibody, monoclonal anti-human IL-15 antibody type MAB647 (R&D Systems, Minneapolis, MN). Store at –20°C.
11. Second antibody, biotinylated monoclonal anti-human IL-15 antibody type BAM247 (R&D Systems). Store at –20°C.
12. Recombinant human IL-15 (R&D Systems). Store at –20°C.
13. Streptavidin HRP (type 43-4323; Zymed, San Francisco, CA). Store at 4°C.
14. Chromogen substrate: TMBSingle Solution (Zymed). Store at 4°C.
15. Stop solution: H$_2$SO$_4$ (1 N).
16. Multichannel pipet, squirt bottle, manifold dispenser, or automated microtiter plate washer.
17. Microtiter plate reader capable of measuring absorbance at 450 nm, with correction wavelength set at 540 or 570 nm.

2.3. IL-15 Biologic Activity

1. Tissue culture facilities (sterile hood, CO$_2$ incubator).
2. Microtiter plate reader capable of measuring absorbance at 450–500 nm, with correction wavelength set at 630–690 nm.

3. PBS.
4. β-Mercaptoethanol (β-ME). Prepare a 50 m*M* stock in PBS, sterilize by filtration (0.45 μm), and store at –20°C.
5. Culture medium: RPMI-1640 supplemented with 10% fetal calf serum (FCS), 2 m*M* L-glutamine, 100 U/mL penicillin, 100 μg/mL streptomycin, and 50 μ*M* β-ME (1:1000 from the stock).
6. 96-well flat-bottomed tissue culture plates.
7. Recombinant human IL-15 (R&D Systems, *see* **Subheading 3.2.2.**).
8. Recombinant human IL-2 (R&D Systems).
9. Anti-human IL-15 monoclonal antibody (R&D Systems; *see* coating antibody in **Subheading 3.2.2.**).
10. Control antibody IgG stock concentration (available from many sources; must be without sodium azide).
11. CTLD cell line (*see* **Note 5**).
12. XTT cell proliferation kit (Biological Industries, Beit-Haemek, Israel; *see* **Note 6**). Included in the kit are XTT and *N*-methyl dibenzopyrazine methyl sulfate (PMS) solutions.

3. Methods
3.1 RT-PCR for IL-15 mRNA
3.1.1. Total RNA Extraction

1. Cells should be seeded in 12-well (1×10^5 cells/well) or 24-well (0.5×10^5 cells) plates. The cells should be allowed to adhere and grow to confluence for 24–72 h. Each experimental set should be in triplicate (*see* **Note 7**).
2. Remove the supernatants by gentle aspiration, or invert the plate sharply over a bin and remove residual fluid by blotting the plate against clean paper towels.
3. Transfer buffer RLT to a 15-mL tube, calculate 350 μL of RLT per well, and then add 10 μL of β-ME per 1 mL RLT buffer (*see* **Note 8**).
4. Add 350 μL buffer RLT + β-ME to each well, and lyse the cells by scraping with a tip and by several up and down pipetations (*see* **Note 9**).
5. Add an equal volume of 70% ethanol, mix gently, and transfer the lysate of each well to RNeasy mini-columns sitting on 2-mL collecting tubes.
6. Centrifuge the minicolumns with the collecting tube in a microcentrifuge, at 14,000*g* for 15 s.
7. Discard the flowthrough, add 700 μL buffer RW1 to the minicolumns, and centrifuge again under the same conditions.
8. Discard the flowthrough and the collecting tube. Put new 2-mL collecting tubes in place, add 500 μL buffer RPE to the minicolumns, and centrifuge again under the same conditions.
9. Discard the flowthrough, add 500 μL buffer RPE to the minicolumns, and centrifuge for 2 min to dry the columns.
10. Transfer the minicolumns to new 1.5-mL collecting tubes, add 30 μL of RNase-free water, and centrifuge for 1 min to elute the RNA. RNA should be kept at –70°C if not used immediately.

3.1.2. Preparation of cDNA

1. Prepare on ice an RT-master reaction buffer for all the RNA samples. Amount per RNA sample should be as follows:
   1 μL MMLV-RT.
   4 μL 5X reverse transcriptase buffer.
   0.5 μL DTT.
   0.5 μL RNase inhibitor.
   1 μL oligo-d(T).
   1 μL dNTP mixture.
2. Label 1.5-mL tubes, and insert 8 μL of the master mix solution per tube.
3. Add 12 μL of the RNA sample, vortex, and spin down the drops by pulse centrifugation.
4. Incubate the reaction tubes for 1 h at 37°C, then inactivate the enzyme at 65°C for 10 min, and place the tubes on ice.
5. Add 40 μL of water, mix, and spin down. Keep the cDNA samples at –20°C.

3.1.3. PCR

1. Prepare on ice a PCR-master reaction buffer for all the cDNA samples and for one negative control (*see* **Note 8**). Amounts per cDNA sample should be as follows:
   32.75 μL H_2O.
   2.5 μL sense primer (20 m*M*).
   2.5 μL antisense primer (20 m*M*)
   2 μL dNTP mixture.
   5 μL 10X reaction buffer.
   0.25 μL *Taq* DNA polymerase.
2. Vortex the master PCR reaction mixture and add 45 μL to labeled 0.6-mL PCR tubes. Keep the tubes on ice.
3. If the thermal cycler is not equipped with a heated cover, add 50 μL of mineral oil to the PCR tubes.
4. Add 5 μL of cDNA to each tube and to the negative control tube add water (*see* **Note 10**).
5. Place the samples in a thermal cycler that has been prewarmed to 95°C, and run the PCR for 20–25 cycles with β-actin primers under the following conditions: 2 min at 95°C, then 5–10 cycles of 45 s each at 95°C, 1 1/2 min at 60°C, and 1 min at 72°C. Program the last 15 cycles to the same conditions, except for the elongation phase, which should be set at 72°C with a 5-s increment each cycle.
6. Load and run the PCR samples (8 μL) on 2% agarose gel containing ethidium bromide (0.5 μg/mL).
7. Make a record of the gel by a video imaging system, and evaluate the intensity of the bands using densitometry software. The expected size of the β-actin product is 237 bp.
8. PCR amplification should be repeated at least once with different cycles to ensure amplification in the exponential phase of PCR. If the intensity of the bands appears high and all the bands have the same intensity, the samples were probably overamplified and reached a plateau. Repeat the PCR amplification

with five cycles less or add five cycles if the intensity of the bands is low and difficult to analyze.

9. Run the PCR with IL-15 primers with the same thermal cycler protocol except set the annealing temperature at 55°C instead of 60°C. Usually, the IL-15 signal is lower than that of the actin, and therefore five additional cycles are needed for optimal amplification. As for β-actin, repeat PCR at different cycle numbers to ensure amplification in the exponential phase of PCR. The expected size of the IL-15 product is 290 bp.

10. Normalize the β-actin samples according to densitometry and run them with the corresponding IL-15 samples adjusted to the same proportion. Ideally, you should get equal loading in the β-actin samples and equal intensity in triplicate of the IL-15 bands.

11. Repeat the densitometry and calculate the IL-15/β-actin ratio. Express the control levels as 1, and normalize the other samples to this value.

3.2. ELISA of IL-15 Protein

3.2.1. Sample Collection and Storage

1. Grow cells in 24-, 12-, or 6-well plates until they are confluent.
2. Wash the cells twice with medium, and allow IL-15 to accumulate in the supernatant for 24–72 h (*see* **Note 11**).
3. Collect the supernatants and store at –20°C; avoid repeated freeze-thaw cycles. You may use medium with 0.1% NP-40 to lyse cells for determination of intracellular IL-15 levels.
4. Alternatively, if the cells produce low IL-15, you may collect total IL-15 (cell associated and secreted) by adding NP-40 to a final concentration of 0.1% to the cell supernatants in the plates. For this purpose, prepare a 10% NP-40 solution, and then dilute 1 to 100 in the well. To ensure complete lysis of the cells, place the cells on ice and shake them in an orbital shaker for 5 min. Collect cell lysates, and store at –20°C.

3.2.2. Reagent Preparation

1. Blocking buffer: To 200 mL PBS add 1% BSA, 5% sucrose and 0.05% sodium azide (*see* **Note 12**). Store for up to 1 mo at 4°C. **Caution:** Sodium azide is a dangerous poison.
2. Wash buffer: Add 0.05% Tween-20 to 500 mL PBS.
3. Diluent: Prepare 500 mL Tris-buffered saline (20 mM Trizma base, 150 mM NaCl, pH 7.3), and add 0.1% BSA and 0.05% Tween-20. Store for up to 1 mo at 4°C.
4. Coating antibody: Reconstitute in sterile PBS to reach a concentration of 500 μg/mL. Prepare aliquots of 40 μL and store at –70°C. Avoid repeated freeze-thaw cycles.
5. Second antibody: Reconstitute in sterile *diluent* to reach a concentration of 50 μg/mL. Prepare aliquots of 20 μL, and store at –70°C. Avoid repeated freeze-thaw cycles.
6. rhIL-15: In a sterile hood reconstitute 5 μg in 1 mL of sterile PBS containing 0.1% BSA (10 μL of a 10% BSA solution). Store in small aliquots at –70°C.

rhIL-15 may be used for bioassay as well as for the ELISA. For ELISA, dilute in your cell medium (containing serum) some of the reconstituted rhIL-15 to a final concentration 5000 pg/mL, and prepare aliquots of 100 µL in 1.5-mL microtubes. Store at –70°C. Avoid repeated freeze-thaw cycles.

3.2.3. Coating ELISA Plates

1. Reconstitute 1 aliquot of coating antibody in 10 mL of PBS (to reach a concentration of 2 µg/mL).
2. Add 100 µL to each well in the microtiter plate.
3. Cover with an adhesive sheet or with parafilm and incubate overnight.
4. Invert the plate sharply over a bin and remove residual fluid by blotting the plate against clean paper towels. Wash by filling each well with 400 µL wash buffer using a multichannel pipet, squirt bottle, or manifold dispenser. Dry wells following each wash by inverting the plate sharply over a bin and blotting against clean paper towels. Repeat the process three times for a total of four washes.
5. Add 300 µL of blocking buffer to each well, and incubate for at least 1 h.
6. Invert the plate sharply over a bin and remove residual fluid by blotting the plate against clean paper towels. To proceed with the assay, continue to wash as in **step 4**.
7. Alternatively, plates can be stored at this stage for future use: Thoroughly dry the wells without washing. Desiccate by vacuum and store in a sealed plastic bag in the presence of a desiccant. Store at 4°C for up to 1 mo.

3.2.4. Assay Procedure

1. Bring all reagents to room temperature (RT) before use.
2. Defrost and put on ice one 100-µL aliquot of rhIL-15 (5000 pg/mL) and add 900 µL of your cell culture medium to reach a concentration of 500 pg/ml (*see* **Note 13**).
3. Pipet 500 µL medium into eight 1.5-mL tubes marked 0, 3.9, 7.9, 15.8, 31.6, 62.5, 125, and 250 pg/mL. Transfer 500 µL from the 500-pg/mL standard tube to the tube labeled 250 and mix. Repeat this process to make serial dilutions of the standards. The zero standard will be medium alone.
4. Thaw the samples, vortex, and centrifuge them to precipitate denatured protein.
5. Add duplicates of 100 µL/well of samples or standards, cover, and incubate at RT for 2 h (*see* **Note 14**).
6. Invert the plate sharply over a bin and remove residual fluid by blotting the plate against clean paper towels. Wash by filling each well with 400 µL wash buffer using a multichannel pipet, squirt bottle, or manifold dispenser. Dry wells following each wash by inverting the plate sharply over a bin and blotting against clean paper towels. Repeat the process three times for a total of four washes.
7. Thaw a second antibody aliquot and dilute in 10 mL diluent to a final concentration of 100 ng/mL.
8. Add 100 µL/well of diluted second antibody to wells and incubate at RT for 2 h (*see* **Note 14**).
9. Wash as in **step 6**.

10. Dilute 3 μL streptavidin-HRP in 3 mL diluent. Dilute again 500 μL in 10 mL diluent to obtain a final 1:20,000 dilution of streptavidin-HRP.
11. Add 100 μL/well streptavidin-HRP, cover, and incubate at RT for 20 min.
12. Wash as in **step 6**.
13. Add 100 μL/well of substrate solution, cover, and incubate for 30 min. A clear blue color gradient should appear in the standard wells.
14. Add 50 μL/well of stop solution and gently tap the plate for thorough mixing, making sure that the blue color thoroughly changes to yellow.
15. Determine the optical density within 30 min in a microtiter plate reader set to 450 nm. If wavelength correction is available, set to 540 or 570 nm.
16. Use ELISA software to calculate the value of the samples. A linear regression fit should be used for the standard curve.

3.2.5. Expected Values

Primary renal tubular cells (10^5 cells/mL) treated with 100 U/mL IFN-γ produce approx 50 pg/mL IL-15 per day.

3.3. Assaying Biologic Activity of IL-15

3.3.1. Maintaining the CTLD Cells

1. Grow the CTLD cells in standing small 25-cm^2 flasks. The CTLD cell line requires the administration of recombinant IL-2 every 3–4 d, which is done by diluting 1 mL of cells in 9 mL RPMI medium containing 5–10 U/mL IL-2 (*see* **Note 15**).

3.3.2. CTLD Bioassay

1. Plan the distribution of the samples and standards in the plate. Take into consideration that you will not use the external wells of the plate for the assay (*see* **Note 16**). Include wells with neutralizing and control antibodies. You can test your antibodies on recombinant IL-15.
2. Prepare IL-15 standards by pipeting 500 μL medium into eight 1.5-mL tubes marked 0, 7.9, 15.8, 31.6, 62.5, 125, 250, and 500 pg/mL. Transfer 500 μL from the 500-pg/mL standard tube to the tube labeled 250, and mix. Repeat this process to make serial dilution of the standards. The zero standard will be medium alone.
3. Add 200 μL RPMI to the marginal wells.
4. Add 100 μL/well of standards and samples in triplicate.
5. As an option, to inhibit the IL-15-dependent proliferation, add 10 μL of neutralizing IL-15 antibody to the samples. You should also add control antibody to noninhibited wells and medium to control wells. Incubate for 60 min at RT.
6. Transfer 8 mL CTLD suspension from their flasks to a 15-mL tube. Centrifuge at 25°C, 200g for 10 min. Remove supernatant and resuspend cells by gently whipping at the bottom of the tube.
7. Add 10 mL PBS and wash the cells twice by centrifugation.
8. Resuspend the CTLD cells with 10 mL RPMI. Count viable cells by trypan-blue staining. Dilute cell suspension to a final concentration of 5×10^4 cells/mL.

Apply 100 μL cell suspension (5×10^3 cells) per well. This should be performed while continuously maintaining homogeneity of the suspension, and with the greatest precision.

9. Incubate for 72 h. Follow daily the reaction of the CTLDs to the treatments by inverted microscope (*see* **Note 17**).

3.3.3. Quantification of CTLD Proliferation: XTT Reaction

1. Follow XTT-kit manufacturer's instructions. Briefly: after mixing the activation solution with the XTT reagent, add 50 μL of the mixture to each well, and incubate for 4–6 h (*see* **Note 18**).
2. Determine the optical density with a microtiter plate reader set at 450–550 nm with reference wavelength set at 630–690 nm.
3. Use ELISA software to calculate the value of the samples. A four-parameter regression fit should be used for the standard curve.

4. Notes

1. Twelve samples can easily be handled in this procedure. The initial three steps are fairly simple. However, it is critical that an experienced technician with a good knowledge of imaging and densitometry software should perform the last step, which consists of video imaging and densitometry of the agarose gel electrophoresis.
2. Human IL-15 ELISA kits are available from R&D Systems and other suppliers. Usually commercial kits are quite reliable; however, the cost per sample using the method we describe is about 5–10 times cheaper.
3. The samples collected for this assay must be sterile. During preparation, detergents or cytotoxic drugs must be avoided to prevent nonspecific effects on the vitality of the CTLDs. To obtain cell lysate it is preferable to lyse the cells without using detergents, e.g., 2–3 cycles of freeze-thawing the cells.
4. For RNA extraction we found the RNeasy Mini Kit (Qiagen) reliable, fast, easy to use, and free of phenol, unlike most RNA extraction reagents. In addition, we obtained a higher RNA yield using this kit, compared with other reagents. We successfully used RNeasy for total RNA extractions from tissue and adherent and nonadherent cells. The protocol described below is for adherent kidney tubular epithelial cells; however, with slight modification, it can be useful for other types of cells.
5. CTLD can be obtained from us or else other IL-2/IL-15-dependent cells like CTLL can be purchased from ATCC.
6. XTT cell proliferation kits are available from other sources. XTT and the activator PMS are available from Sigma, and their solutions can be prepared at the lab. However, home-made preparation of the reagents needed for this assay is tricky and time consuming, and reproducibility of the assay might be affected.
7. IL-15 mRNA reached peak levels approx 6 h following IFN-γ stimulation. Therefore, 6 h is a good time point to harvest cells for RNA analysis. Nevertheless, we recommend finding optimal conditions for specific experimental procedures.
8. ***Important:*** To prevent-false positive PCR results from contamination of the PCR reaction mixture by PCR products, the pre-PCR working place should be in a

separate room or far as possible from the area of analysis of PCR products. Also, the extraction of RNA and the preparation of the PCR reaction mixture must be performed using a *separate set of pipets and reagents.*

9. At this time point it is possible to freeze the plate at –70°C and continue with RNA extraction when convenient.

10. To prevent high background and nonspecific amplification resulting from mispriming, it is important to add the cDNA to a cold PCR reaction buffer just before amplification and to prewarm the thermal cycler to the denaturation temperature (95°C).

11. Treatment with human IFN-γ (5–500 U/mL) may be used as a positive control for induction of IL-15 production in many types.

12. Sodium azide is an inhibitor of HRP and should be avoided in other solutions.

13. The diluent used for standards preparation should be similar to the samples being assayed. If you assay cell supernatants, use medium; if you assay serum samples, dilute the standards in FCS.

14. Incubation for 1 h is sufficient if you shake the plate (200 rpm) on an orbital shaker.

15. Avoid long intervals between IL-2 administrations, which may lead to the development of an IL-2-independent cell population and hence deficient sensitivity of the assay. The CTLDs must be well "starved" for growth factor before being included in the assay; avoid using CTLDs within the first or second day of IL-2 administration.

16. Do not use the marginal wells of the plate since they tend to dehydrate during long incubations.

17. Follow the bioassay; usually at 24 h you will observe some proliferation clamps in the high standards. At 48–72 h you should not see proliferating cells in the control wells without IL-15. In contrast, you should see an IL-15 dose-dependent proliferation. The duration of incubation may vary due to assay conditions and requirements. Long duration may achieve higher assay sensitivity due to decreased background in the IL-15-poor wells and an increasingly significant population mass in the proliferating wells.

18. The standard incubation time is 4–6 h; however, optimal incubation time may vary from 2 to 24 h. Following the addition of the XTT reagent, the medium changes its color from orange to dark red in correlation to cell numbers. Short XTT incubation might give low sensitivity of the assay. Long exposure might bring the high standards to plateau levels. We recommend reading the assay when the color signal in the 125-pg/mL standard is clearly higher than that of the control. In any case, after reading, the plate can be incubated again and read several times until optimal sensitivity is reached.

References

1. Waldmann, T., Tagaya, Y., and Bamford, R. (1998) Interleukin-2, interleukin-15, and their receptors. *Int. Rev. Immunol.* **16**, 205–226.
2. Grabstein, K. H., Eisenman, J., Shanebeck, K., Rauch, C., Srinivasan, S., Fung, V., et al. (1994) Cloning of a T cell growth factor that interacts with the beta chain of the interleukin-2 receptor. *Science* **264**, 965–968.

3. Bamford, R. N., Battiata, A. P., Burton, J.D., Sharma, H., and Waldmann, T. A. (1996) Interleukin (IL) 15/IL-T production by the adult T-cell leukemia cell line HuT-102 is associated with a human T-cell lymphotrophic virus type I R region/IL-15 fusion message that lacks many upstream AUGs that normally attenuate IL-15 mRNA translation. *Proc. Natl. Acad. Sci. USA* **93,** 2897–2902.
4. Tagaya, Y., Bamford, R. N., DeFilippis, A. P., and Waldmann, T. A. (1996) IL-15: a pleiotropic cytokine with diverse receptor/signaling pathways whose expression is controlled at multiple levels. *Immunity* **4,** 329–336.
5. Weiler, M. R. B., Einbinder, T., Hausmann, M. J., Kaneti, J., Chaimovitz, C., and Douvdevani, A. (1998) Interleukin-15, a leukocyte activator and growth factor, is produced by cortical tubular epithelial cells. *J. Am. Soc. Nephrol.* **9,** 1194–201.
6. Scudiero, D. A., Shoemaker, R. H., Paull, K. D., Monks, A., Tierney, S., Nofziger, T. H., et al. (1988) Evaluation of a soluble tetrazolium/formazan assay for cell growth and drug sensitivity in culture using human and other tumor cell lines. *Cancer Res.* **48,** 4827–4833.

III

Assaying Interleukins in Particular Pathologies

18

Assaying Interleukin-6 in Breast Cancer

Judith Harmey, Amanda Haverty, Deirdre Foley, and David Bouchier-Hayes

1. Introduction

Interleukin-6 (IL-6) is a 21–28 kDa glycoprotein produced by T and B cells, monocytes, macrophages, fibroblasts, endothelial cells, and tumor cells *(1)*. Elevated IL-6 has been identified in the serum of breast cancer patients *(2)*. IL-6 has been implicated in breast cancer metastasis *(3)*, and IL-6 was produced by a breast cell line of metastatic origin but not by a cell line derived from a primary lesion *(4)*. Furthermore, IL-6 is elevated in the serum of breast cancer patients with visceral metastases *(5)*, and a reduction in serum IL-6 is associated with clinical response to treatment in advanced breast cancer patients *(6)*.

An IL-6 immunoassay was used to assay IL-6 in serum and plasma samples from breast cancer patients, IL-6 levels in tumor and normal breast tissue, and IL-6 production by cultured breast cancer cells. To optimize detection of circulating IL-6 levels in breast cancer, we compared IL-6 concentrations in serum and plasma and in samples that had been frozen, thawed, and refrozen. We measured IL-6 production from cultured cells in the presence of varying concentrations of fetal calf serum to determine optimum culture conditions for IL-6 detection. In the case of tissue homogenates, IL-6 measurements were normalized against total cell protein.

The principles of the IL-6 immunoassay are outlined in **Fig. 1**. The IL-6 immunoassay is essentially a sandwich enzyme-linked immunosorbent assay (ELISA). In essence, the microtiter plate is coated with a monoclonal antibody specific for IL-6. The sample is applied, and the immobilized antibody binds IL-6 present in the sample. Washing removes unbound molecules. A polyclonal second antibody specific for IL-6 and conjugated to horseradish peroxidase (HRP) enzyme then binds to IL-6 molecules bound to the first antibody.

From: *Methods in Molecular Medicine, vol. 60: Interleukin Protocols*
Edited by: L. A. J. O'Neill and A. Bowie © Humana Press Inc., Totowa, NJ

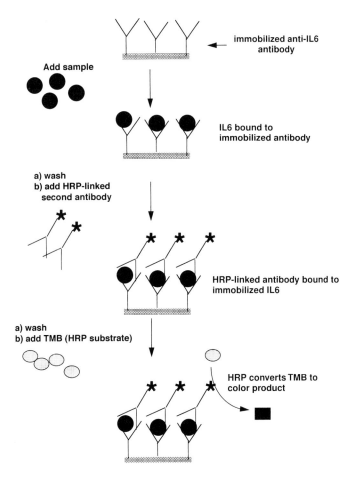

Fig. 1. Sandwich immunoassay.

Unbound antibody is again removed by washing. Bound antibody is detected using a color substrate. In the presence of hydrogen peroxide (H_2O_2), HRP cleaves tetramethylbenzidine (TMB) to a blue colored product. The color development reaction is stopped by the addition of sulfuric acid. The amount of color is detected by reading the absorbance at 450 nm. The color developed is proportional to the amount of HRP-conjugated antibody and therefore is an indirect measurement of the amount of IL-6 present in the sample.

2. Materials

Plasma or serum samples were collected in heparinized or serum collection tubes, respectively (Sarstedt). R&D Systems Quantikine human IL-6 immunoassay (code D6050) was used to measure IL-6 in serum, plasma, tissue homogenates, and cell culture supernatants. All kit components were stored at 4°C except recombinant IL-6, which was stored in aliquots at –20°C. Diluent buffers RD1A, RD6F, and RD5A, microtiter plates precoated with a murine monoclonal antibody specific for IL-6, wash buffer, polyclonal HRP-conjugated anti-IL-6 antibody, color reagents (H_2O_2 and TMB chromogen), stop solution (2 *N* sulfuric acid), and recombinant IL-6 are provided in the kit. RD6F is an animal serum used to dilute serum and plasma samples and standards for serum/plasma immunoassays. RD5A buffer is used to dilute cell culture supernatants and standards for culture supernatant and tissue homogenate assays. Bicinchoninic acid (BCA) protein assay was provided by Pierce (Rockford, IL). Phosphate-buffered saline (PBS), pH 7.4, bovine serum albumin (BSA), and phenyl methyl sulfonyl flouride (PMSF) were obtained from Sigma. A stock solution of 100 m*M* PMSF in methanol was prepared immediately before use. Cell culture reagents, Dulbecco's modified Eagle's medium (DMEM), L15, fetal calf serum (FCS), penicillin, and streptomycin were obtained from GIBCO-BRL.

3. Methods
3.1. IL-6 Immunoassay

Depending on the type of samples to be assayed, two diluent buffers are provided in the kit to prepare the standards. A standard curve was prepared (300, 100, 50, 25, 12.5, 6.25, and 3.12 pg/mL) by making serial dilutions from a 300-pg/mL stock of recombinant human IL-6 provided in the kit in either RD5A (cell culture supernatants and tissue homogenates) or RD6F (serum and plasma samples). If both serum/plasma and cell culture samples are to be assayed, a separate standard curve must be carried out for each sample type. All samples and standards were measured in duplicate (*see* **Note 1**).

1. Diluent buffer RD1A (100 µL) and sample (100 µL) are pipetted into wells, and the plate is sealed and incubated on a shaking table at room temperature for 2 h.
2. Samples are removed and unbound molecules washed away by washing the plate three times with 400 µL/well of wash buffer. To prevent nonspecific binding during the IL-6 immunoassay, it is important that all solution changes be carried out by inverting the plate, shaking vigorously to remove liquid, and then vigorously blotting the inverted plate on tissue paper until no more liquid comes off, usually 2 or 3×.
3. Horseradish peroxidase (HRP)-conjugated anti-IL-6 antibody (200 µL) is added to each well, and the plate is sealed and incubated at room temperature for 2 h on a shaker table.
4. After incubation, antibody is removed and the plate washed three times as before with wash buffer. During the last wash, the substrate solution should be prepared by mixing equal volumes of TMB and H_2O_2 solutions. The substrate solution should be used within 15 min of preparation.
5. Substrate solution (200 µL) is added to each well and incubated for 20 min at room temperature.

6. Following color development, 50 µL of sulfuric acid is added to stop the reaction. To ensure even color development within the wells, the plate is tapped gently. Any bubbles in the well can be broken with a needle tip.

7. The optical density is read in a microtiter plate reader set at 450 nm with a 570-nm wavelength correction. This corrects for optical imperfections in the plate. The standard curve is prepared by plotting mean absorbance against concentration using Microsoft Excel Version 5.0 or its equivalent. The correlation coefficent between the fitted data and actual data should be greater than 0.95. IL-6 concentrations of samples were determined using the curve fit equation ($y = mx + c$) generated. Statistical analysis was carried out using DataDesk 5.0 (Data Description, Ithaca, NY). Data were taken to be significant where $p > 0.05$. Serum and plasma IL-6 levels were analyzed by unpaired Student's t-test. Matched normal and breast tumor tissue IL-6 was analyzed by paired t-test. IL-6 production by cultured breast cancer cells in different FCS concentrations were analyzed by ANOVA with Scheffe's post hoc correction.

3.2. IL-6 Levels in Serum and Plasma Samples

Whole blood (10 mL) was collected by venopuncture from healthy human volunteers and breast cancer patients, in either heparin tubes for plasma or serum collection tubes for serum. Blood was collected from breast cancer patients prior to surgery, or chemo- or radiotherapy. All blood samples were processed within 1 h of collection. Serum was allowed to allowed to clot for 30 min prior to centrifugation. Both plasma and serum samples were centrifuged at 300g for 30 min at room temperature. Plasma and serum were recovered and stored in aliquots at –80°C.

Patients with breast cancer had significantly higher levels of serum IL-6 than healthy volunteers ($p < 0.05$) **(Fig. 2)**. In healthy volunteers IL-6 levels were between 0 and 7.63 pg/mL compared with 44.57 and 197.53 pg/mL in breast cancer patients. These values are similar to those previously reported: Healthy control serum values were 11 ± 2 and ovarian cancer patients were 125 ± 10 pg/mL *(7)*. We compared IL-6 levels in serum and plasma samples from the same patient; although there was a trend for slightly higher IL-6 (pg/mL) in serum samples (133.32 vs 118.32, 27.32 vs 25.0, and 27.33 vs 23.32 serum vs plasma), this difference was not statistically significant **(Fig. 3)**. However, it is not advisable to compare plasma and serum IL-6 from different patients, that is, all blood samples should be prepared identically. We assessed the effect of refreezing serum **(Fig. 4A)** and plasma **(Fig. 4B)** on IL-6 levels. Blood samples were processed as described and frozen at –80°C. Refrozen samples were stored at –80°C, incubated at room temperature for 1 h, and refrozen at –80°C. We found that refreezing samples once had no effect ($p = $ ns) on either serum or plasma IL-6 compared with samples frozen once. However, repeated cycles of freezing and thawing resulted in a complete loss of detectable IL-6. For any set of experiments, all samples should be processed identically.

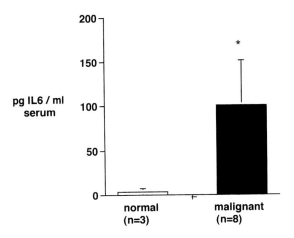

Fig. 2. IL-6 in serum. Serum from healthy volunteers ($n = 3$) and patients with malignant breast disease ($n = 8$) were assayed for IL-6 by ELISA. Data are expressed as mean ± SD. Statistical analysis is by unpaired t-test. *$p < 0.05$ malignant vs controls.

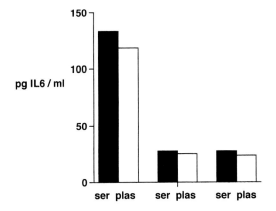

Fig. 3. Comparison of IL-6 levels in plasma and serum. IL-6 in serum (ser) and plasma (plas) of three cancer patients was assayed by ELISA. Statistical analysis is by paired t-test. p = ns plasma vs serum.

Hemolyzed samples often give false readings in cytokine ELISAs. We assessed the effects of hemolysis on IL-6 detection in serum and plasma samples **(Fig. 5)**. Hemolysis was achieved by passing blood samples twice through a 26-G needle. In the IL-6 immunoassay described here, hemolysis reduced plasma IL-6 levels by 3 or 5% and serum IL-6 by 6 or 11%. (25.66 vs 27.32 and 118.32 vs 133.62 pg IL-6/mL hemolysed vs nonhemolysed serum; 24.33 vs 25 and 112.32 vs 118.32 pg IL-6/mL hemolysed vs nonhemolysed plasma).

A

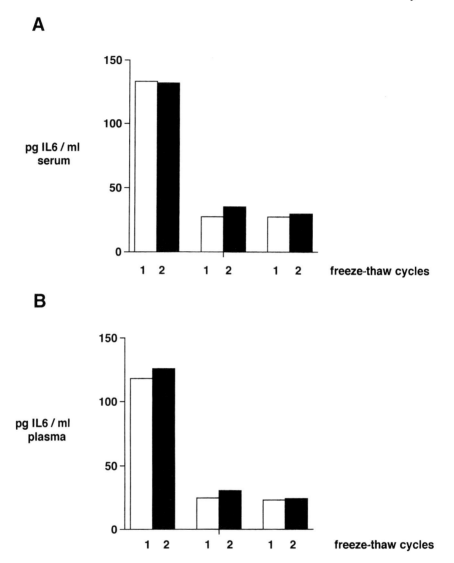

Fig. 4. Effect of repeated freezing on serum (**A**) and plasma (**B**) levels of IL-6. Samples were stored frozen at $-80°C$, thawed, and assayed for IL-6 immediately (1) or refrozen and thawed and assayed for IL-6 (2). Three samples are shown. Statistical anlaysis was by paired t-test. p = ns 1 vs 2 freeze-thaw cycles.

In summary, although plasma or serum samples are suitable for the IL-6 immunoassay, all samples in a given study should be prepared identically. Repeated freeze-thawing of serum and plasma samples should be avoided, and hemolyzed samples should be excluded from analysis, when possible.

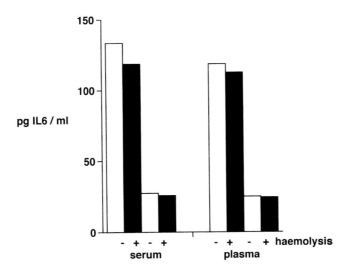

Fig. 5. The effect of hemolysis on serum and plasma IL-6 measurements. Hemolyzed samples were prepared by passing whole blood twice through a 26-G needle. Two samples for serum and plasma are shown.

3.3. IL-6 Levels in Breast Tissue Homogenates

1. Breast tumor and adjacent histologically normal tissue were flash frozen in liquid nitrogen within 1 h of resection and then stored at –80°C.
2. Specimens (0.5–1.0 cm³)were diced in liquid nitrogen in a ceramic dish. Diced tissues were then homogenized in 0.5–1 mL of PBS containing 1 m*M* PMSF on ice using a Polytron homogenizer (*see* **Note 2**).
3. Debris was pelleted by centrifugation at 12,000*g* for 5 min and the supernatant (below the level of the upper lipid-rich layer and above the pellet) was recovered. Samples were maintained on ice.
4. IL-6 in tissue homogenates was assayed by ELISA as above (*see* **Subheading 3.1.**).
5. Total protein in homogenates was estimated using the BCA assay (*see* **Note 3**).
6. Data are expressed as pg IL-6/µg protein.

We assayed IL-6 levels in matched normal and malignant breast tissue from seven patients (**Fig. 6**). IL-6 was not detected in any of the normal breast tissue. However, significant levels of IL-6, 13.19 ± 6.6 pg IL-6/µg protein (range 4.2–21.3 pg IL-6/µg protein), were found in malignant tissue.

3.4. IL-6 Production by MDA-MB-231 Breast Cancer Cells

MDA-MB-231 cells (ECACC92020424), a breast cancer cell line derived from a malignant pleural effusion, were maintained in L15 culture medium containing 10% FCS, 50 IU/mL penicillin, and 50 µg/mL streptomycin in sealed flasks at 37°C.

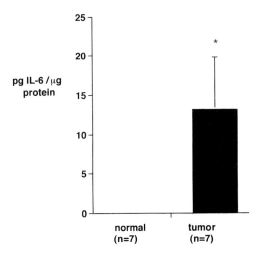

Fig. 6. Levels of IL-6 in homogenates prepared from matched histologically normal and malignant breast tissue ($n = 7$) were assayed by ELISA. Data are expressed as mean ± SD. Statistical analysis was by paired t-test. *, $p < 0.05$ normal vs malignant breast tissue.

1. To assay IL-6 production, 10,000 cells were plated in 96-well plates in 200 μL of DMEM containing 0, 1, 5, or 10% FCS, 50 IU/mL penicillin, and 50 μg/mL streptomycin.
2. Cells were incubated at 37°C for 24 h in a humidified atmosphere of 5% CO_2/ 95% air. Supernatants were collected and stored at –80°C.
3. IL-6 was assayed by ELISA (*see* **Subheading 3.1.**).
4. Data were expressed as pg IL-6/10^4 cells/ 24 h (*see* **Note 4**).

The amount of IL-6 produced by MDA-MB-231 cells varied according to the amount of FCS in the growth medium (47.89 ± 4.11, 49.21 ± 9.86, 67.01 ± 2.09, 89.41 ± 4.15 pg IL-6/10^4 cells/24 h in 0, 1, 5, and 10% FCS, respectively) (**Fig. 7**). DMEM supplemented with 10% FCS contained 8.25 pg IL-6/mL. Increasing IL-6 production with increasing FCS could be due to either increased stability of IL-6 in FCS-containing medium or stimulation of the cells by factors present in FCS. The higher levels of IL-6 detected in supernatants from cells in increasing FCS is most likely due to increased stability of the IL-6 produced, since when FCS is replaced by BSA, IL-6 values increase with increasing BSA concentration (27.63 ± 7.95, 46 ± 15.56, 63.13 ± 7.25, and 67.25 ± 13.79 pg IL-6/10^4 cells/24 h in 0, 1, 5, and 10% BSA, respectively). Therefore, when assaying IL-6 production by cultured cells, the inclusion of either FCS or BSA in the growth medium as a protein stabilizer is recommended.

4. Notes

1. The IL-6 immunoassay, including sample preparation and dilution, can be carried out in approx 6 h. To prevent nonspecific binding during the IL-6 immunoassay, it is

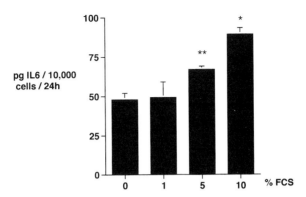

Fig. 7. Effect of varying concentrations of FCS on IL-6 production by MDA-MB-231 cells. Cells were incubated for 24 h, and IL-6 was assayed by ELISA. Data are expressed as mean ± SD and represent three independent experiments. Statistical analysis is by ANOVA with Scheffe's post hoc correction. *, $p < 0.05$ vs 5%, 1% or 0% FCS. **, $p < 0.05$ vs 1% or 0% FCS.

important that all solution changes be carried out by inverting the plate, shaking vigorously to remove liquid, and then vigorously hitting the inverted plate on tissue paper until no more liquid comes off, usually two or three times. To ensure accuracy, it is essential that a standard curve be carried out for each immunoassay, with the standards prepared in the appropriate diluent for samples to be assayed. To minimize the number of standard curves, samples are collected, stored at –80°C, and assayed in bulk.

This method is sensitive in the range 0–300 pg IL-6/mL. When assaying samples in which the likely range of IL-6 concentrations is unknown, or when high levels are anticipated, a diluted sample (1 in 5 or 1 in 10) should also be assayed to ensure that the IL-6 concentration falls within the range of the standard curve. IL-6 concentrations of samples that have an absorbance reading higher than the standards cannot be accurately measured. If samples do exceed the standards, the sample should be diluted further and reassayed. Cell culture supernatants should be diluted in cell culture medium, tissue homogenates should be diluted in PBS containing 1 m*M* PMSF, and serum or plasma samples should be diluted in the diluent RD6F (animal serum) provided in the immunoassay kit. It is possible to design an ELISA using antibody pairs. However, using antibody pairs for a range of cytokines, we have never achieved the same sensitivity as with commercial ELISAs.

2. Tissues can also be homogenized using a Dounce homogenizer if a Polytron is not available. It is important, however, that tissue be maintained at 4°C during the homogenization step to minimize protein degradation. IL-6 expression in breast tissue can also be assessed by immunohistochemistry of paraffin-embedded sections or Western blotting of tissue homogenates. However, whereas immunohistochemistry allows identification of individual cells expressing IL-6, it provides qualitative rather than quantitative information. Similarly, Western blotting is a semiquantitative technique and can only identify gross differences in protein levels.

3. To ensure accuracy, it is essential that a standard curve be carried out for each protein assay. The standard curve range is 0–1000 µg/mL. To ensure that cell lysates or tissue homogenates fall within this range, both concentrated and diluted samples should be assayed. Cell lysates and tissue homogenates should be diluted 1 in 10 with PBS prior to estimating total protein. This assay can be carried out at either room temperature or 37°C. The samples should be incubated for 30 min at 37°C or 1 h at room temperature.

   To control for interfering substances in the sample buffer, a control sample containing buffer only should be included in the protein assay. Alternatively, the standards can be prepared in the same buffer as the samples. Total protein can also be assayed using a Coomassie assay. However, this method is not as sensitive as the BCA assay.

4. In the experiments shown here, IL-6 production by cultured cells is expressed as pg IL-6/10^4 cells/24 h. Alternatively, IL-6 production can be expressed as pg IL-6/µg cell protein. In this case, cell supernatants are recovered, and the cells are washed three times in PBS. PBS (100 µL) is added and the cells lysed by three cycles of freeze-thawing. Total protein can then be estimated by the BCA total protein assay.

References

1. Kishimoto, T. (1989) The biology of interleukin-6. *Blood* **74,** 1–10.
2. Jablonska, E. and Pietruska, Z. (1998) Changes in soluble IL-6 receptor and IL-6 production by polymorphonuclear cells and whole blood cells of breast cancer patients. *Arch. Immunol. Ther. Exp.* **46,** 25–29.
3. Sierra, A., Price, J. E., Garcia-Ramirez, M., Mendez, O., Lopez, L., and Fabra, A. (1997) Astrocyte-derived cytokines contribute to the metastatic brain specificity of breast cancer cells. *Lab. Invest.* **77,** 357–368.
4. Mobus, V. J., Moll, R., Gerharz, C. D., Kieback, D. G., Merk, O., Runnebaum, I. B., et al. (1998) Differential characteristics of two new tumorgenic cell lines of human breast carcinoma origin. *Int. J. Cancer* **77,** 415–423.
5. Abe, M., Ouchi, N., Harada, Y., Mori, S., Rishiki, H., and Kumagai, K. (1992) Elevated serum levels of interleukin-6 in breast cancer patients with visceral metastases. *Nippon Geka Gakkai Zasshi* **93,** 107.
6. Barak, V., Kalikman, I., Nisman, B., Farbstein, H., Fridlender, Z.G., Baider, L., et al. (1998) Changes in cytokine production of breast cancer patients treated with interferons. *Cytokine* **10,** 977–983.
7. Maccio, A., Lai, P., Santona, M. C., Pagliara, L., Melis, G. B., and Mantovani, G. (1998) High serum levels of soluble IL-2 receptor, cytokines, and C reactive protein correlate with impairment of T cell response in patients with advanced epithelial ovarian cancer. *Gynecol. Oncol.* **69,** 248–252.

19

Cytokines, Stress, and Depressive Illness

Hymie Anisman, Shawn Hayley, Arun V. Ravindran, Zul Merali, and Jenna Griffiths

1. Introduction

Stressors may instigate a series of hormonal variations, coupled with neurochemical alterations within the brain that promote cognitive alterations and favor the development of depressive illness. Indeed, it appears that in many respects the effects of stressors are reminiscent of the presumed neurochemical disturbances thought to be associated with depression, including elevated hypothalamic-pituitary-adrenal (HPA) functioning, as well as altered monoamine activity within hypothalamic and limbic areas of the brain. With respect to the latter, it has become clear that stressors reliably induce variations of brain norepinephrine (NE), dopamine (DA), and serotonin (5-HT) and that the behavioral disturbances associated with stressors are alleviated by treatments that attenuate the amine alterations, including antidepressant agents (1).

Although it has typically been assumed that psychological (psychogenic) and physical (neurogenic) stressors are most closely aligned with depression, the suspicion has arisen that systemic stressors, including immune alterations, may also act in such a provocative capacity (2). In this respect, it has become clear that communication occurs among the immune, endocrine, autonomic, and central nervous systems (CNS) (3,4), and that psychosocial factors (e.g., stressors) that impact on CNS processes and hormonal functioning also come to affect immune system functioning. Conversely, immune activation may affect hormonal processes and the activity of central neurotransmitters. Thus, the position has been entertained that by virtue of the neurochemical effects imparted, immune activation may come to affect behavioral outputs and may even be related to behavioral pathology such as depressive illness (2,5–7).

From: *Methods in Molecular Medicine, vol. 60: Interleukin Protocols*
Edited by: L. A. J. O'Neill and A. Bowie © Humana Press Inc., Totowa, NJ

This chapter describes the presumed relationship between cytokines and depressive illness in humans, as well as some of the presumed mechanisms that may underlie this relationship. Particular attention will be devoted to describing caveats and pitfalls (listed under Notes) that may be encountered in conducting research to assess the cytokine abnormalities associated with depressive illnesses (and these apply, of course, to other psychiatric disorders). These will be given in the context of a particular study.

1.1. Cytokines as Immunotransmitters

Although several potential routes of communication exist between the immune and central nervous systems, increasing attention has been devoted to the possibility that signaling molecules of an activated immune system, namely, cytokines, may also play a fundamental role in alerting the CNS to immunologic challenge *(8,9)*. For instance, it was suggested that cytokines, such as interleukin-1β (IL-1β), stimulate cytokine receptors present on the dendrites of the vagal nerve at visceral locations or at the level of the nodose ganglion *(10–12)*, culminating in the activation of brainstem regions, such as the nucleus of the solitary tract (NTS). A second view has been that macrophage-derived cytokines, such as IL-1β, IL-6, and tumor necrosis factor-α (TNF-α), as well as IL-2 secreted from T cells, gain access to the brain, promoting the release of various neurotransmitters. Although cytokines are fairly large molecules, entry into the brain may occur where the blood-brain barrier is less restrictive (e.g., the organum vasculosum laminae terminalis), or via a saturable transport system *(13)*. Also, entry into the brain may occur particularly readily under some pathologic conditions (e.g., seizure) *(4,13)*.

In addition to gaining entry to the brain following antigenic challenge, cytokines may be constitutively expressed in the brain. Bioactivity and mRNA expression of several cytokines and their receptors have been documented in several brain regions, including the hypothalamus and numerous extrahypothalamic sites—the hippocampus, cerebellum, forebrain regions, basal ganglia, several circumventricular regions, and brainstem nuclei (e.g., NTS, ventrolateral medulla). Moreover, bioactivity of cytokines within the brain may be provoked by various challenges, including systemic or central bacterial endotoxin administration, and by neuropathologic conditions, including brain injury, cerebral ischemia, and seizure *(4,14,15)*. The functional role of central cytokine activation has yet to be fully elucidated. On the one hand, proinflammatory cytokines such as IL-1β may function in a reparative capacity in neurologic diseases or brain trauma, and on the other hand, it is possible that they actually promote neuronal damage following central insults *(14,15)*.

1.2. Neurochemical Consequences of Cytokine Challenge
1.2.1. Immediate Effects of Cytokines

Neurogenic stressors increase IL-1β mRNA expression and IL-1β protein within the brain *(16–18)*, and pretreatment with an IL-1 receptor antagonist (IL-1RA) attenuated the hypothalamic monoamine and the neuroendocrine effects otherwise observed (e.g., increased pituitary adrenocorticotropic hormone [ACTH] and adreneal glucocorticoid release) *(19)*. In contrast, however, when a psychogenic (psychological) stressor was administered either acutely or chronically (in this instance exposing rats to a predator, the ferret), mRNA expression of IL-1β, IL-1R-I, IL-1R-II, IL-1RA, IL-1 accessory proteins, and TNF-α, was not altered *(20)*. It may be that this stressor was simply not sufficiently severe to elicit such effects, or that psychological stressors do not promote central cytokine variations. After all, CNS cytokine activation after everyday insults may be maladaptive. Nevertheless, it is possible that in animals (or in some strains) that are particularly vulnerable to stressors, altered CNS cytokine functioning would be realized.

Paralleling the effects of traditional psychological or physical stressors, both central and systemic IL-1β administration increases the release of hypothalamic neuropeptides. For instance, IL-1β is particularly effective in activating neurons of the paraventricular nucleus that contain corticotropin-releasing hormone (CRH) and arginine vasopressin (AVP) *(21,22)*. The CRH and AVP synergistically stimulate pituitary ACTH release, which then stimulates release of adrenal corticosterone *(9)*. There is reason to believe that NE may promote IL-1β-induced HPA changes, whereas nitric oxide restrains HPA responses to proinflammatory stimuli *(23)*.

In addition to affecting neuropeptide release, systemic administration of IL-1β or the endotoxin lipopolysaccharide (LPS), increased NE activity and/or affected the levels of the amine in several hypothalamic nuclei, including the paraventricular nucleus (PVN) and median eminence *(24–26)*. Likewise, in vivo analyses confirmed that systemic IL-1β increased the release of hypothalamic NE and DA *(19,27–31)* and hippocampal 5-HT *(32–34)*. Cytokine treatment has also been shown to increase the use of NE at several extrahypothalamic sites *(25)* and has induced variations in tryptophan in the brainstem, hypothalamus, and prefrontal cortex (PFC) *(24)*. The hormonal and central neurotransmitter alterations were not only elicited by IL-1β, but could also be induced by TNF-α. For instance, TNF-α stimulated plasma corticosterone secretion *(24)* and provoked central monoamine alterations at several central sites *(35)*. Although these cytokines had stressor-like actions, in some respects their actions could be distinguished from those of stressors. For instance, in contrast to stressors, IL-1β did not induce marked DA changes within the prefrontal cortex and nucleus accumbens *(25,33,34,36)*. Interestingly, however, systemic administration of LPS increased in vivo accumbal DA release *(37)*, raising the possibility that immune activation and the sequential (or concurrent) release of several cytokines are necessary to mimic the effects of stressors.

1.2.2. Sensitization of Cytokine Effects

In addition to the immediate effects of stressors, aversive stimuli may augment the neurochemical response to later challenges (sensitization), and may consequently influence vulnerability to subsequent stressor-related behavioral and physical disturbances *(1)*. Likewise, IL-1β may provoke a "sensitization-like" effect *(38)*, and, as in the case of stressors, this effect may be dependent on the passage of time *(39)*. In particular, IL-1β increases the costorage of CRH and AVP within CRH terminals at the external zone of the median eminence; however, this effect only becomes evident with the passage of time, peaking during the second week after treatment and declining thereafter *(38,40)*. Interestingly, among animals treated with the cytokine, later exposure to a neurogenic stressor (footshock) or to the cytokine itself, augmented later plasma ACTH and corticosterone secretion. It would appear that acute administration of IL-1β increases the availability of secretagogues, thereby enhancing the response to later challenges.

The neurochemical consequences of TNF-α have received less attention than those of IL-1β, but it appears that this cytokine also exerts relatively protracted actions on HPA activity, central monoamine functioning, and behavior. Once again, it was reported that in mice exposed to recombinant human TNF-α, at doses that elicited little behavioral effect (1.0–4.0 μg), subsequent reexposure to a subthreshold dose of TNF-α induced marked reductions in consumption of highly favored foods, motor activity, and social exploration, coupled with a degradation of the animal's general appearance. However, whereas these effects were not apparent in mice reexposed to the cytokine 1 or 7 d after the initial treatment, they were marked on reexposure after a 14–28 d interval *(35)*. Likewise, the increased plasma corticosterone associated with systemic injection of TNF-α was greatly augmented on reexposure to the cytokine 14–28 d later. Interestingly, cytokine reexposure 1 d after initial TNF-α administration provoked a significant desensitization, such that plasma corticosterone levels were reduced relative to those of acutely treated mice. Evidently, reexposure to TNF-α may provoke either a desensitization or sensitization effect, depending on the time of reexposure.

Just as TNF-α promotes the sensitization of HPA activity, this cytokine proactively increased the utilization of NE within the PVN, and this effect was progressively greater with the passage of time since the initial cytokine challenge. In contrast, within the prefrontal cortex and the central amygdala, a marked sensitization effect was only evident upon reexposure to the cytokine at the 1-d interval. Clearly, TNF-α may engender a sensitization effect wherein the response to later neurochemical functioning is increased in a brain region-specific fashion. Although the mechanisms governing these varied effects remains to be elucidated, it seems that cytokine treatment may instigate a series of dynamic processes involving different temporal patterns and may subserve different behavioral sequelae. In view of the similarity between the effects of cytokines and stressors, the possibility exists that depressive-like behaviors may be provoked by virtue of the neurochemical alterations imparted by cytokine challenges.

1.3. Cytokines and Depressive Illness

As observed in response to severe stressors, there have been reports indicating that major depression is associated with alterations of various aspects of the immune response, including a reduction in mitogen-stimulated lymphocyte proliferation, as well as reduced natural killer (NK) cell activity (*see* reviews in **refs. 5** and *41–44*). It appears that these effects are most pronounced in severely depressed patients (i.e., those exhibiting melancholia) *(5,44)*, and the altered immunity may be attenuated with symptom remission *(45)*. In contrast to these findings, however, there have been reports that depression was associated with neither reduced NK cell activity nor suppression of the mitogen response *(44,46)*.

In contrast to the assumption that depression was associated with the suppression of nonspecific immunity, it has been argued that the compromised immunity may actually be secondary to an initial immune *activation*, not unlike an acute-phase response *(2,5,6)*. Products of an activated immune system (cytokines), may come to promote variations of HPA functioning and central monoamine activity, and these in turn subserve depressive symptoms. Indeed, depressed patients were found to display signs of immune activation, including increased plasma concentrations of complement proteins, C3 and C4, and immunoglobulin (Ig) M, as well as the positive acute-phase proteins haptoglobin, α_1-antitrypsin, and α_1, and α_2-macroglobulin, coupled with reduced levels of negative acute phase proteins *(2,47)*. Major depressive illness was also accompanied by an increased number of activated T cells (CD25$^+$ and HLA-DR$^+$) and secretion of neopterin, prostaglandin E$_2$, and thromboxane *(2,5)*. Furthermore, among depressed subjects the levels of circulating cytokines or their soluble receptors were elevated, including IL-2, soluble IL-2 receptors (sIL-2R), IL-1β, IL-1RA, IL-6, soluble IL-6 receptor (sIL-6R), and interferon-γ (IFN-γ) *(2,5,48–59)*. There have also been reports of increased mitogen-elicited production of the proinflammatory cytokines IL-1β, IL-6, and TNF-α *(2,5,50,51,60–63)*. Although the elevated levels of IL-1β, IL-6, and α_1-acid glycoprotein normalized with antidepressant medication *(49,59)*, such treatment did not affect the upregulated production of sIL-2R, IL-6, and sIL-6R in major depression *(2)* or that of IL-1 in patients suffering from chronic low-grade depression (dysthymia) *(60)*. Thus, these data raise the possibility that these cytokines may be trait markers of the illness *(2,5)*, although it is possible that more sustained treatment is necessary to realize normalization of the cytokine levels or activity *(64)*.

The data presently available concerning cytokine elevations in depressive illness are largely correlational. Thus, it is unclear whether the cytokine elevations are secondary to the illness (i.e., being directly or indirectly brought on by the depression) or play an etiologic role in the provocation of the disorder. However, high doses of IL-2, IFN-α, and TNF-α in humans undergoing immunotherapy induce neuropsychiatric symptoms, including depression, and these effects were related to the cytokine treatment rather than to the primary illness *(65–68)*. Furthermore, in animals the administration of cytokines such as IL-1β and TNF-α results in a constellation of symptoms referred to as sickness behaviors (which include not only soporific effects and reduced locomotor activity) and provokes an apparent anhedonia (reduced pleasure obtained from otherwise rewarding stimuli), which is a key symptom of depression. Of particular relevance is that the behavioral changes exerted by cytokines are not simply a reflection of malaise engendered by the treatments but are thought to arise owing to alterations of a centrally mediated motivational state *(10)*. In fact, in rodents, reward processes are disrupted by systemic treatment with LPS, independent of potential motoric factors or physical malaise *(37,69)*. Likewise, endotoxin administration reduces consumption of a palatable substance (again possibly reflecting anhedonia), and this effect was modifiable by antidepressant administration *(70)*. Together, these findings provide *prima facie* evidence in favor of the supposition that cytokines may play a provocative role in the elicitation of depressive symptoms.

Given the apparent contribution of cytokines to depressive illness, as well as to other psychiatric illnesses such as schizophrenia, increasing efforts have been devoted to the analysis of cytokines in psychiatric populations. **Subheading 3.** is typical of manuscripts dealing with cytokine functioning in depressive illnesses. Inasmuch as depression is associated with hormonal variations, and these hormonal factors may impact on immune and cytokine functioning, neuroendocrine factors are also determined. The procedural description is followed by a discussion of numerous caveats that need to be considered in the analysis of the biologic underpinnings of depressive illness (as well as other psychiatric conditions).

2. Materials

1. Radioimmunoassay kits for ACTH and cortisol (ICN Biomedicals).
2. High Sensitivity Quantikine kits for IL-1β, Il-2, IL-6, and their soluble receptors (R&D Systems, Minneapolis, MN).
3. Histopaque-1077 (Sigma).
4. Cell culture medium: RPMI, fetal calf serum, streptomycin (Gibco).

3. Methods

1. Subjects were amassed according to the following criteria. Patients were consecutive referrals to the Mood Disorders Program at the Royal Ottawa Hospital. Patients, 18–60 yr of age, with a diagnosis of major depression or dysthymia. Clinical assessments included a Structured Clinical Interview (SCID) *(71)*, conducted by a psychiatrist and confirmed by a second psychiatrist blind as to the initial diagnosis. During an initial screen visit, when written informed consent was obtained, demographic information was recorded, as were characteristics of the current depressive episode, as well as past history and family history of psychiatric illness. The major depressive patients fulfilled the *Diagnostic and Statistical Manual of Mental Disorders*, 4th ed. (DSM-IV) criteria for unipolar major depression and had mild-moderate severity on the Clinical Global Impressions scale (CGI) *(72)* and a score of 16–24 on the first 17 items of the 29-item Hamilton Depression Inventory (HAM-D) *(73)*. The dysthymic patients had a diagnosis of primary dysthymia and a score of 13–20 on the first 17 items of the HAM-D. Patients diagnosed with atypical depression were those who scored >6 on items 23–28 of the 29-item HAM-D and fulfilled the Columbia criteria for atypical depression with a score of ≥4 on the Atypical Depression Diagnostic Scales (ADDS) *(74)*. In addition to the HAM-D, depression scores were also obtained using the Montgomery-Asberg Depression Rating Scale *(75)* (*see* **Notes 1–8**).

2. Patients had no other Axis I diagnosis nor any physical or organic disorders. The presence of personality disorder was determined using the Millon Clinical Multiaxial Inventory-II (MCMI) *(76)*. Additionally, clinical evaluation included a full physical examination, as well as routine clinical investigations (full blood count, urinalysis, and electrocardiogram). The urinalysis was also used to ascertain the presence of drugs (e.g., alcohol or illicit drugs) that may influence either affective state or the behavioral, endocrine, or immune measures. Pregnant or lactating women or those of childbearing potential not using reliable contraception were not included. Exclusion criteria also included self-reported viral illness during the preceding 2 wk, severe allergies, multiple adverse drug reactions, or hypertension, significant recurrent dermatitis, malignant, hematologic, endocrine, pulmonary, cardiovascular, renal, hepatic, gastrointestinal, or neurologic disease (*see* **Notes 2–6**).

3. Nondepressed subjects, comprising volunteers obtained from large commercial and government organizations and community groups, served as normative controls. Subjects, matched for age, sex, and socioeconomic status, were screened using a structured clinical interview (M.I.N.I.) *(77)* to exclude past or present DSM-IV axis I disorders, had a Beck Depression Inventory (BDI) score of <4, and scored 0 on the first question of this scale "I do not feel sad" *(78)*. None of the control subjects had ever been treated with psychotropic medications or received behavioral therapy for depressive illness.

4. After clinical measures were obtained, patients underwent a washout period of at least a week, during which they received single-blind placebo. In addition, patients on prior psychoactive therapy had a further washout period, long enough so that the total duration off psychoactive medication before starting double-blind therapy was at least five half-lives of the medication (e.g., 5-wk wash-out for

fluoxetine, 4 wk for monoamine oxidase inhibitors [MAO-Is], 1 wk for most other antidepressant agents; *see* **Note 9**).

5. In addition to the clinical measures, at the commencement of the study, and following 12 wk of treatment, subjects completed a series of questionnaires to determine stressful life experiences encountered and coping styles used. These include a Life Events Scale to measure major stressors encountered *(79)*, the Daily Hassles and Uplifts Scales to assess ongoing minor stressors and uplifting experiences *(80)*, the Ways of Coping Questionnaire to determine the various coping strategies employed by subjects *(81)*, and the Batelle Quality of Life scale, which assesses quality of life across several domains *(82)*. Additionally, since the reliability of self-report questionnaires may be problematic owing to either over- or underreporting, a structured interview was administered *(83)* by one of the investigators well trained in this procedure. Finally, life style data were collected, including alcohol and cigarette consumption.

6. After washout and collection of blood samples, patients were treated with either placebo or a selective serotonin reuptake inhibitor (SSRI), sertraline (Zoloft), commencing with a dose of 50 mg (with 50-mg increments every 2 wk, to a maximum dose of 200 mg, as determined by treatment response and adverse events). The drug treatments were administered in a double-blind fashion, such that neither the treating physician nor the patient was aware of the treatment administered. The only concurrent psychotropic medication permitted during the study period was temazepam up to 30 mg at night as a hypnotic on an as-needed basis. Although the study was conducted as a double-blind, if patients exhibited obvious side effects or if their psychological condition worsened noticeably, the protocol required that patients be taken off the study and alternative drug therapy instituted. Patients were maintained on their respective drug schedules for a 12-wk period, after which the drug was downtitrated over 3 d; 4 d afterward blood samples were collected. Control subjects did not receive pharmacotherapy but were otherwise treated like the patient groups. Several patients dropped out of the study over the 12-wk trial. Their baseline measures were compared with those of subjects who completed the study to determine whether they were characteristic of the group as a whole.

7. Following the initial washout period, as well as after the washout following 12 wk of treatment, blood samples were collected from fasting subjects. To avoid potential confounding effects associated with diurnal hormonal variations, experimental procedures began between 0700 and 0830 h. Subjects had a catheter inserted into the antecubital fossa of their arm, while they sat comfortably in a sofa chair watching a neutral videotape. Using a Dakmed ambulatory pump, 60 mL blood of blood was withdrawn over a 2-h period (the lengthy interval precluded variability associated with pulsatile release of hormones) commencing 30 min after catheter insertion (to permit adaptation to the stress of catheter insertion: This duration was not sufficient to cause inflammation, which might have influenced the results). Each control subject was tested in tandem with a depressed patient so that the immunologic measures, which were performed using fresh blood, would not be unduly biased by between-days differences that may occur in the assay. (This is less problematic for endocrine measures, for which batches of plasma are assayed at once.)

8. Blood samples were processed within 1 h of being taken. Aliquots of blood pooled over this period were used to assay the various hormones, as well as mitogen-stimulated cytokine production. Tubes used for cortisol, ACTH, and amine determinations contained EDTA; samples used for mitogen-stimulated cytokine production contained sodium heparin. Serum cytokine levels were determined from the initial 10 min of blood collected (i.e., 30–50 min after catheter insertion). Samples used for serum cytokines were collected in tubes that contained a clot activator. Plasma samples used for endocrine analyses were quickly frozen and stored at –70°C, and those used for mitogen-stimulated lymphocytes were processed while fresh.

9. Plasma ACTH and cortisol levels were determined (in duplicate) using commercially available radioimmunoassay (RIA) kits (ICN Biomedicals). Using this method and crosschecking with internal standards, intra- and interassay variations were <10% for both hormones. The ACTH antiserum showed negligible (<0.1%) crossreactivity with β-endorphin, α-melanocyte stimulating hormone (α-MSH), β-MSH, α-lipotropin, or β-lipotropin. The cortisol antiserum showed crossreactivity of 6.1% with desoxycorticosterone, 0.29% with progesterone, and negligible (<0.1%) with other steroids including aldosterone, dihydroprogesterone, testosterone, and estradiol (*see* **Note 10**).

10. Plasma amines (NE and epinephrine [Epi]) were determined via high-performance liquid chromatography (HPLC) with coulometric detection, using a modification of the procedure of Seegal et al. *(84)*. Amine standards were dissolved in standard diluent (100 µg/mL stock solution). At the time of analysis an aliquot was diluted with 5% trichloroacetic acid (TCA) to 50 ng/mL (NE, Epi, and MHPG). To about 200 µL of thawed plasma was added an equal volume of 10% TCA for protein precipitation. The solution was shaken and microcentrifuged for 3 min (13,500 rpm), and the supernatant was placed in an HPLC vial. Using a Waters M-6000 pump, guard column, and radial compression column (5 µm, C_{18} reverse phase, 8 mm × 10 cm) and a three-cell coulometric electrochemical detector (ESA model 5100A), 20 µL of the supernatant was passed through the system at a flow rate of 1.5 mL/min (1400–1600 psi). The mobile phase consisted of 850 mL deionized H_2O, 1.3 g 1-heptane sulfonic acid, Na salt, 0.1 g EDTA, and 7.3 mL thiethylamine; the pH was adjusted to 2.45 using H_3PO_4. To this 60 mL acetonitrile was added, and the solution was made up to 1 L with deionized water, filtered using 0.22-µm filter paper, and then degassed. Area and height of curves was determined by a Hewlett-Packard integrator.

11. For determination of IL-1β, IL-2, IL-6, and their soluble receptors in serum, blood samples were spun for 10 min at 2000 rpm (700g), and then pipeted into Eppendorf tubes and stored at –80°C. The quantitative measurement of serum cytokines was later determined, in duplicate, using a commercially available High Sensitivity Quantikine kit (R&D Systems).

12. To determine mitogen-stimulated IL-1β and IL-2 production, mononuclear cells were isolated by layering whole blood onto Histopaque-1077 (Sigma) in a 1:1 dilution in a conical tube and centrifuged (400g) for 30 min at room temperature. The mononuclear fraction was washed in PBS containing streptomycin (3×), and centrifuged at 400g for 10 min at 4°C. The supernatant was discarded and the

cells resuspended in 5.0 mL of complete RPMI (containing 10% FCS). Mononuclear cells were counted and adjusted to 1×10^6/mL in complete RPMI. Mitogen was added (2.0, 4.0, or 6.0 µg LPS together with 1.0 µg phytohemagglutin (PHA) in a volume of 100 µL) to 1×10^6 cells in RPMI containing 10% FCS, penicillin-streptomycin (10,000 IU/L), streptomycin (10,000 µg/L), and sodium pyruvate (0.5 mL/L). The plates were incubated for 72 h in 5% CO_2 at 37°C and then centrifuged; the supernatant was then removed and stored at –80°C. For determination of IL-2 concentrations, a monoclonal antibody, anti-tac, was added to the cultures to prevent binding of IL-2 to receptors on activated T-cells *(85)*. Cytokines and their soluble receptors were determined, in duplicate, by ELISA in 96-well flat-bottomed titer plates, using kits obtained from R&D Systems (*see* **ref. 86** for a one-stage procedure).

13. Earlier studies in this laboratory demonstrated powerful treatment effects in dysthymic and major depressive patients. In fact, behavioral measures, as well as alterations of IL-1β, were observed with as few as 15 subjects per group. Allowing for a 10–15% dropout rate (based on our past studies), a sample of 25 subjects in each condition should provide sufficient power (80%) to detect a 65% improvement in the treatment groups (the rate that we and others have typically demonstrated in treating dysthymic and major depressive patients). It was of interest to ascertain whether behavioral/endocrine/cytokine measures of depressive and control patients could be distinguished from one another and whether placebo and drug treatment differentially influenced these variables (*see* **Notes 11–15**). It was also of particular interest to establish whether drug nonresponders could be distinguished from those of patients who showed a favorable treatment response (defined as a 50% decline in HAM-D scores and a 17-item HAM-D score <10; *see* **Notes 16–18**).

4. Notes

1. In evaluating the relationship between depression and cytokine changes, several factors need to be considered relating either to depressive illnesses, factors comorbid with or secondary to the depression, or characteristics of the depressed individual. Irwin *(43)* has described many of these direct or interactive effects and their implications for immune activity. Before setting out to analyze the relationship between mood and cytokines, it is of course essential to obtain a reliable diagnosis of the disorder. To this end, it is recommended that patients be assessed by a trained diagnostician, using the SCID for DSM-IV Axis I Disorders, which provides guidelines for a diagnosis of depression and also distinguishes subtypes of depression *(71)*. For research purposes a quantitative index of the illness is required, and several different scales are available such as the HAM-D (21- or 29-item) *(73)*, the Montgomery Asberg Depression Rating Scale (MADRS) *(75)*, or scales specialized for subtypes of depression, such as the Cornell Dysthymia Scale (for assessing dysthymic illness) *(87)* or the Atypical Depression Diagnostic Scales (ADDS) to assess atypical vs typical features of depression *(74)*.

2. In addition to the clinical features required for a diagnosis of depression, numerous functional and psychosocial features should be considered, since these may impact on cytokine levels or activity. For instance, all subtypes of depression

that we have examined are associated with increased stressor perception, inadequate or ineffective methods of coping with the stressor, reduced perception of uplifting events, diminished quality of life, and increased feelings of loneliness *(88)*. Psychosocial and financial stresses may also evolve secondary to the depression, and interpersonal skills may be greatly impaired; hence social buffering of stresses may be limited. Given that stressor experiences or perception may impact on immune and cytokine functioning *(42,89)*, it is obvious that cytokine changes may not be related to the mood disturbance *per se*, but may be secondary to the real or perceived stress associated with the illness.

3. Numerous comorbid features are often present in depressed individuals, including high levels of anxiety and personality disturbances; personal hygiene (neglect) may even be affected. Depressive illness may also be associated with increased drug use (including nicotine, alcohol, and illicit drugs), possibly in an effort to self-medicate. As indicated by Irwin *(43)*, a history of alcoholism may be associated with altered immune functioning, and still greater alterations of NK cell activity may be apparent in depressed patients with comorbid alcoholism *(90)*. Likewise, it appeared that smoking (tobacco) in depressed patients was associated with a greater reduction of NK cytotoxicity than would be expected from either depression or smoking alone. Irwin *(43)* suggested that such factors may affect cell proliferation, and the possibility ought to be considered that the altered levels of serum cytokines and acute-phase proteins might be related to these comorbid features.

4. In addition to the influence of the aforementioned features, it is important to consider that depressive illnesses tend to occur more frequently in women than in men. Thus, hormonal factors, or psychosocial factors related to sex (e.g., coping styles, stress and uplift perception), could potential affect the immune and cytokine processes. The relative importance of these factors remains to be deduced, but there is some suggestive evidence that immune functioning may differ in depressed men and women *(43)*.

5. The contribution of age to the immune changes associated with depression is difficult to gauge. Although several reviews have cited age of the depressed individual as one of the fundamental features indicating immune dysregulation *(41,44)*, it has been reported that among inpatient depressive subjects the degree of immunosuppression was unrelated to age *(91)*. Of course, as all patients in this study were severely depressed, the influence of the age variable may have been obfuscated. However, in studies conducted in our laboratory that involved outpatients suffering from depression of moderate severity, age was likewise found not to be related to either circulating NK cells *(92)* or the production of either IL-1β or IL-2 *(60)*. Interestingly, the duration of illness, and particularly the age of illness onset, may play a greater role in cytokine activity *(60)*.

6. As in the case of many pathologies, the selection of subjects can be an onerous task. Frequently patients may be prescribed medications unrelated to depression, which may impact on immune or cytokine functioning. These cover a wide range of agents, including antihistamines, analgesics, antihypertensives, and so forth. In a study of cytokine functioning such patients cannot be included, yet it should be considered that the comorbid features may be part of the depressive pathology

(heart disease, for instance, is associated with depression) or may either provoke or exacerbate depressive illness *(6)*. Thus, in excluding these patients, an important segment of the study population may be lost. This may be particularly important if it is considered that the stress of a pathology (or the pathology itself) may act synergistically with depressive state to promote cytokine alterations.

7. Several subtypes of depression exist that may differ with respect to etiology, neuro-chemical concomitants, course, symptoms, treatment, and hence the potential involvement of cytokine processes. The symptoms characterizing "typical" major depression comprise either depressed mood or loss of interest or pleasure (anhedonia), coupled with four of the following: feelings of worthlessness/guilt, diminished ability to think or concentrate, recurrent thoughts of death or suicidal ideation, and neurovegetative features such as weight loss, insomnia, psychomotor agitation/retardation, fatigue, or loss of energy. In a variant of the illness termed atypical depression, the symptoms comprise mood reactivity, coupled with reversed neurovegetative symptoms (hyperphagia, significant weight gain, hypersomnia), extreme fatigue, and persistent rejection sensitivity *(74,93)*. Furthermore, hypersecretion of CRH may be less prominent in atypical than in typical major depression *(94)*, and desipramine-elicited plasma cortisol secretion was greater in atypical patients, suggesting a less dysfunctional NE system *(95)*. Additionally, atypical patients, particularly women, responded preferentially to MAO-Is relative to tricyclic agents *(96)*. In typical major depression, neurovegetative symptoms can be marked, and it is certainly possible that these characteristics of the illness, quite apart from the mood disturbances, may support altered cytokine functioning. Indeed, sleep disturbance alone may promote altered cytokine activity *(97)*, and it is likewise possible that the reduced food intake and weight loss in typical major depression may come to provoke cytokine alterations. It was, in fact, reported that the altered NK cell activity in major depressive illness was correlated with two symptom clusters, namely, motor retardation and sleep disturbance *(98)*.

8. Given that sleep disturbances might contribute to the altered cytokine activity in depression, it ought to be considered that changes in circadian rhythms may likewise play a role in this respect. To be sure, depression is associated with a shift of the circadian pattern of HPA functioning, as well as that of cytokine production *(99)*. In fact, peak production of IFN-γ, TNF-α, IL-1, and IL-12 occurs at night and early morning, corresponding to the nadir of cortisol production. Such findings have implications not only for the variations seen with respect to symptoms of inflammatory disorders but also be for the apparent cytokine elevations in depressive illness. Although diurnal changes of NK cell activity were less profound in major depressive than controls, this did not reflect a shift of the circadian cycle *(43)*. As indicated by Irwin *(43)*, to obtain adequate information regarding phase shifts, multiple daily blood samples would be required. Whether such phase shifts occur with respect to cytokine production among depressive populations remains to be determined.

9. Typically, patients suffering depression (particularly severe depression or recurrent depressive illness) will not reach the point of a drug trial or a study of

depression until they have seen their family physicians or have visited a psychiatrist in hospital or private practice. Thus, these patients may previously have undergone some sort of treatment involving either pharmacologic or behavioral manipulations. In effect, these patients are not treatment-naïve, and the efficacy of the medication being applied in a given study may be confounded by expectancies on the part of the patients. Furthermore, if the subject has been taking any sort of psychotropic medication, then a washout period would be necessary to downtitrate medications. The duration of the washout is typically five half-lives of the drug, followed by a 1 wk placebo washout period (i.e., all patients receive placebo for a 1-wk period to ascertain whether any are rapid placebo responders).

10. In addition to the differing symptomatology, the two subtypes of depression may also be associated with different neurochemical processes. Thus, typical major depressive illness may involve elevated ACTH and cortisol, and atypical depression (or illnesses with atypical components, such as chronic fatigue syndrome, bulimia, or seasonal affective disorder) may be characterized by reduced basal plasma cortisol, increased basal ACTH, and reduced ACTH release following CRH challenge *(100–103)*. As indicated earlier, HPA functioning is affected by cytokines and conversely may affect cytokine functioning. These neuroendocrine differences form yet another reason to suspect that cytokine and immune differences might be expected in differing subtypes of depression.

11. Commensurate with the aforementioned proposition, we observed greater reductions in T-cell proliferation in typical than in atypical depressive patients *(104)*. Although typical vs atypical features did not influence the production of IL-1β in lymphocytes stimulated with PHA *(60)*, we observed that IL-1β in the serum of atypical depressive patients was elevated, and this was not the case in typical major depressive patients *(103)*. The mechanisms underlying the various characteristics of depression remain to be identified; however, it may be the case that the elevated levels of IL-1β contributed to the atypical symptomatology. Although high levels of IL-1β would be expected to reduce eating, a characteristic not seen in atypical patients, this cytokine may have contributed to the increased sleep and muscle fatigue, an effect consistent with the well-documented soporific effects of IL-1β *(10,12)*.

12. It appears that NK changes, as well as the elevations of cytokines and their soluble receptors, were dependent on the severity of the depressive illness *(2,5)*. Marked variations were observed in melancholic (severely depressed) patients but were less notable in moderately depressed patients. As the symptoms of melancholic depression are more profound that in typical major depression and the HPA disturbances are more common, the possible contribution of neurovegetative features, as well as hormonal dysregulation, to altered cytokine levels and production is still more likely. Additionally, as severe depression often requires hospitalization, it has been considered that this (and related factors such as change of diet, diurnal factors, social buffering, etc.) may be responsible for the altered immune and cytokine alterations *(41)*.

13. Related to symptom severity is the issue of those patients who are treatment resistant, that is, despite three or more pharmacologic attempts to alleviate the

symptoms, the depression persists. In terms of understanding the neurochemical (and cytokine) underpinnings of the disorder, one must question whether treatment-resistant patients reflect the same population (involving the same mechanisms) as those patients that respond to therapy.

14. In animals, many of the neurochemical and neuroendocrine effects of acute stressors are attenuated following a chronic stressor regimen *(93)*. This adaptation may be of limited effectiveness, and it is possible that the wear and tear on the system associated with a chronic stressor (referred to as allostatic load) may have particularly adverse consequences *(106)*. In a like fashion, it may be important to distinguish between the effects of acute and chronic depressive illness. In fact, it may be that chronic depression of a relatively mild nature (dysthymia) may have particular effects. This form of depression persists for at least 2 yr and is often associated with early onset (<20 yr of age). Interestingly, dysthymic patients have a heightened comorbidity for numerous psychiatric conditions, such as anxiety and personality disorders, as well as alcohol abuse, and are at risk for the development of a major depression superimposed on the dysthymic state (double depression). It has been found that among dysthymic patients, mitogen-stimulated production of IL-1β is appreciably increased, and the extent of the increase is positively correlated with the duration of illness. Thus, it seems that even in the absence of a severe depressive episode, altered cytokine activity may occur, provided that the depressive illness is sufficiently long-lasting.

15. It has been suggested that certain peptides such as CRH and thyroid-releasing hormone (TRH) may play an integral role in subserving the depression *(107,108)* and that alterations in peptide release provoked by stressors may influence mood states. Although the peptide variations elicited by an acute stressor were fairly transient, with repeated challenges the release of some peptides would be more readily induced and might also be more persistent. The initial episode of depression may stem from stressor-provoked peptidergic alterations. However, with each subsequent stressor experience, or with each episode of depression, the peptidergic systems may become sensitized so that progressively less intense psychosocial stressors provoke the onset of a depressive episode. Ultimately, the depressive episodes may become manifest even in the absence of obvious stress triggers. Given the interrelationships between neuropeptides and cytokine functioning, the possibility should be explored that cytokine alterations might likewise vary with first vs subsequent depressive episodes.

16. If depressive illness and altered cytokine levels or production are related to one another (even if this relationship is an indirect one, such as being secondary to the stress associated with the illness), then it might be expected that successful alleviation of the illnesses would eliminate or reduce the aberrant cytokine levels. Not surprisingly, numerous caveats need to be considered in assessing the sequelae of pharmacologic intervention in depression.

17. Only a subset of patients exhibit beneficial effects following treatment with a given agent. The view has often been expressed that depression is a biochemically heterogeneous disorder, and hence it would be expected that a positive effect would be most likely if the drug acts on neural systems associated with the disorder. Given the

potential biochemical diversity underlying depression, considerable variability would be expected with respect to cytokine correlates of depression. Moreover, it follows that attenuation of cytokine abnormalities would only occur if the pharmacologic agent were effective in alleviating the illness. In effect, the appropriate comparison condition would not be that of drug- vs placebo-treated patients, but instead drug responders vs nonresponders vs placebo-treated patients. Parenthetically, a positive response is obtained in a substantial portion of placebo-treated patients (approx 30%). In a proportion of these subjects, the positive response is transient, lasting a week or so; in others the effect is long-lasting. It has been suggested that in placebo-treated patients functional disturbances (e.g., diminished quality of life) may persist despite apparent clinical improvement and hence, relapse and recurrence may be particularly high *(109)*. By the same token, among drug-treated subjects that display a positive response, it would be reasonable to suspect that a proportion actually are displaying a placebo response rather than a genuine drug-related improvement. As relapse/recurrence in these patients will probably occur at a high rate, it is questionable whether the mechanisms associated with their improvement are the same as those of "genuine responders," and hence it might be expected that the cytokine correlates of their illness would differ from those of the true responders.

18. As indicated earlier, some pharmacologic studies indicated that aspects of cytokine functioning are normalized with symptom alleviation, and other studies reported that such effects did not occur *(29)*. One should not conclude from this that cytokines are not involved in depressive illness. First, it is possible that abnormal cytokine levels represent trait markers, rather than state markers of the illness. That is, those individuals vulnerable to depression have high levels of the cytokine(s), which may or may not play a provocative role in the illness. Alleviation of depression would thus not result in normalization of cytokine levels. If they do play a role in the illness, the persistence of the abnormal cytokine levels may be an important marker in identifying individuals at risk for relapse. At this point it is important to note, as well, that if cytokine changes were associated with depression, it is not necessarily the case that normalization would be evident contemporaneously with symptom alleviation, particularly for chronic depression: Biologic sequelae of the illness lag behind symptom alleviation *(63)*. Even if one observes that a pharmacologic treatment influences depression and also alters cytokine functioning, it cannot be concluded that the cytokine changes were secondary to alleviation of depression. After all, the drug treatment may have multiple effects, one of which involves its antidepressant actions, and a second independent action may be that of attenuating immune and cytokine activity. If cytokine alterations result directly from alleviation of depression, then it might be expected that attenuation of the cytokine actions would be apparent using nonpharmacologic treatment of the disorder. In the case of depressive illness, it would be expected that treatment such as cognitive therapy would likewise result in normalization of the cytokine changes following symptom remission. To date, we are unaware of any studies that assessed nonpharmacologic agents to evaluate cytokine correlates of depressive illness.

Acknowledgments

This work was supported by the Medical Research Council of Canada. H.A. is an Ontario Mental Health Senior Research Fellow.

References

1. Anisman, H., Zalcman, S., Shanks, N., and Zacharko, R. M. (1991) Multisystem regulation of performance deficits induced by stressors: An animal model of depression, in *Neuromethods: Animal Models of Psychiatry, II, vol. 19.* (Boulton, A., Baker, G., Martin-Iverson, M., eds.), Humana Press, Totowa, NJ, pp. 1–59.
2. Maes, M. (1999) Major depression and activation of the inflammatory response system. *Adv. Exp. Med. Biol.* **461,** 25–46.
3. Blalock, J. E. (1994) The syntax of immune-neuroendocrine communication. *Immunol. Today* **15,** 504–511.
4. Rothwell, N. J. and Hopkins, S. J. (1995) Cytokines and the nervous system. II: Actions and mechanisms of action. *Trends Neurosci.* **18,** 130–136.
5. Maes, M. (1995) Evidence for an immune response in major depression: a review and hypothesis. *Prog. Neuropsychopharmacol. Biol. Psychiatry* **19,** 11–38.
6. Licinio, J. and Wong, M. L. (1999) The role of inflammatory mediators in the biology of major depression: central nervous system cytokines modulate the biological substrate of depressive symptoms, regulate stress-responsive systems, and contribute to neurotoxicity and neuroprotection. *Mol. Psychiatry* **4,** 317–327.
7. Yirimaya, R., Weidenfeld, J., Pollak, Y., Morag, M., Morag, A., Avitsur, R., et al. (1999) Cytokines, "depression due to a general medical condition," and antidepressant drugs. *Adv. Exp. Med. Biol.* **461,** 283–316.
8. Anisman, H., Zalcman, S., and Zacharko, R. M. (1993) The impact of stressors on immune and central neurotransmitter activity: bidirectional communication. *Rev. Neurosci.* **4,** 147–180.
9. Dunn, A. J. (1995) Interactions between the nervous system and the immune system, in *Psychopharmacology: The Fourth Generation of Progress* (Bloom, F. E. and Kupfer, D. J., eds.), Raven, NY, pp. 719–731.
10. Dantzer, R., Bluthe, R. M., Aubert, A., Goodall, G., Bret-Dibat, J.-L., Kent, S., et al. (1996) Cytokine actions on behavior, in *Cytokines and the Nervous System.* (Rothwell, N. J., ed.), Landes, London, pp. 117–144.
11. Ek, M., Kurosawa, M., Lundenberg, T., and Ericsson, A. (1998) Activation of vagal afferents after intravenous injection of interleukin-1β: role of endogenous prostaglandins. *J. Neurosci.* **18,** 9471–9479.
12. Maier, S. F. and Watkins, L. R. (1998) Cytokines for psychologists: implications of bidirectional immune-to-brain communication for understanding behavior, mood, and cognition. *Psychol. Rev.* **105,** 83–107.
13. Banks, W. A., Ortz, L., Plotkin, S. R., and Kasten, A. J. (1991) Human interleukin (IL) 1 alpha, murine IL-1 alpha and murine IL-2 beta are transported from blood to brain in the mouse by a shared saturable mechanism. *J. Pharmacol. Exp. Ther.* **259,** 988–996.

14. Plata-Salaman, C. and Turrin, N. (1999) Cytokine interactions and cytokine balance in the brain: relevance to neurology and psychiatry. *Mol. Psychiatry* **4**, 303–306.
15. Rothwell, N. J. (1999) Cytokines—killers in the brain. *J. Physiol.* **514**, 3–17.
16. Minami, M., Kuraishi, Y., Yamaguchi, T., Nakai, S., Hirai, Y., and Satoh, M. (1991) Immobilization stress induces interleukin-1β mRNA in rat hypothalamus. *Neurosci. Lett.* **123**, 254–256.
17. Nguyen, K. T., Deak, T., Owens, S. M., Kohno, T., Fleshner, M., Watkins, L. R., and Maier, S. F. (1998) Exposure to acute stress induces brain interleukin-1β protein in the rat. *J. Neurosci.* **18**, 2239–2246.
18. Nguyen K. Y., Deak, T., Hunsaker, B., Fleshner, M., Watkins, L. R., and Maier, S. (1999) Effects of stress on interleukin-1β and interleukin-6 protein in the brain and periphery. PNIRS Meeting P1. 37, Abst #98.
19. Shintani, F., Nakaki, T., Kanba ,S., Sato, K., Kato, R., and Asai, M. (1995) Role of interleukin-1 in stress responses. *Mol. Neurobiol.* **10**, 47–71.
20. Plata-Salamán, C. R., Ilyin, S. E., Gayle, D., Flynn, M. C., Turrin, N. P., Bedard, T., et al. (2000) Neither acute nor chronic exposure to a naturalistic (predator) stressor influences the IL-1β system, TNF-α, TGF-β1, and neuropeptide mRNAs, CRH or bombesin content in specific brain regions. *Brain Res. Bull.* **51**, 187–193.
21. Ericsson, A., Kovacs, K. J., and Sawchenko, P. E. (1994) A functional anatomical analysis of central pathways subserving the effects of interleukin-1 on stress-related neuroendocrine neurons. *J. Neurosci.* **14**, 89–91.
22. Rivest S. and Rivier C. (1994) Stress and interleukin-1 beta-induced activation of c-Fos, Ngfi-B and CRF gene expression in the hypothalamic PVN—comparison between Sprague-Dawley, Fisher-344 and Lewis rats. *J. Neuroendocrinol.* **6**, 101–117.
23. Turnbull, A. V. and Rivier, C. (1996) Cytokine effects on neuroendocrine axes: influence of nitric oxide and carbon monoxide, in *Cytokines in the Nervous System* (Rothwell, N. J., ed.), R. G. Landes, London, pp. 93–116.
24. Dunn, A. J. (1992) Endotoxin-induced activation of cerebral catecholamine and serotonin metabolism: comparison with interleukin-1. *J. Pharmacol. Exp. Ther.* **261**, 964–969.
25. Lacosta, S., Merali, Z., and Anisman, H. (1998) Influence of interleukin-1 on exploratory behavior, plasma ACTH and corticosterone, and central biogenic amines in mice. *Psychopharmacology* **137**, 351–361.
26. Lacosta, S., Merali, Z., and Anisman, H. (1999) Behavioral and neurochemical consequences of lipopolysaccharide in mice: anxiogenic-like effects. *Brain Res.* **818**, 291–303.
27. Anisman, H. and Merali, Z. (1999) Anhedonic and anxiogenic effects of cytokine exposure. *Adv. Exp. Med. Biol.* **461**, 199–233.
28. Gemma, C., Ghezzi, P., and De Simoni, M. G. (1991) Activation of the hypothalamic serotonergic system by central interleukin-1. *Eur. J. Pharmacol.* **209**, 139–140.
29. Mohankumar, P. S. and Quadri, S. K. (1993) Systemic administration of interleukin-1 stimulates norepinephrine release in the paraventricular nucleus. *Life Sci.* **52**, 1961–1967.

30. Mohankumar, P. S., Thyagarajan, S., and Quadri, S. K. (1991) Interleukin-1 stimulates the release of dopamine and dihydroxyphenylacetic acid from hypothalamus in vivo. *Life Sci.* **48,** 925–930.
31. Smagin, G. N., Swiergiel, A. H., and Dunn, A. J. (1996) Peripheral administration of interleukin-1 increases extracellular concentrations of norepinephrine in rat hypothalamus: comparison with plasma corticosterone. *Psychoneuroendocrinology* **21,** 83–93.
32. Linthorst, A. C. E., Flachskamm, C., Muller-Preuss, P., Holsboer, F., and Reul, J. M. H. M. (1995) Effect of bacterial endotoxin and interleukin-1β on hippocampal serotonergic neurotransmission, behavioral activity, and free corticosterone levels: an in vivo microdialysis study. *J. Neurosci.* **15,** 2920–2934.
33. Merali, Z., Lacosta, S., and Anisman, H. (1997) Effects of interleukin-1β and mild stress on alterations of central monoamines: a regional microdialysis study. *Brain Res.* **761,** 225–235.
34. Song, C., Merali, Z., and Anisman, H. (1998) Variations of nucleus accumbens dopamine and serotonin following systemic interleukin-1, interleukin-2 or interleukin-6 treatment. *Neuroscience* **88,** 823–836.
35. Hayley, S., Brebner, K., Merali, Z., and Anisman, H. (1999) Sensitization to the effects of tumor necrosis factor-α: neuroendocrine, central monoamine, and behavioral variations. *J. Neurosci.* **19,** 5654–5665.
36. Deutch, A. Y. and Roth, R. H. (1990) The determinants of stress-induced activation of the prefrontal cortical dopamine system. *Prog. Brain Res.* **85,** 367–403.
37. Borowski, T., Kokkinidis, L., Merali, Z., and Anisman, H. (1998) Lipopolysaccharide, central in vivo amine alterations, and anhedonia. *Neuroreport* **9,** 3797–3802.
38. Tilders, F. J. H. and Schmidt, E. D. (1998) Interleukin-1-induced plasticity of hypothalamic CRH neurons and long-term stress hyperresponsiveness. *Ann. NY Acad. Sci.* **840,** 65–73.
39. Tilders, F. J. H., Schmidt, E. D., and De Goeij, D. C. E. (1993) Phenotypic plasticity of CRF neurons during stress. *Ann. NY Acad. Sci.* **697,** 39–52.
40. Schmidt, E. D., Janszen, A. W. J. W., Wouterlood, F. G., and Tilders, F. J. H. (1995) Interleukin-1 induced long-lasting changes in hypothalamic corticotropin-releasing hormone (CRH) neurons and hyperresponsiveness of the hypothalamic-pituitary-adrenal axis. *J. Neurosci.* **15,** 7417–7426.
41. Herbert T. B. and Cohen, S. (1993) Depression and immunity: a meta-analytic review. *Psychol. Bull.* **113,** 472–486.
42. Herbert, T. B. and Cohen, S. (1993) Stress and immunity in humans: a meta-analytic review. *Psychosom. Med.* **55,** 364–379.
43. Irwin, M. (1999) Immune correlates of depression. *Adv. Exp. Med. Biol.* **461,** 1–24.
44. Weisse, C. S. (1992) Depression and immunocompetence: a review of the literature. *Psychol. Bull.* **113,** 475–586.
45. Irwin, M. R., Smith, T. L., and Gillin, J. C. (1992) Electroencephalographic sleep and natural killer cell activity in depressed patients and control subjects. *Psychosom. Med.* **54,** 10–21.
46. Stein, M., Keller, S. E., and Schleifer, S. J. (1982) The role of brain and the neuroendocrine system in immune regulation-potential links to neoplastic

diseases, in *Biological Mediators of Behavior and Disease: Neoplasia* (Levy, S. M., ed.), Elsevier, NY, pp. 147–174.

47. Sluzewska, A. (1999) Indicators of immune activation in depressed patients. *Adv. Exp. Med. Biol.* **461**, 59–74.

48. Berk, M., Wadee, A. A., Kuschke, R. H., and O'Neill-Kerr, A. (1997) Acute phase proteins in major depression. *J. Psychosom. Res.* **43**, 529–534.

49. Frommberger, U. H., Bauer, J., Haselbauer, P., Fraulin, A., Riemann, D., and Berger, M. (1997) Interleukin-6 (IL-6) plasma levels in depression and schizophrenia: comparison between the acute state and after remission. *Eur. Arch. Psychiatry. Clin. Neurosci.* **247**, 228–233.

50. Maes, M., Bosmans, E., Meltzer, H. Y., Scharpe, S., and Suy, E. (1993) Interleukin-1β: a putative mediator of HPA axis hyperactivity in major depression? *Am. J. Psychiatry* **150**, 1189–1193.

51. Maes, M., Bosmans, E., Suy, E., Vandervorst, C., de Jonckheere, C., Minner, B., et al. (1991) Depression-related disturbances in mitogen-induced lymphocyte responses and interleukin-1β and soluble interleukin-2 receptor production. *Acta Psychiatr. Scand.* **84**, 379–386.

52. Maes, M., Lambrechts, J., Bosmans, E., Jacobs, J., Suy, E., Vandervorst, C., et al. (1992) Evidence for a systemic immune activation during depression: results of leukocyte enumeration by flow cytometry in conjunction with monoclonal antibody staining. *Psychol. Med.* **22**, 45–53.

53. Maes, M., Meltzer, H. Y., Bosmans, E., Bergmans, R., Vandoolaeghe, E., Ranjan, R., et al. (1995) Increased plasma concentrations of interleukin-6, soluble interleukin-6, soluble interlcukin 2 and transferrin receptor in major depression. *J. Affect. Disord.* **34**, 301–309.

54. Mullar, N. and Ackenheil, M. (1998) Psychoneuroimmunology and the cytokine action in the CNS: implications for psychiatric disorders. *Prog. Neuropsychopharm. Biol. Psychiatry* **22**, 1–33.

55. Nassberger, L. and Traskman-Bendz, L. (1993) Increased soluble interleukin-2 receptor concentrations in suicide attempters. *Acta Psychiatr. Scand.* **88**, 48–52.

56. Smith, R. S. (1991) The macrophage theory of depression. *Med. Hypoth.* **35**, 298–306.

57. Song, C., Dinan, T., and Leonard, B. E. (1994) Changes in immunoglobulin, complement and acute phase protein levels in depressed patients and normal controls. *J. Affect. Disord.* **30**, 283–288.

58. Maes, M., Bosmans, E., De Jongh, R., Kenis, G., Vandoolaeghe, E., and Neels, H. (1997) Increased serum IL-6 and IL-1 receptor antagonist concentrations in major depression and treatment resistant depression. *Cytokine* **9**, 853–858.

59. Sluzewska, A., Rybakowski, J. K., Laciak, M., Mackiewicz, A., Sobieska, M., and Wiktorowicz, K. (1995) Interleukin-6 serum levels in depressed patients before and after treatment with fluoxetine. *Ann. NY Acad. Sci.* **762**, 474–476.

60. Anisman, H., Ravindran, A. V., Griffiths, J.. and Merali, Z. (1999) Endocrine and cytokine correlates of major depression and dysthymia with typical or atypical features. *Mol. Psychiatry* **4**, 182–188.

61. Anisman, H., Ravindran, A. V., Griffiths, J., and Merali, H. (1999) Interleukin-1 variations associated with dysthymia prior to and following antidepressant medication. *Biol. Psychiatry* **46**, 1649–1655.

62. Maes, M., Scharpe, S., Meltzer, H. Y., Bosmans, E., Suy, E., Calabrese, J., and Cosyns, P. (1993) Relationships between interleukin-6 activity, acute phase proteins, and function of the hypothalamic-pituitary-adrenal axis in severe depression. *Psychiatry Res.* **49,** 11–27.

63. Seidel, A., Arolt, V., Hunstiger, M., Rink, L., Behnisch. A., and Kirchner, H. (1995) Cytokine production and serum proteins in depression. *Scand. J. Immunol.* **41,** 534–538.

64. Griffiths, J., Ravindran, A. V., and Merali, Z., and Anisman, H. (2000) Dysthymia: neurochemical and behavioral perspectives. *Mol. Psychiatry* **5,** 242–261.

65. Capuron, L., Ravaud, A., Radat, F., Dantzer, R., and Goodall, G. (1998) Affects of interleukin-2 and alpha-interferon cytokine immunotherapy on the mood and cognitive performance of cancer patients. *Neuroimmunomodulation* **5,** 9.

66. Caraceni, A., Martini, C., Belli, F., Mascheroni, L., Rivoltini, L., Arienti, F., et al. (1992) Neuropsychological and neurophysiological assessment of the central effects of interleukin-2 administration, *Eur. J. Cancer* **29A,** 1266–1269.

67. Denicoff, K. D., Rubinow, D. R., Papa, M. Z., Simpson, L., Seipp, L. A., Lotze, M. T., et al. (1987) The neuropsychiatric effects of treatment with interleukin-2 and lymphokine-activated killer cells. *Ann. Intern. Med.* **107,** 293–300.

68. Meyers, C. A. and Valentine, A. D. (1995) Neurological and psychiatric adverse effects of immunological therapy. *CNS Drugs* **3,** 56–68.

69. Anisman, H. and Merali, Z. (1999) Cytokines and stress in relation to anxiety and anhedonia, in *Cytokines, Stress and Depression* (Dantzer, R., Wollmann, E. E., and Yirmiya, R., eds.), Plenum, London, pp. 199–223.

70. Yirmiya, R. (1996) Endotoxin produces a depressive-like episode in rats. *Brain Res.* **711,** 163–174.

71. First, M. B., Gibbon, M., Soitzer, R. L., and Williams, J. B. W. (1996) *User's Guide for the Structured Clinical Interview for DSM-IV Axis I Disorders— Research Version.* Biometrics Research, NY.

72. Guy, W. (1976) *ECDEU Assessment Manual for psychopharmacology.* NIMH, Psychopharmacology Research Branch, Bethesda, MD.

73. Hamilton, M. (1967) Development of a rating scale for primary depressive illness. *Br. J. Soc. Clin. Psychol.* **6,** 278–298.

74. Liebowitz, M. R., Quikin, F. M., Stewart, J. W., McGrath, P. J., Harrison, W. M., Markowitz, J. S., et al. (1988) Antidepressant specificity in atypical depression. *Arch. Psychiatry* **45,** 129–137.

75. Montgomery, S. A. and Asberg, M. (1979) A new depression scale designed to be sensitive to change. *Br. J. Psychiatry* **134,** 382–389.

76. Millon, T. (1987) *Manual for the Millon Clinical Multiaxial Inventory-II,* 2nd ed. National Computer Systems, Minneapolis.

77. Sheehan, D., Lecrubier, Y., Janavs, J., Knapp, E., Weiller, E., Sheehan, M., et al. (1998) *Mini-international Neuropsychiatric Interview. Clinician-Rated.* Version 2. 1. University of South Florida Institute for Research in Psychiatry, Tampa, Florida, and INSERM-Hôpital de la Salpêtrière, Paris, France.

78. Beck, A. T., Ward, C. H., Mendelson, M., Mock, J., and Erbaugh, J. (1961) An inventory for measuring depression. *Arch. Gen. Psychiatry* **4,** 561–569.

79. Paykel, E. S., Prusoff B. A., and Uhlenhuth, E. H. (1971) Scaling of life events. *Arch. Gen. Psychiatry* **25,** 340–347.
80. Kanner, A. D., Coyne, J. C., Schaefer, C., and Lazarus, R. S. (1981) Comparison of two modes of stress measurement: daily hassles and uplifts versus major life events. *J. Behav. Med.* **4,** 1–39.
81. Beckham, E. E. and Adams, R. L. (1984) Coping behavior in depression: report on a new scale. *Behav. Res. Ther.* **22,** 71–75.
82. Ravicki, D. A., Turner, R., Brown, R., and Martindale, J. J. (1992) Batelle Quality of Life Scale. *Qual. Life. Res.* **1,** 257–266.
83. Brown, G. W. and Harris, T. O. (1978) Social *Origins of Depression: A Study of Psychiatric Disorder in Women.* Free Press, NY.
84. Seegal, R. F., Brosch, K. O., and Bush, B. (1986) High-performance liquid chromatography of biogenic amines and metabolites in brain, cerebrospinal fluid, urine and plasma. *J. Chromatogr.* **377,** 141–144.
85. Baroja, M. L. and Cueppens, J. L. (1987) More exact quantification of interleukin-2 production by addition of anti-Tac monoclonal antibody to cultures of stimulated lymphocytes. *J. Immunol. Methods* **98,** 267–270.
86. De Groote, D., Gevaert, Y., Lopez, M., Gathy, R., Fauchet, F., Dehart, I., et al. (1993) Novel method for the measurement of cytokine production by a one-stage procedure. *J. Immunol. Methods* **163,** 259–267.
87. Mason, B. J., Kocsis, J. H., Leon, A. C., Thompson, S., Frances, A. J., Morgan, R. O., and Parides, M. K. (1993) Measurement of severity and treatment response in dysthymia. *Psychiatr. Ann.* **23,** 625–631.
88. Ravindran, A., Griffiths, J., Waddell, C., and Anisman, H. (1995) Stressful life events and coping styles in dysthymia and major depressive disorder: variations associated with alleviation of symptoms following pharmacotherapy. *Prog. Neuropsychopharmacol. Biol. Psychiatry.* **19,** 637–653.
89. Kiecolt-Glazer, J. K. and Glazer, R. (1991) Stress and immune function in humans, in *Psychoneuroimmunology* (Ader, R., Felten, D. L., and Cohen, N., eds.), Academic, San Diego, CA, pp. 849–867.
90. Irwin, M. R., Caldwell, C., Smith, T. L., Brown, S., Schuckit, M. A., and Gillin, J. C. (1990) Major depressive disorder, alcoholism, and reduced natural killer cytotoxicity: role of severity of depressive symptoms and alcohol consumption. *Arch. Gen. Psychiatry* **47,** 713–719.
91. Irwin, M. R., Patterson, T. L., Smith, T. L., Caldwell, C., Brown, S., Gillin, J. C., et al. (1990) Reduction of immune function in life stress and depression. *Biol. Psychiatry* **27,** 22–30.
92. Ravindran, A. V., Griffiths, J., Merali, Z., and Anisman, H. (1998) Circulating lymphocyte subsets in major depression and dysthymia with typical or atypical features. *Psychosom. Med.* **60,** 283–289.
93. Quitkin, F. M., Harrison, W. M., Stewart, J. W., McGrath, P. J., Tricamo, E., Ocepek-Welikson, K., et al. (1991) Response to phenelzine and imipramine in placebo responders with atypical depression. *Arch. Gen. Psychiatry* **48,** 319–323.
94. Nemeroff, C. B. (1996) The corticotropin-releasing factor (CRF) hypothsesis of depression: new findings and new directions. *Mol. Psychiatry* **1,** 336–342.

95. McGinn, L. K., Asnis, G. M., and Rubinson, E. (1996) Biological and clinical validation of atypical depression. *Psychiat. Res.* **60,** 191–198.

96. McGrath, P. J., Stewart, J. W., Harrison, W. M., Ocepek-Wilekson, K., Rabkin, J. G., Nunes, E. N., et al. (1992) Predictive value of symptoms of atypical depression for differential drug treatment outcome. *J. Clin. Psychopharmacol.* **12,** 197–202.

97. Moldofsky, H. (1995) Sleep and the immune system. *Int. J. Immunopharmacol.* **17,** 649–654.

98. Cover, H. and Irwin, M. (1994) Immunity and depression: insomnia, retardation and reduction of natural killer cell activity. *J. Behav. Med.* **17,** 217–223.

99. Petrovsky, N. and Harrison, L. C. (1997) Diurnal rhythmicity of human cytokine production. *J. Immunol.* **158,** 5163–5168.

100. Demitrack, M. A., Dale, J. K., Straus, S. E., Laue, L., Listwak, S. J., Kruesi, M. J. P., et al. (1991) Evidence for impaired activation of the hypothalamic-pituitary-adrenal axis in patients with chronic fatigue syndrome. *J. Clin. Endocrinol. Metab.* **148,** 337–344.

101. Gold, P. W., Licinio, J., Wong, M. L., and Chrousos, G. P. (1995) Corticotropin releasing hormone in pathophysiology of melancholic and atypical depression and in the mechanism of action of antidepressant drugs. *Ann. NY Acad. Sci.* **771,** 716–729.

102. Joseph-Vanderpool, J. R., Rosenthal, N. E., Chrousos, G. P., Wehr, T. A., Skwerer, R., Kasper, S., and Gold, P. W. (1991) Abnormal pituitary-adrenal responses to corticotropin-releasing hormone in patients with seasonal affective disorder: clinical and pathophysiological implications. *J. Clin. Endocrinol. Metab.* **72,** 1382–1387.

103. Levitan, R. D., Kaplan, A. S., Brown, G. M., Joffe, R. T., Levitt, A. J., Vaccarino, F. J., et al. (1997) Low plasma cortisol in bulimia nervosa patients with reversed neurovegetative symptoms of depression. *Biol. Psychiatry* **41,** 366–368.

104. Zaharia, M. D., Ravindran, A. V., Griffiths, J., Merali, Z., and Anisman, H. (2000) Lymphocyte proliferation among major depressive and dysthymic patients with typical or atypical features. *J. Affect. Disord.* **58,** 1–10.

105. Griffiths, A. V. Ravindran, Z., Merali, Z., and Anisman, H. (1996) Immune and behavioral correlates of typical and atypical depression. *Soc. Neurosci.* (Abst) **22,** 1350.

106. Schulkin, J., Gold, P. W., and McEwen, B. S. (1998) Induction of corticotropin-releasing hormone gene expression by glucocorticoids: implication for understanding the states of fear and anxiety and allostatic load. *Psychoneuroendocrinology* **23,** 219–243.

107. Post, R. M. (1992) Transduction of psychosocial stress into the neurobiology of recurrent affective disorder. *Am. J. Psychiatry* **149,** 999–1010.

108. Post, R. M. and Weiss, S. R. B. (1995) The neurobiology of treatment-resistant mood disorders, in *Psychopharmacology: The Fourth Generation of Progress* (Bloom, F. E. and Kupfer, D. J., eds.), Raven, NY, pp. 1155–1170.

109. Ravindran, A. V., Anisman, H., Merali, Z. Charbonneau, Y., Telner, J., Bialik, R. J., et al. (1999) Treatment of primary dysthymia with cognitive therapy and pharmacotherapy: clinical symptoms and functional Impairments. *Am. J. Psychiatry* **156,** 1608–1617.

20

Measurement of Interleukins in Cutaneous Disorders

Competitive RT-PCR for Determination of IL-10 mRNA Expression in Psoriasis

Khusru Asadullah, Antje Haeussler-Quade, Wolf Dietrich Doecke, Wolfram Sterry, and Hans-Dieter Volk

1. Introduction

Cytokines are considered to be of major importance for the pathogenesis of several cutaneous disorders. Their considerable impact may result from autocrine, paracrine, or endocrine effects. Consequently, numerous investigations aim to measure cytokines, including interleukins. Since reliable determination of cutaneous interleukin expression at the protein level is problematic (*see* **Notes 1–7**), determination of mRNA expression came to the forefront of scientific interest. Such approaches, however, are associated with difficulties in the quantification of gene transcripts.

1.1. Cytokines and Psoriasis

Psoriasis is a common cutaneous disorder characterized by inflammation and abnormal epidermal proliferation, with a prevalence of 2–3% in the general population (*1*). Several reports indicate that T cells and cytokines (*2–8*) are of major importance in the pathogenesis of this chronic skin disease. These observations are supported by the beneficial effects of systemic administration of immunosupressive drugs like cyclosporin A, FK506, and fumaric acid esters, known to act on T cells and to influence the cytokine pattern. According to the predominant expression of interleukin (IL)-2 and interferon (IFN)-γ and the lack of IL-4 in skin lesions, psoriasis is believed to be characterized by a type 1 cytokine pattern (*4,5*). Moreover, the involvement of other proinflammatory cytokines like IL-1, IL-6, IL-8, and tumor necrosis factor (TNF)-α has been

From: *Methods in Molecular Medicine, vol. 60: Interleukin Protocols*
Edited by: L. A. J. O'Neill and A. Bowie © Humana Press Inc., Totowa, NJ

demonstrated *(9–12)*. In contrast to proinflammatory cytokines, there was only limited knowledge regarding the role of antiinflammatory cytokines, in particular IL-10, in psoriasis. Thus, conflicting data have been published. Whereas IL-10 mRNA was detected rarely or not at all by some authors *(4,5)*, overexpression has been reported by others *(10,13)*. This may partly result from the different polymerase chain reaction (PCR) techniques used. Obtaining reliable data regarding IL-10 expression seems to be of particular importance, however, since IL-10 has great impact on immunoregulation. It promotes the development of a type 2 cytokine pattern by inhibiting the IFN-γ production of T-lymphocytes and natural killer cells, particularly via the suppression of IL-12 synthesis in accessory cells *(14)*. Moreover, it suppresses proinflammatory cytokine production and the antigen-presenting capacity of monocytes/macrophages and dendritic cells *(15,16)*.

1.2. Measurement of Cytokines by Competitive RT-PCR

For measurement of intracutaneous cytokine gene expression level in psoriasis and other dermatoses, we established a competitive reverse transcriptase (RT-PCR) technique *(17,18)*. This technique was developed according to the technique already introduced by Wang et al. *(19)* and was adapted for measurement of the cytokine gene transcription by Platzer et al. *(20)* and Siegling et al. *(21)*. Quantification of cytokine cDNA derived from mRNA was carried out using multispecific control fragments as an internal standard for competitive PCR in multiple-step analyses and the oligonucleotides indicated in **Table 1**. First, the cDNA samples to be compared were equilibrated according to their glyceraldehyde-3-phosphate-dehydrogenase cDNA housekeeping gene expression content. Then, the relative concentrations of IL-10 or TNF-α cDNA in each sample were estimated from the concentration of control fragment DNA that achieved equilibrium between its own amplification and that of the target cDNA. The concentrations were determined in arbitrary units (AU). One AU was defined as the lowest concentration of control fragment that yielded a detectable amplification product given the primer pair and the PCR conditions used. Thus the technique allows us to compare the cDNA concentrations of a set of samples. This method, using an internal standard with similar amplification conditions, seems more reliable than absolute concentrations (molecules per tube) based on calculations of values obtained from an external standard.

1.3. Conclusions from Cytokine mRNA Expression Results in Psoriasis

Using the competitive RT-PCR technique, we demonstrated significantly lower cutaneous IL-10 mRNA expression in psoriasis compared with other

Table 1
Oligonucleotides Used to Amplify Target cDNA and Control Fragment DNA and Lengths (bp) of PCR Products (20)

	cf	5' Sense 3'	5' Antisense 3'	Sample cDNA 3' (bp)	CF (bp)	Annealing temp.	Cycles
GADPH	1/2	GCAGGGGGGAGCCAAAAGGG	TGCCAGCCCCAGCGTCAAAG	567	477/438[a]	68	28
IL-2	1	CCTCAACTCCTGCCACAATG	TTGCTGATTAAGTCCCTGGG	340	232	60	42
IL-2 Rp55	1	CCTGCCTCGTCACAACAACA	AAAACGCAGGCAAGCACAAC	312	182	68	40
IL-4	1	GCTTCCCCCTCTGTTCTTCC	TCTGGTTGGCTTCCTTCACA	371	289	60	40
IL-6	2	TAGCCGCCCCACACAGACAG	GGCTGGCATTTGTGGTTGGG	408	358	60	42
IL-7	1	TTTTATTCCGTGCTGCTCGC	GCCCTAATCCGTTTTGACCA	429	316	58	40
IL-8	2	GGGTCTGTTGTAGGGTTGCC	TGTGGATCCTGGCTAGCAGA	403	298	60	40
IL-10	1	CTGAGAACCAAGACCCAGACATCAAGG	CAATAAGGTTTCTCAAGGGGCTGG	351	196	68	42
IFN-γ	1	TCGTTTTGGGTTCTCTTGGC	GCAGGCAGGACAACCATTAC	477	357	60	40
TNF-α	2	CTCTGGCCCAGGCAGTCAGA	GGCGTTTGGGAAGGTTGGAT	519	358	60	40
Granzyme A	1	TGAACAAAAGGTCCCAGGTC	ATTCATTCCAATCACAGGGT	368	289	61	41
CD3δ	1	CTGGACCTGGGAAAACGCATC	GTACTGAGCATCATCTCGATC	309	233	60	42

[a]Control fragments DNA 1 and 2, respectively.

inflammatory dermatoses, whereas a marked overexpression of proinflammatory cytokines was found in psoriasis lesions. Without a quantitative approach, these differences would not have been detectable since IL-10 mRNA molecules were detectable in all samples investigated, in considerably different concentrations, however. Thus our findings indicated relative IL-10 deficiency in psoriasis. Moreover, using the competitive RT-PCR approach, we could show that established antipsoriatic treatment protocols are associated with enhanced IL-10 mRNA expression in PBMC. Since this suggested that IL-10 induction may have antipsoriatic activity, we performed the first administration of IL-10 in psoriasis in three patients *(18)*. Based on the very promising observations from this pilot trial, we subsequently performed a phase II study strongly suggesting the safety and efficiency of IL-10 therapy in psoriasis *(22)*.

Using the competitive RT-PCR technique, we were able to quantify cutaneous cytokine expression. In the case of IL-10 mRNA determination in psoriasis, this led to discovery of the key role for this cytokine in this frequent immune disease and to IL-10 treatment as a promising new therapeutic approach in psoriasis.

2. Materials

2.1. RNA Isolation

1. Denaturing solution: 47% (w/v) guanidinium thiocyanate, 0.7% (w/v) sodium citrate, pH 7.0, 0.5% (w/v) *N*-lauroylsarcosine (store at 4°C); before use add 0.7% β-mercaptoethanol.
2. Dispersing system (Ultra Turrax, Janke and Kunkel, Germany).
3. 2 *M* Sodium acetate, pH 4.0.
4. Water-saturated phenol.
5. Chloroform-isoamyl alcohol, 24:1.
6. RNA-Matrix and RNA-wash solution (RNaid PLUS Kit, Dianova, Hamburg, Germany).
7. DEPC-treated water, 0.1% (v/v).

2.2. Reverse Transcription of RNA

1. 5X First strand buffer: 250 m*M* Tris-HCl, 375 m*M* KCl, 15 m*M* $MgCl_2$, pH 8.3 (Life Technologies GIBCO/BRL Paisley, GB).
2. 100 m*M* Dithiothreitol.
3. 10 m*M* dNTPs.
4. Oligo dT primers: 0.1 mg/mL 5'-pd(T)$_{12-18}$-3'.
5. RNasin® ribonuclease-inhibitor, 40 U/μL (Promega, Madison, WI).
6. Moloney murine leukemia virus (MMLV) reverse transcriptase, 200 U/μL (Gibco BRL).

2.3. Competitive Polymerase Chain Reaction

1. 10X PCR buffer II: 500 m*M* KCl, 100 m*M* Tris-HCl, pH 8.3 (Perkin-Elmer, Foster City, CA).

2. 25 m*M* MgCl$_2$ solution.
3. 10 m*M* dNTPs.
4. 10 µ*M* Oligonucleotides used as primer pairs (**Table 1**).
5. AmpliTaq DNA polymerase, 5 U/µL (Perkin Elmer).
6. 10 ng/µL Control fragment.
7. Thermocycler (GeneAmp PCR-system 9600, Perkin Elmer).

2.4. Measurement of the PCR Product by Gel Electrophoresis and Videoimaging

Agarose:

1. 10 mg/mL Ethidium bromide.
2. 10X TBE buffer, pH 8.3.
3. 10X TAE buffer, pH 8.3.
4. Gel loading solution: 0.25% (w/v) bromophenol blue, 15% (w/v) Ficoll.
5. 1 µg/µL 100-bp ladder (Pharmacia Biotech, Uppsala, Sweden).
6. Videoimaging system (WinCam 2.2, Cybertech, Berlin, Germany).

3. Methods

The gene quantification method described here consists of the following separate procedures:

1. Total RNA isolation from skin specimens based on Chromczynski and Sacchi *(23)*.
2. Reverse transcription of mRNA in cDNA.
3. PCR amplification of the desired cDNA in competition to an internal standard.
4. Quantification of the PCR product by gel electrophoresis and Videoimaging.

3.1. RNA Isolation

The RNA isolation procedure has been used successfully with material from skin punch biopsies as small as 3–4 mm in diameter.

1. Tissue specimens have to be snap-frozen (liquid nitrogen) in RNAase-free plastic tubes *immediately after biopsy*. Store the samples at temperatures below –60°C and take care that stable temperature is guaranteed (*see* **Note 1**).
2. Add 500 µL of denaturing solution to every tube. Homogenize the samples during thawing. Take care that the samples do not become warm. Fifty microliters of sodium acetate, 500 µL of water-saturated phenol, and 100 µL of chloroform-isoamyl alcohol are added to the lysate. Mixtures are vortexed and stored on ice for a further 20 min prior to centrifugation (1000*g*, 20 min, 4°C).
3. The aqueous phase is incubated with 8 µL RNA matrix at room temperature for 5 min and then centrifuged (1000*g*, 1 min, 20°C). The RNA-bound matrix is washed three times with 200 µL RNA wash solution, and total RNA is eluted with 20 µL DEPC-treated water. Therefore, the samples are incubated at 55°C for 10 min.
4. The quality of total RNA should be estimated by electrophoresis on ethidium bromide (0.5 µg/mL) stained 0.7% agarose gel in 1X TBE buffer. Good-quality

RNA is characterized by sharp bands of both 28S RNA and 18S RNA. Staining of 28S should be twice as intensive as the 18S RNA.

5. Quantification of RNA is possible by comparison with standard RNA.

3.2. Reverse Transcription of mRNA in cDNA

The mRNA has to be reverse transcribed into cDNA using oligo dT primers *(24)* in 40-µL reaction mixtures containing about 0.2–1 µg of total RNA.

1. Prepare a reverse transcription master solution by adding the following: 80 µL 5X first-strand buffer, 40 µL dithiothreitol, 40 µL dNTPs, 20 µL oligo dT-primers, 10 µL RNasin ribonuclease inhibitor, and 10 µL MMLV reverse transcriptase. This is sufficient for 10 reactions.
2. Dilute the RNA to final volume of 20 µL and denature RNA at 95°C for 5 min.
3. The mixture is incubated at room temperature for 10 min, and thereafter for 1 h at 42°C. Denature at 95°C for 5 min.
4. Store cDNAs at –20°C.

3.3. Competitive RT-PCR Amplification
3.3.1. Principles/General Aspects

1. The multispecific competitor control fragment (cf), "a synthetic gene," is always used together with sample cDNA in the same reaction mixtures. Sample and control cDNAs are amplified with the same primers as indicated in **Table 1**, which also includes the appropriate number of cycles. A cDNA equivalent of about 5 ng total RNA should be taken for each RT-PCR analysis.
2. Control RT-PCR without template cDNA should be performed in all experiments to exclude contamination (water-negative control). As an additional control, the RT-PCR reaction should be performed as described, but reverse transcriptase has to be omitted in the reaction mixture for each specimen to distinguish the amplification of contaminating genomic DNA from that of reverse transcribed mRNA (second negative control). Finally, a tube containing cf without sample cDNA should be included as a positive control.
3. Variations in amplification efficiency between reactions can be estimated because the control fragment serves as an internal control. The control and sample PCR products are distinguished by gel electrophoresis due to length differences. With the input concentration of the control fragment known and amplification of both PCR products occurring proportionally, it is possible to quantify the sample cDNA. Measurement of the PCR product is performed by gel electrophoresis and Videoimaging (*see* **Subheading 3.3.2.**).

3.3.2. Adjusting Samples to Equal GAPDH-cDNA Concentrations

First, to equilibrate the input cDNA amounts of the samples studied, the concentration of the housekeeping gene GAPDH cDNA has to be determined in dilution series using competitive RT-PCR with the GAPDH-specific

Table 2
PCR Amplification for GAPDH Determination

Cycles	Temperature (°C)	Time	Step
1	94	5 min	Denaturation
28	94	15 s	Denaturation
	68	15 s	Annealing
	72	15 s	Extension
1	72	5 min	Final extension
1	4	—	Storage

primers. Therefore, an appropriate fixed concentration of the control fragment (in a dilution of $1:10^3–1:10^5$) is added to dilution series from the tissue samples. For each sample, the concentration of GAPDH cDNA that yields an equilibration with the cf after amplification is determined. Based on these results the input cDNA is calculated (*see* **Note 2**).

Example: If equilibration between target cDNA and cf is reached with a sample dilution of 1:100 in tube A whereas this is the case in tube B when using a cf dilution of 1:10, a 10-fold higher GAPDH-cDNA content in sample A is indicated. Consequently, the input of cDNA for the subsequent experiments has to be 10 times higher for sample B than for sample A.

1. Prepare a PCR master solution under DANN-free conditions (*see* **Subheading 4.**) by adding the following: 178 μL water, 26 μL 10X PCR buffer II, 15 μL MgCl$_2$, 10 μL dNTPs, 10 μL primer mix, 10 μL control fragment, and 1 μL AmpliTaq DNA polymerase. This is sufficient for 10 reactions.
2. Place 25 μL of PCR master solution in a PCR reaction tube and add 1 μL of cDNA.
3. Amplify by PCR using the cycle profile as shown in **Table 2**.

3.3.3. Proof of the Adjustment of all Samples to Equal GAPDH-cDNA Concentrations

After the concentrations that should result in an equal GAPDH-cDNA amplification have been calculated for each sample, this is proved in a subsequent PCR. A constant cf concentration is added to all samples. The PCR products from all samples should be found in equal density by the Videoimaging. If not, the adjusting of samples to equal GAPDH-cDNA concentrations has to be repeated.

3.3.4. Determination of the Relative Cytokine cDNA Amount

After adjusting all samples to equal GAPDH-cDNA concentrations, the relative cytokine cDNA amount is determined in a second competitive RT-PCR using different cf dilutions, the appropriate cytokine-specific primers, cycles, and annealing temperatures (*see* **Table 1**).

3.4. Measurement of the PCR Product by Gel Electrophoresis and Videoimagining

Electrophoresis is performed on ethidium bromide (0.5 mg/mL) stained 1.5% agarose gel.

1. Add 2 µL of gel loading solution to tubes containing the PCR product.
2. Place the mixture in one well of an agarose gel (MBT Brand, Gießen, Germany; tray: 18.5 × 24 cm; well: 0.5 cm).
3. Perform electrophoresis (120 V, 1 h).

Density of the PCR products is determined by an Videoimagining program (Herolab). The relative concentration of the cytokine cDNA in each sample is expressed in AU. One arbitrary unit is defined as the lowest concentration of control fragment that gives a detectable amplification product for one particular primer pair given and the PCR conditions used *(20)*.

4. Notes

1. The quality of the samples is crucial for the results. Use only skin biopsies that were collected and stored appropriately (e.g., shock-frozen within seconds and stored continuously below –70°C). Take care that the work is carried out under RNAase free conditions (e.g., hand gloves).
2. The most difficult but essential part is the adjustment of the samples to equal GAPDH-cDNA concentrations. The difficulty of this task increases with the number of samples to be compared. Once this has been reached, it is relatively easy to determine the cytokine mRNA content. From a practical point of view, it is possible to handle up to about 40 different samples for comparison of cytokine expression. In our experience, the time between adjustment to equal GAPDH-cDNA content and analyses of cytokine cDNA content should not exceed 3 wk. Otherwise the GAPDH-cDNA equilibration has to be proved by PCR again.
3. It does not seem appropriate to compare values obtained for cytokine expression in one experiment with those obtained from an other. This means that 1 AU from one calculation is not 100% identical with 1 AU from another experiment since the concrete PCR conditions might have changed in the meantime (minor changes, e.g., in the efficiency of the primers, temperature of the PCR machine, activity of the enzymes, etc.). Consequently, only samples analyzed in the same series of experiments should be compared. If you want to compare "old" and "new" data directly, you have to adjust the new samples with some "old" samples.
4. Contaminations are a serious danger and have to be strictly avoided. It is recommended to do (a) preparation of the PCR reaction mix; (b) PCR itself; and (c) analyses of the PCR product in different rooms with separate equipment (pipets).
5. Control RT-PCR without template DNA should be performed in all experiments to exclude contamination. As an additional control, reverse transcriptase should be omitted from the reaction mixture during cDNA synthesis to prove the absence of genomic DNA.

Methods for Determination of the Cellular Source of Cutaneous Cytokine Expression

Method	Characteristics
Immunohistology	Frequently used. However, often an intercellular pattern is found. Since the majority of cutaneous cytokines can be produced by very different cell types (including lymphocytes, keratinocytes, fibroblasts, and macrophages), a possible intercellular detection could not provide sufficient evidence concerning the cellular source. Moreover, cytokines might be washed out, and nonspecific binding can frequently occur resulting in false-positive or -negative results.
In situ hybridization	Fluorescence *in situ* hybridization is only successful if very high cytokine mRNA concentrations are present. Thus, many cytokines cannot be detected by this method, although they are clearly demonstrable by RT-PCR. When using more sensitive radioactive *in situ* hybridization, it might be difficult to determine the cell type of a positive cutaneous cell.
In vitro cytokine secretion of purified cutaneous cells	In short-term cultures of isolated cells from mechanically (better than enzymatically) disaggregated skin biopsies, the cytokine secretion into the supernatants can be measured. However, many fresh cutaneous cells rapidly die ex vivo. Cytokine secretion under this artificial conditions does not necessarily reflect their cytokine formation in vivo. Magnetic beads separation of purified lymphocytes from skin biopsies is difficult.
Intracellular cytokine formation	Recently such protocols have been developed for cutaneous T cells. The bases are FACS analysis of stimulated, permeabilized cells after mechanically or enzymatic disaggregation and subsequent isolation (*see* above).
Purification of circulating skin homing cells	In certain cutaneous disorders (e.g., in Sezary syndrome), the crucial skin homing T cells temporarily circulate in the blood. These cells can be isolated for subsequent analysis by FACS or in culture. However, their cytokine pattern does not necessarily represent the cytokine pattern the cells when homing in the skin. Thus, compartment-associated shifts might be possible.
Correlation with histology/immunohistology	Neither the simple presence of a particular cell population nor its frequency allow us to draw a reliable conclusion as to which population is responsible for which cytokine formation. Consequently, only speculation based on these new data might be possible.
In situ RT-PCR	This method is not yet sufficiently established for cutaneous cytokine mRNA detection.
Single cell techniques	Using micromanipulation, it recently became possible to analyze the DNA of single cutaneous cells. This technique, however, has not been successfully adopted for mRNA analyses so far (sensitivity problems; mostly only nuclei are collected).

247

6. Competitive RT-PCR gives reliable data only regarding the cytokine gene expression level in total, i.e., within the skin. Differentiation between epidermal and dermal cytokine expression might be possible after splitting the biopsies using appropriate methods. It is likely, however, that such procedures influence the quality of the mRNAs. Therefore, we would not recommend this. The cellular origin of the cutaneous cytokines found to be overexpressed remains unclear. Several methods might be used for this approach; however, their limitations must be considered (**Table 3** [*see* p. 247]).

7. Competitive RT-PCR gives data regarding the mRNA expression. This is not necessarily equal with cytokine expression on protein level. Thus posttranscriptional processes might influence the final protein production, which is of biologic importance. In fact, for some cytokines the correlation between mRNA and protein formation is quite weak (e.g., IL-15, TGF-β).

Acknowledgments

This work was supported by a grant from the Deutsche Forschungsgemeinschaft (Ste 366/7). We thank Dr. T. Hansen-Hagge, Berlin, for critically reading the manuscript.

References

1. Christophers, E. and Sterry, W. (1993) Psoriasis, in *Dermatology in General Medicine*. (Fitzpatric, T. B., Eisen, A. Z., Wolff, K., Freedberg, I. M., and Austen, K. F., eds.), McGraw-Hill, New York, pp. 489–515.
2. Valdimarsson, H., Baker, B. S., Johnsdottir, I., and Fry, L. (1986) Psoriasis: a disease of abnormal keratinocyte proliferation induced by T lymphocytes. *Immunol. Today* **7**, 256–259.
3. Nickoloff, B. J. (1991) The cytokine network in psoriasis. *Arch. Dermatol.* **127**, 871–884.
4. Uyemura, K., Yamamura, M., Fivenson, D. F., Modlin, R. L., and Nickoloff, B. J. (1993) The cytokine network in lesional and lesion-free psoriatic skin is characterized by a T-helper type 1 cell-mediated response. *J. Invest. Dermatol.* **101**, 701–705.
5. Schlaak, J. F., Buslau, M., Jochum, W., Hermann, E., Girndt, M. (1994) T cells involved in psoriasis vulgaris belong to the Th 1 subset. *J. Invest. Dermatol.* **102**, 145–149.
6. Wrone-Smith, T. and Nickoloff, B. J. (1996) Dermal injection of immunocytes induces psoriasis. *J. Clin. Invest.* **98**, 1878–1887.
7. Krueger, J. G., Krane, J. F., Carter, D. M., and Gottlieb, A. B. (1990) Role of growth factors, cytokines, and their receptors in the pathogenesis of psoriasis. *J. Invest. Dermatol.* **94**, 135S–140S.
8. Boehncke, W. H., Dressel, D., Manfras, B., Zollner, T. M., Wettstein, A., Böhm, B. O., et al. (1995) T-cell-receptor repertoire in chronic plaque-stage psoriasis is restricted and lacks enrichment of superantigen-associated Vβ regions. *J. Invest. Dermatol.* **104**, 725–728.

9. Ohta, Y., Katayama, I., Funato, T., Yokozeki, H., Nishiyama, S., Hirano, T., et al. (1991) In situ expression of messenger RNA of interleukin-1 and interleukin-6 in psoriasis: interleukin-6 involved in formation of psoriatic lesions. *Arch. Derm. Res.* **283,** 351–356.

10. Lemster, B. H., Carroll, P. B., Rilo, H. R., Johnson, N., Nikaein, A., and Thomson, A. W. (1995) IL-8/IL-8 receptor expression in psoriasis and the response to systemic tacrolimus (FK506) therapy. *Clin. Exp. Immunol.* **99,** 148–154.

11. Ettehadi, P., Greaves, M. W., Wallach, D., Aderka, D., and Camp, R. D. (1994) Elevated tumor necrosis factor-alpha (TNF-alpha) biological activity in psoriatic skin lesions. *Clin. Exp. Immunol.* **96,** 146–151.

12. Asadullah, K., Prösch, S., Audring, H., Volk, H. D., Sterry, W., and Döcke, W. D. (1999) A high prevalence of cytomegalovirus antigenaemia in patients with moderate to severe psoriasis: an association with systemic TNF-overexpression. *Br. J. Dermatol.* **141,** 94–102.

13. Olaniran, A. K., Baker, B. S., Paige, D. G., Garioch, J. J., Powles, A. V., and Fry, L. (1996) Cytokine expression in psoriatic skin lesions during PUVA therapy. *Arch. Derm. Res.* **288,** 421–425.

14. D'Andrea, A., Aste-Amezaga, M., Valiante, N. M., Ma, X., Kubin, M., and Trinchieri, G. (1993) Interleukin 10 (IL10) inhibits human lymphocyte interferon gamma-production by suppressing natural killer cell stimulatory factor/IL-12 synthesis in accessory cells. *J. Exp. Med.* **178,** 1041–1048.

15. De Waal Malefyt, R., Abrams, J., Bennett, B., Figdor, C. G., and de Vries, J. E. (1991) Interleukin 10 (IL10) inhibits cytokine synthesis by human monocytes: an autoregulatory role of IL-10 produced by monocytes. *J. Exp. Med.* **174,** 1209–1220.

16. Fiorentino, D. F., Zlotnik, A., Mosmann, T. R., Howard, M., and O´Garra, A. (1991) IL-10 inhibits cytokine production by activated macrophages. *J. Immunol.* **147,** 3815–3822.

17. Asadullah, K., Döcke, W. D., Haeußler, A., Sterry, W., and Volk, H. D. (1996) Progression of *Mycosis fungoides* is associated with increasing cutaneous expression of IL-10 mRNA. *J. Invest. Dermatol.* **107,** 833–837.

18. Asadullah, K., Sterry, W., Stephanek, K., Leupold, M., Jasulaitis, D., Audring, H., et al. (1998) IL-10 is a key cytokine in psoriasis: proof of principle by IL-10 therapy—a new therapeutic approach. *J. Clin. Invest.* **101,** 783–794.

19. Wang, A. M., Doyle, M. V., and Mark, D. F. (1989) Quantitation of mRNA by the polymerase chain reaction. *Proc. Natl. Acad. Sci. USA* **86,** 9717–9721.

20. Platzer, C., Ode Hakim, S., Reinke, P., Döcke, W. D., Ewert, R., and Volk, H. D. (1994) Quantitative PCR analysis of cytokine transcription patterns in peripheral mononuclear cells after anti-CD3 rejection therapy using two novel multispecific competitor fragments. *Transplantation* **58,** 264–268.

21. Siegling, A., Lehmann, M., Platzer, C., Emmrich, F., and Volk, H. D. (1994) A novel multispecific competitor fragment for quantitative PCR analysis of cytokine gene expression in rats. *J. Immunol. Methods* **177,** 23–28.

22. Asadullah, K., Döcke, W. D., Ebeling, M., Friedrich, M., Belbe, G., Audring, H., et al. (1999) IL-10 treatment of psoriasis—clinical results of a Phase II trial, *Arch. Dermatol.* **135,** 187–192.

23. Chomczynski, P. and Sacchi, N. (1987) Single-step method of RNA isolation by acid guanidinium thiocyanate-phenol-chloroform extraction. *Anal. Biochem.* **162,** 156–159.

24. Murphy, E., Hieny, S., Sher, A., and O'Garra, A. (1993) Detection of in vivo expression of interleukin-10 using a semi-quantitative polymerase chain reaction method in *Schistosoma mansoni* infected mice. *J. Immunol. Methods* **162,** 211–223.

21

Interleukins in Graves' Disease

Jan Komorowski

1. Introduction

The pathogenesis of Graves' disease, an autoimmune thyroid disorder, remains incompletely understood. Increasing clinical and experimental evidence shows that genetic predisposition, disturbances of the immune system function and environmental factors affecting thyroid gland activity appear to play crucial roles. Graves' disease is characterized by hyperthyroidism and/or ophthalmopathy related to retroorbital tissue infiltration by autoreactive T-lymphocytes (1). The hallmarks of the disorder, which have been considered to be responsible for ophthalmopathy, hyperthyroidism, acropachy, pretibial dermopathy, and goiter are factors such as circulating antibodies against thyroid autoantigens (mainly to thyrotropin [TSH] receptor) (2,3), association with immune response (HLA-DR) genes (4–8), and an intermittent clinical course of exacerbations and remissions. It has been also proved that in Graves' disease autoantibodies are capable of stimulating the synthesis of hormones in thyrocytes via the central autoimmune target—TSH receptor, which has been cloned and sequenced (9). Most patients with Graves' disease are hyperthyroid. The availability of free thriiodothyronin (fT$_3$), free thyroxin (fT$_4$), and highly sensitive TSH techniques has vastly simplified the diagnosis of the early subclinical form of hyperthyroidism (7). Development of TSH receptor autoantibody assays (10) has enhanced the ability of the clinician to identify subtle presentation of this autoimmune thyroid disease (7).

Thyroid Graves' ophthalmopathy (TAO) is generally considered to represent an autoimmune process of the retroorbital space that is closely associated with immunogenic hyperthyroidism, but the target antigen has yet to be identified. Retroorbital tissues display lymphocytic infiltration, a characteristic sign of an autoimmune response. Histologic examination of the ocular tissues of patients

From: *Methods in Molecular Medicine, vol. 60: Interleukin Protocols*
Edited by: L. A. J. O'Neill and A. Bowie © Humana Press Inc., Totowa, NJ

with thyroid-associated ophthalmopathy reveals the presence of infiltration by activated T-lymphocytes, B cells, macrophages (which may act as antigen-presenting cells) and excessive amounts of hydrophilic glycosaminoglycans (GAG) *(8,11–13)*. Patients with TAO typically describe a gritty sensation in their eyes, blurring of vision, photophobia, increased lacrimation, double vision, or deep orbital pressure *(11)*.

The signs and symptoms of endocrine orbitopathy can be explained by the pathologic changes in the orbit. Swelling of the eye muscles and the presence of fat cause proptosis and inhibit venous drainage, leading to the edema of periorbital tissues and eyelids. Periorbital swelling is also because of prolapse of the orbital fat through the orbital septum. Swelling of the muscles impairs their function, which results in diplopia. Overexposure of the cornea can cause keratitis. Visual impairment can be the result of direct pressure of the enlarged muscle on the optic nerve or the indirect effect of a general increase in the retrobulbar pressure *(14)*. Ophthalmologic and imaging (ultrasonography, computed tomography, or nuclear magnetic resonance) studies show that the extraocular muscles are enlarged and that much of this enlargement is related to the excess of GAG and water accumulation in the interstitial space. The treatment of patients with hyperthyroidism usually (but not always) improves the TAO features. Sometimes optic neuropathy develops, with decreased visual acuity, dulling of color perception, and visual field defects. There is currently no way to prevent thyroid-associated ophthalmopathy, and the condition is usually treated when the symptoms become serious or vision is affected. In severe orbitopathy, our management aims at reducing the pressure and volume of ocular tissues, which can be achieved by corticosteroid immunosuppression, retrobulbar irradiation, decompressive surgery, and the application of somatostatin analogs, pentoxyfiline, nicotinamide, or immunoglobulins.

The human immune system function is designed to recognize the myriad of molecules in the world around us. Three types of molecules are involved: immunoglobulins (antibodies), T-cell receptors, and products of the major histo-compatibility complex (MHC). Aberrant expression of MHC class II antigens, heterodimeric transmembrane glycoproteins encoded by the human leukocyte antigen-D (HLA-D) region on chromosome 6, is associated with autoimmune thyroid disease *(15)*. These antigens play a central role in the immune reaction *(16)*. MHC class II molecules are usually expressed on antigen-presenting cells such as macrophages, B-lymphocytes, and dendritic cells, but not on thyreocytes *(6)*. The MHC class II antigens present antigenic peptides to CD-positive T-lymphocytes, causing T-cell activation *(16)*. Aberrant or abnormal expression of MHC class II glycoproteins on thyroid epithelial cells has been documented in Graves' disease patients *(17)*.

Interferon-γ (IFN-γ) produced and released into the circulation from T-lymphocytes during bacterial or viral infections is the most potent inducer of class

II gene expression on lymphoid and thyroid cells *(6,17,18)*. This phenomenon suggests that nonspecific inflammation can result in the autoimmune response. Therefore, many soluble signals called T-cell-derived cytokines or interleukins often act as peptide messengers between cells and play a pivotal role in normal or abnormal immune activity. Chronic stimulation of T cells leads to the development of T helper (Th)0 cells, which release a wide range of cytokines and may differentiate into Th1 or Th2 cells with production of various cytokines.

This phenomenon (Th1 or Th2 cell development) is regulated by the interaction of a wide array of cytokines, co-stimulatory molecules, antigens, and certain types of antigen-presenting cells. The predominance of Th1 or Th2 CD4+ cells promotes different immunopathologic reactions. Th1 lymphocytes produce IFN-γ, tumor necrosis factor-β (TNF-β), and interleukin-2 (IL-2), mediating delayed-type hypersensitivity and T-cell cytotoxicity, as well as macrophage activation and opsonizing antibody production (IgG). Th2 cells, which release IL-4, IL5, IL-6, IL-10, and IL-13, facilitate IgA and IgE and nonopsonizing antibody production and also augment the degranulation of mast cells and eosinophils. Both types of CD4+ lymphocytes (Th1 and Th2) have the ability to secrete TNF-α, granulocyte-macrophage colony-stimulating factor (GM-CSF), and IL-3 *(19,20)*.

The interactions between interleukins and immune cells are very important in the immune response, resulting in the progression or remission of the autoimmune disease. It has been documented that IL-4 promotes the differentiation of Th2 cells and, similar to IL-10, inhibits cytokine secretion by Th1 cells. IL-12 and IFN-γ promote the proliferation and generation of Th1 cells and downregulate Th2 cell responses *(3,20)*. In autoimmune diseases, the local production of cytokines tends to increase the accumulation and activation of immunocompetent cells but may also affect the target organ directly. The inhibitory role of IL-10 (produced by Th0, Th1, and Th2 lymphocyte clones) in macrophage activation and T-cell proliferation shows that the proinflammatory or antiinflammatory function of Th1 lymphocytes may depend on the ratio of IFN-γ or IL-2 to IL-10 *(21)*.

The evaluation of cytokine expression by the mononuclear cell infiltrate in autoimmune thyroid disease gives ambiguous and often controversial results *(22)*. In thyroid gland tissue (obtained by surgery) from Graves' disease patients the predominance of antigen-specific T cells with the Th0 and Th1 phenotype has been shown *(3,22)*. These T cells produce mainly IL-2, IFN-γ, and IFN-α, but no IL-4 mRNA. Thyroid epithelial cells are also the source of many cytokines. They produce IL-1, IL-6, IL-8, TNF, TGF-β, and intercellular adhesion molecules 1 and 3 and express antigen HLA classes I and II *(3,22)*.

The relative contribution of cellular and humoral immunity in the pathogenesis of Graves' ophthalmopathy is also unknown, but it is possible that both mechanisms are important for the clinical expression and propagation of the autoimmune process within the orbit. The nature of the autoantigen that links the thyroid gland and the orbit is still uncertain *(23)*. Lymphocytic infiltration of the muscular and connective tissues of the retroorbital space, and the presence of humoral and cellular immune reactions directed against the putative orbital antigens are human defence system abnormalities documented in the TAO condition. In the orbital tissue various growth factors and cytokines (platelet-derived growth factor [PDGF], insulin-like growth factor-1 [IGF-1], IFN-γ, TNF-α, IL-1α, IL-1β, IL-2, IL-4, IL-5, IL-6, IL-8, IL-10, IL-13, IL-15, and transforming growth factor-β [TGF-β]) are produced and secreted by infiltrating autoreactive T cells, macrophages, and fibroblasts in a paracrine and autocrine fashion *(8,24)*. The cytolytic T cells with a Th1-like cytokine profile (IL-2, IFN-γ, and TNF-α) predominate in the retroorbital lymphocytic infiltrates of Graves' ophthalmopathy *(25)*.

Proinflammatory cytokines induce and stimulate the expression of various immunomodulatory peptides including HLA-DR, adhesion molecules (ICAM-1, ELAM-1, VCAM-1, CD44, and LFA-1), and stress proteins. These peptides are of central importance in the recruitment and targeting of activated lymphocytes in the retroocular space and in the processing and presentation of antigenic epitopes to the T cell *(8)*. It is well known that certain growth factors, cytokines, and oxygen free radicals, released from both the infiltrating inflammatory and residential cells, act on retroorbital fibroblasts in a paracrine and autocrine manner to stimulate cell proliferation, GAG synthesis, and the expression of immunomodulatory molecules *(8,26)*.

In the last decade the evaluation of certain cytokines in peripheral blood (plasma or serum) has had important clinical implications for patients with autoimmune thyroid disease. Increased serum concentrations of soluble IL-2 receptor (sIL-2R, also termed α, Tac, or p55), known as an antagonist of IL-2-mediated cell responses, were present in patients with hyperthyroidism and ophthalmopathy *(27,28)*. SIL-2R levels showed a strong correlation with thyroid hormone concentrations (fT_3, fT_4) as markers of Graves' disease hormonal activity *(29,30)*. Naturally occurring IL-1 receptor antagonist (IL-1Ra) also plays a prominent role in the evolution of the immune process in Graves' orbitopathy, and its measurements in the peripheral blood may predict the therapeutic response to orbital irradiation *(31)*. Blood serum changes in concentrations of IL-6, IL-8, and TNF-α may be the markers of the functional state of thyroid cells in hyperthyroidism, as well as after strumectomy and treatment with radioactive iodine, propylothiouracil, or carbimazole *(32–35)*. Recently, elevated serum levels of granulocyte colony-stimulating factor (G-CSF) *(36)* and IL-5 *(37)* IL-12, IL-18 *(38)* have been documented in patients with Graves' disease.

Serum or supernatant concentrations of interleukins are generally determined by a highly sensitive sandwich enzyme-linked immunoassay technique using commercially manufactured kits. A typical procedure (for the Quantikine kit) is as follows:

A monoclonal antibody specific for the interleukin tested is precoated onto a microtiter plate provided with the kit. Standards, samples, and conjugate are pipetted into the wells, and any cytokine present is bound (sandwiched) by the immobilized antibody and the enzyme-linked polyclonal antibody specific for the interleukin tested. After washing away any unbound components, an enzyme-linked polyclonal antibody specific for a given cytokine is added to the wells. Following a wash to remove any unbound antibody-enzyme reagent, a substrate solution is added to the wells, and color develops in proportion to the amount of interleukin bound in the initial step. The color development is stopped, and the intensity of the color is evaluated.

2. Materials

1. Serum: Use a serum separator tube and allow samples to clot for 30 min (at room temperature) before centrifugation for 10 min at approx 100g. Remove serum and store frozen at $-20°C$ (or colder) until assay. Avoid repeated freeze-thaw cycles.
2. Collect plasma using EDTA (recommended), heparin, or citrate as an anticoagulant. Rapid separation of plasma after collection, for less than 30 min, will ensure optimal recovery. Remove particulates by centrifugation and store frozen at $-20°C$ (or colder) until assay. Avoid repeated freeze-thaw cycles.
3. Cell culture supernatants: Centrifuge to remove any particulate material and store frozen at £ $-20°C$ (or colder) until assay. Avoid repeated freeze-thaw cycles.
4. Interleukin microtiter plate: 96-well plate made from polystyrene (12 strips of 8 wells) coated with a murine monoclonal antibody against the interleukin tested. After opening, unused wells may be stored for up to 1 mo at 2–8°C, resealed in the foil pouch containing the desiccant pack (*see* **Notes 1–6**).
5. Interleukin conjugate: A solution of polyclonal antibody against the cytokine tested conjugated to horseradish peroxidase, with preservative. It may be stored for up to 1 mo at 2–8°C after reconstitution) (*see* **Note 1**).
6. Standard of tested interleukin: Lyophilized human cytokine in a buffered protein base with preservative, which it may be stored for up to 1 mo at $-20°C$ or below after reconstitution. Reconstitute the standard in adequate calibrator diluent that reflects the composition of the samples being assayed. It is important that the diluent selected for reconstitution and dilution of the standard reflect the environment of the samples being measured. Allow the standard to sit for a minimum of 30 min with gentle agitation prior to making dilutions. Use this stock solution to produce a dilution series as described in the kit booklet. It may be stored for to up 1 mo at $-20°C$ or below without repeated freeze-thaw cycles. Use the stock solution to produce a dilution series in polypropylene test tubes. Pipet the same volume of calibrator diluent into each tube. Pipet interleukin standard into the "maximum standard" tube. Transfer the same volume of the standard solution to the next tube. Repeat this process successively to complete the twofold dilution series. Mix each tube thoroughly before each subsequent transfer. The undiluted standard serves as the high standard (maximum). Calibrator diluent serves as the zero standard (*see* **Notes 1**, **4**, **6–8**).

7. Assay diluent: A buffered protein base with preservative, which may be stored for up to 1 mo at 2–8°C after reconstitution (*see* **Note 1**).

8. Two different calibrator diluents: For serum/plasma samples and for cell culture supernatant samples, which may be stored for up to 1 mo at 2–8°C after reconstitution (*see* **Note 9**).

9. Wash buffer concentrate: A concentrated solution of buffered surfactant with preservative, which may be stored for up to 1 mo at 2–8°C after reconstitution. If crystals have formed in concentrate, warm it in a 36–38°C water bath and mix before dilution. Dilute into deionized or distilled water, and mix thoroughly. Wash buffer should be kept at room temperature prior to use in the assay. If running partial plates, store the reconstitute for up 1 mo at 2–8°C (*see* **Notes 1** and **7**).

10. Color reagent A: A solution of stabilized hydrogen peroxide (stable for up 1 mo at 2–8°C after reconstitution (*see* **Note 1**).

11. Color reagent B: A solution of stabilized chromogen (tetramethylbenzidine). It may be stored for up 1 mo at 2–8°C after reconstitution. Color reagents A and B should be mixed together in equal volumes within 15 min of use to prepare substrate solution (*see* **Note 10**).

12. Stop solution: A solution of 2 N sulfuric acid. It may be stored for up 1 mo at 2–8°C after reconstitution.
    Caution: *Caustic material. Wear eye, hand, face, and clothing protection.*

13. Plate covers: Four adhesive strips.

14. Spectrophotometer (microtiter plate reader) usually capable of measurements at 450 nm, preferably configured for microtiter plates, capable of using a dual wavelength. (Correction wavelength is 540 or 570 nm.)

15. Pipets: 50, 100, and 200 µL for running the assay; adjustable 1, 5, 10, or 25 mL for reagent preparation.

16. Deionized or distilled water.

17. Pipet, squirt bottle, manifold dispenser, or automated microtiter plate washer.

18. 12 × 75 mm Propylene test tubes.

3. Methods

3.1. Assay Procedure

The example given here is for Quantikine IL-6 immunoassay. Bring all the reagents and samples to room temperature before use. It is recommended that all samples and standards be assayed in duplicates.

1. Determine the number of strips you wish to run. Leave these strips in the plate frame. Place the remaining unused strips back in the foil pouch with the desiccant provided. Store these reserved strips at 2–8°C, making sure that the foil pouch is sealed tightly. After running the assay, retain the plate frame for a second partial plate. When running the second partial plate, place the reserved strips securely in the plate frame.

2. Add 100 µL (usually) of assay diluent to each well (*see* **Notes 4** and **9**).

3. Add 100 µL of standard or sample per well. Cover with the adhesive strip provided. Incubate for 2 h at room temperature (*see* **Notes 11–15**).

4. Aspirate each well and wash, repeating the process three times for a total of four washes. Wash by filling each well with the wash buffer using a squirt bottle, multichannel pipet, mainfold dispenser, or autowasher. Complete removal of liquid at each step is essential for good performance. After the last wash, remove any remaining wash buffer by aspirating or by inverting the plate and blotting it against clean paper toweling.
5. Add 200 μL of interleukin conjugate to each well. Cover with a new adhesive strip. Incubate for 2 h at room temperature (*see* **Note 16**).
6. Repeat the aspiration/wash as in **step 4**.
7. Add 200 μL of substrate solution to each well. Incubate for 20 min at room temperature (*see* **Note 17**).
8. Add 50 μL of stop solution to each well. If color change does not appear uniform, gently tap the plate to ensure thorough mixing (*see* **Note 18**).
9. Determine the optical density (absorbance) of each well within 30 min, using the microtiter plate reader (ELISA reader) set to 450 nm. If wavelength correction is available, set it to 540 or 570 nm. If wavelength correction is not available, subtract the readings at 540 or 570 nm from the readings at 450 nm. This subtraction will correct for optical imperfections in the plate. Readings made directly at 450 nm without correction may be higher and less accurate (*see* **Note 19**).

3.2. Calculation of Results

Average the duplicate readings for each standard, control, and sample and subtract the average zero standard optical density.

Create a standard curve by reducing the data using computer software capable of generating a four-parameter curve-fit. As an alternative, construct a standard curve by plotting the mean absorbance for each standard on the *y*-axis against the concentration of the *x*-axis and draw a best fit curve through the points on the graph. The data may be linearized by plotting the log of the interleukin concentrations vs the log of the optical density; the best fit line can then be determined by regression analysis. This procedure will produce an adequate but less precise fit of the data.

3.3. Assay Parameters and Performance Characteristics

3.3.1. Sensitivity

The sensitivity of the assay (lower limit of detection [LLD]), is determined by assaying replicates of zero and the standard curve. The mean signal of zero + 2 standard deviations read in the dose from the standard curve is the LLD. This value is the smallest dose that is not zero with 95% confidence.

3.3.2. Reproducibility

Intraassay precision (precision within an assay, CV). Three samples of known concentrations (high, medium, and low) are assayed 20 times on one plate to assess intraassay precision. (For interleukin measurements by ELISA, CV% should be <10%.)

Interassay precision (precision between assays, CV). Three samples of known concentrations (high, medium, and low) are assayed in 20 separate assays to assess interassay precision. (For interleukin measurements by ELISA, CV% should be <10%.)

3.3.3. Linearity of Dilution

Linearity of dilution is determined by serially diluting ten different positive samples. The dilutions are run in the ELISA and the observed doses are plotted against the expected doses.

3.3.4. Recovery

The recovery (%) of interleukin spiked to three different levels in five samples throughout the range of the assay in various matrices is evaluated.

4. Notes

1. Store all reagents refrigerated at 2–8°C.
2. Refer to the expiration data on the kit box.
3. Some components of the kits contain sodium azide, which may react with lead and copper plumbing to form explosive metallic azides.
4. Bring all the reagents to room temperature before use.
5. The kit should not be used beyond the expiration date on the kit label.
6. Propylene tubes must be used for sample preparation. Do not use glass tubes.
7. When mixing or reconstituting protein solutions, always avoid foaming.
8. To avoid cross-contamination, change pipet tips between additions of each standard level, between sample additions, and between reagent additions. Also use separate reservoirs for each reagent.
9. Remember to use the same calibrator diluents for cytokine standards and samples (for supernatant or serum/plasma samples).
10. Some kits contain a compound with mercury.
11. Samples that are to be assayed within 24 h should be stored at 2–8°C. When storing samples for longer periods, aliquot and freeze them at –20°C or below.
12. Test samples should be assayed at least in duplicate.
13. Avoid freezing and thawing samples more than once.
14. Samples containing sodium azide should not be used in some assays, because this compound may inactivate horseradish peroxidase and may lead to spurious results.
15. Bring samples gently to room temperature before running the assay (minimum 1 h before starting procedures). Mix samples by gently inverting the tubes. Do not use 37°C or 56°C water baths to thaw samples.
16. To ensure accurate results, proper adhesion of plate sealers during incubation steps is necessary.
17. Substrate solution should remain colorless when added to the plate. Substrate solution should change from colorless to a gradation of blue. The color developed in the wells will turn from blue to yellow upon addition of the stop solution.
18. Stop solution should be added to the plate in the same order as the substrate solution.

19. The plate must be read within 30 min of stopping the reactions. Optical density values obtained for duplicates should be within 10% of the mean. Duplicate values than differ from the mean by greater than 10% should be considered suspect and should be repeated.

References

1. Margolick, J. B., Hsu, S. M., Volkman, D. J., Burman, K. D., and Fauci, A. S. (1984) Immunohistochemical characterization of intra-thyroid lymphocytes in Graves' disease. *Am. J. Med.* **76**, 815–821.
2. Rotella, C. M., Manucci, M., and Di Mario, U. (1992) Autoantigens in thyroid and islet auto-immunity: Similarities and differences. *Autoimmunity* **12**, 223–237.
3. Fisfalen, W. E., Palmer, E. M., Van Seventer, G. A., Soltani, K., Sawai, Y, Kaplan, E., et al. (1997) Thyrotropin-receptor and thyroid peroxidase-specific T cell clones and their cytokine profile in autoimmune thyroid disease. *J. Clin. Endocrinol. Metab.* **82**, 3655–3663.
4. Svejgaard, A., Platz, P., and Ryder L. P. (1984) HLA and disease susceptibility: clinical implications. *Clin. Immunol. Allergol.* **4**, 567–580.
5. Escobar-Morreale, H., Serrano-Gotarredona, J., Villar, L. M., Garcia-Robles, R., Gonzales-Porque, P., Sancho, J. M., et al. (1996) Methimazole has no dose-related effect on the serum concentrations of soluble class I major histocompatibility complex antigens, soluble interleukin-2 receptor, and beta2-microglobulin in patients with Graves' disease. *Thyroid* **6**, 29–36.
6. Montani, V., Shong, M., Taniguchi, S.-I., Suzuki, K., Giuliani, C., Napolitano, G., et al. (1998) Regulation of major histocompatibility class II gene expression in FRTL-5 thyrocytes: opposite effects of interferon and methimazole. *Endocrinology* **139**, 290–302.
7. Burch, H. B. and Wartofsky, L. (1993) Graves' ophtalmopathy: current concepts regarding pathogenesis and management. *Endocr. Rev.* **14**, 747–793.
8. Heufelder, A. E. (1995) Pathogenesis of Graves' ophthalmopathy: recent controversies and progress. *Eur. J. Endocrinol.* **132**, 532–541.
9. Liebert, F., Lefort, A., Gerard, C., Parmentier, M., Perret, J., Ludgate, M., et al. (1989) Cloning sequencing, expression of the human thyrotropin receptor: evidence for binding of antibodies. *Biochem. Biophys. Res. Commun.* **165**, 1250–1255.
10. Rees Smith, B., McLachlan, S. M., and Furmaniak, J. (1988) Autoantibodies of the thyrotropin receptor. *Endocr. Rev.* **9**, 106–121.
11. Bahn, R. S. and Heufelder, A. E. (1993) Pathogenesis of Graves' ophtalmopathy. *N. Engl. J. Med.* **329**, 1468–1475.
12. Heufelder, A. E. (1994) Immunopathogenesis of endocrine orbitopathy. *Eur. J. Endocrinol.* **140(Suppl. 2)**, 67.
13. Volpe, R. (1992) A perspective of human autoimmune thyroid disease: is there an abnormality of the target cell which predisposes the disorder? *Autoimmunity* **13**, 3–9.
14. Prummel, M. F. (19940 Clinical perpectives of endocrine orbitopathy. *Eur. J. Endocrinol.* **130(Suppl. 2)**, 67–68.
15. Baker, J. R. (1997) Autoimmune endocrine disease. *JAMA* **278**, 1931–1937.

16. Ting, J. P.-Y. and Baldwin, A. S. (1993) Regulation of MHC gene expression. *Curr. Opin. Immunol.* **5,** 8–16.

17. Piccinini, L. A., Roman, S. H., and Davies, T. F. (1987) Autoimmune thyroid disease and thyroid cell class II major histocompatibility complex antigens. *Clin. Endocrinol.* **26,** 253–272.

18. Yue, S. J., Enomoto, T., Matsumoto, Y., Kawai, K., and Volpe, R. (1998) Thyrocyte class I and class II upregulation in a secondary phenomenon and does not contribute to the pathogenesis of autoimmune thyroid disease. *Thyroid* **8,** 755–763.

19. Mosmann, T. R. and Coffman, R. L. (1989) Heterogeneity of cytokine secretion patterns and functions of helper T cells. *Adv. Immunol.* **136,** 2348–2357.

20. Paul, W. E. and Seder, R. A. (1994) Lymphocytes responses and cytokines. *Cell* **76,** 241–251.

21. Katsikis, P. D., Cohen, S. B., Londei, M., and Feldman, M. (1995) Are CD4+Th1 cells pro-inflammatory or antiinflammatory? The ratio of IL-10 IFN-γ or IL-2 determines their function. *Int. Immunol.* **7,** 1287–1294.

22. Watson, P. F., Pickerill, A. P., Davies, R., and Weetman, A. P.(1994) Analysis of cytokine gene expression in Graves' disease. *J. Clin. Endocrinol. Metab.* **79,** 335–360.

23. Crisp, M. S., Lane, C., Halliwell, M., Wynford-Thomas, D., and Ludgate, M. (1997) Thyrotropin receptor transcripts in human adipose tissue. *J. Clin. Endocrinol. Metab.* **82,** 2003–2005.

24. Pappa, A., Calder, V., Ajjan, R., Fells, P., Ludgate, M., Weetman, A. P., and Lighman, S. (1997) Analysis of extraocular muscle-infiltrating T cells in thyroid associated ophthalmopathy (TAO). *Clin. Exp. Immunol.* **109,** 362–369.

25. De Carli, M., D'Elios, M. M., Mariotti, S., Pinchera, A., Ricci, M., Romagnani, S., et al. (1993) Cytolytic T cells with Th1-like cytokine profile predominate in retroorbital lymphocytic infiltrates of Graves' ophthalmopathy. *J. Clin. Endocrinol. Metab.* **77,** 1120–1124.

26. Imai, Y., Ibaraki, K., Odajima, R., and Shishiba, Y. (1994) Analysis of proteoglycan synthesis by retro-ocular tissue fibroblasts under the influence of interleukin 1β and transforming growth factor-β. *Eur. J. Endocrinol.* **131,** 630–638.

27. Chow, C. C., Lai, K. N., Leung, J. C. K., Chan, J. C. N., and Cockram, C. S. (1990) Serum soluble interleukin-2 receptor in hyperthyroid Graves' disease and effect of carbimazole therapy. *Clin. Endocrinol.* **33,** 317–321.

28. Prummel, M. F., Wiersinga, M. W., Van der Gaag, R., Mourits, M. P., and Koorneef, L. (1992) Soluble IL-2 receptor levels in patients with Graves' ophthalmopathy. *Clin. Exp. Immunol.* **88,** 405–409.

29. Escobar-Morreale, H. F., Serrano-Gotarredona, J., Villar, L. M., Garcia-Robles, R., Gonzales- Porque, P., Sancho, J. M., and Varela, C. (1996) Methimazole has no dose-related effect on the serum concentrations of soluble class I major histocompatibility complex antigens, soluble interleukin-2 receptor, and beta2-microglobulin in patients with Graves' disease. *Thyroid* **6,** 29–36.

30. Komorowski, J., Jankiewicz, J., Robak, T., Blasínska-Morawiec M., and Stepien H. (1998) Cytokine serum levels as the markers of thyroid activation in Graves' disease. *Immunol. Lett.* **60,** 143–148.

31. Hofbauer, L. C., Muhlberg, T., Konig, A., Heufelder, G., Schworm, H.-D., and Heufelder, A. E. (1997) Soluble interleukin-1 receptor antagonist serum levels in smokers and nonsmokers with Graves' ophthalmopathy undergoing orbital radiotherapy. *J. Clin. Endocrinol. Metab.* **82,** 2244–2247.

32. Bartalena, L., Brogioni, S., Grasso, L., Rago, T., Vitti, P., Pinchera, A., et al. (1994) Interleukin-6: a marker of thyroid-destructive processes?. *J. Clin. Endocrinol. Metab.* **79,** 1412–1427.

33. Celik, I., Alakin, S., and Erbas, T. (1995). Serum levels of interleukin 6 and tumor necrosis factor-α in hyperthyroid patients before and after propylothiouracil treatment. *Eur. J. Endocrinol.* **132,** 668–672.

34. Murai, H., Murakami, S., Ishida, K., and Sugawara, M. (1996) Elevated serum interleukin-6 and decrease thyroid hormone levels in postoperative patients and effects of IL-6 on thyroid cell function in vitro. *Thyroid* **6,** 601–606.

35. Siddiqi, A., Monson, J. P., Wood, D. F., Besser, G. M., and Burrin, J. M. (1999) Serum cytokines in thyrotoxicosis. *J. Clin. Endocrinol. Metab.* **84,** 435–439.

36. Iitaka, M., Noh, J. Y., Kitahama, S., Fukasawa, N., Miura, S., Kawakami, Y., et al. (1998) Elevated serum granulocyte colony-stimulating factor levels in patients with Graves' disease. *Clin. Endocrinol.* **48,** 275–280.

37. Hidaka, Y., Okamura, M., Shimaoka, Y., Takeoka, K., Tada, H., and Amino, N. (1998) Increased serum concentration of interleukin-5 in patients with Graves' disease and Hashimoto's thyroiditis. *Thyroid* **8,** 235–239.

38. Miyauchi, S., Matsuura, B., and Onji, M. (2000) Increased levels of serum interleukin-18 in Graves' disease. *Thyroid* **10,** 815–819.

22

Evaluation of Cytokines in Migraine Patients by ELISA

Irene Munno, Mariarosaria Marinaro, Giuseppe Lacedra,
Antonia Bassi, and Vincenzo Centonze

1. Introduction

The history of laboratory testing closely follows developments in the field of immunology in general. Serologic investigations were a natural outgrowth of the study of immunity, and the period from 1900 to 1950 has been called the era of international serology (*1*). Serology is the study of the noncellular components in the blood. At this time, attention turned to research on the production and use of serum to control disease, and several scientific institutes were created for this purpose. Many of the tests performed in today's clinical laboratory fall into the category of serologic tests. The need to develop rapid, specific and sensitive assays to determine the presence of important biologically active molecules ushered in a new era of testing in the clinical laboratory.

Labeled immunoassays are designed to detect antigens and antibodies that are not involved in precipitation or agglutination reactions either because they are too small or because they are present in very low concentrations. The presence of such antigens and antibodies has to be determined indirectly using a labeled reactant to ascertain whether specific binding has taken place.

Yalow and Berson's development of the radioimmunoassay (RIA) in 1959 (*2*), based on the use of a new toll, i.e., an antigen labeled with a radioactive tracer, made it possible to measure a substance with accuracy and high specificity. Although the RIA is highly sensitive and versatile and has been applied with success in various fields, its further extension has been hampered by the inherent drawbacks encountered with radioisotopes. To overcome these, several alternative procedures based on the use of other marker substances (such as free radicals, chemiluminescent or fluorescent labels, bacteriophages, and enzymes) have been proposed. Enzyme immunoassays were first reported in 1971 by Avrameas and Guilbert in France (*3*), and by Engvall and Perlmann in Sweden (*4*). These assays

From: *Methods in Molecular Medicine, vol. 60: Interleukin Protocols*
Edited by: L. A. J. O'Neill and A. Bowie © Humana Press Inc., Totowa, NJ

were employed to quantitate antigens and subsequently to titrate antibodies, based on principles similar to those of radioimmunoassays; they therefore required the use of antigen or antibody immobilized on a solid phase, i.e., an immunoadsorbent, to separate the free antigen or antibody from the antigen-antibody immune complex. These heterogeneous or solid-phase enzyme immunoassays were termed enzyme-linked immunosorbent assays (ELISAs) by Engvall and O' Beirne (5).

The principles of ELISA are similar to those developed for quantitative RIAs, but measurement of enzyme activity replaces radioactivity counting.

The *enzyme immunoassay* has been extensively developed during the past 15 yr, probably because of the high amplifying capacity of enzyme markers and the relatively simple laboratory equipment they require. ELISA has replaced RIA in many clinical and basic science laboratories.

Enzymes are naturally occurring substances that catalyze certain biochemical reactions. They react with suitable substrates to produce breakdown products that may be chromogenic, fluorogenic, or luminescent (6). The changes involved can then be measured by some type of spectroscopy. As labels for immunoassay, they are readily available, have a long shelf life, are easily adapted to automation, and cause changes that can be measured using inexpensive equipment (7,8). Sensitivity can be achieved without disposal problems or the health hazards of radiation (9). Since one molecule of enzyme can generate many molecules of product, little reagent is necessary to produce high sensitivity (10).

Enzymes used as labels for immunoassay are chosen according to the following criteria: (1) number of substrate molecules converted per molecule of enzyme; (2) purity; (3) sensitivity; (4) ease and speed of detection; (5) stability; and (6) absence of interfering factors in test fluids (7). In addition, the availability and cost of enzyme and substrate play a role in the choice of a particular enzyme as reagent. Typical enzymes that have been used as labels include horseradish peroxidase, glucose oxidase, glucose-6-phosphate dehydrogenase, alkaline phosphatase, and β-D-galactosidase (11).

For peroxidase, several chromogens are employed, yielding various colors that allow its spectrophotometric measurement. The results obtained indicate that *o*-phenylene diamine (giving an orange color) is the chromogen that provides the most sensitive and reliable measurement. The fluorometric assays of peroxidase are neither as sensitive nor as reliable as those using chromogens. Alkaline phosphatase and β-galactosidase are easily and accurately measured spectrophotometrically using *p*-nitrophenyl phosphate and *o*-nitro-phenyl-β-D-galactoside, respectively, as substrates; minute amounts of these enzymes are measured by spectrofluorimetry using 4-methyl-umbelliferylphosphate or 4-methyl-umbelliferyl- β-D-galactoside as substrates. Several other enzymes, like urease, glucose oxidase, acetylcholinesterase, penicillase, and catalase, for example, have been tried as labels in ELISA, but they are rarely used.

End products of glucose-6-phosphate dehydrogenase activity need to be determined by fluorimetric means. Alkaline phosphatase and horseradish peroxidase have the highest turnover (conversion of substrate) rates and high sensitivity and are easy to detect, so they are most often employed in such assays *(10)*. Alkaline phosphatase, however, is expensive, whereas horseradish peroxidase is readily available, is easily coupled to proteins, and reacts with a number of available chromogens (substrates that produce a colored end product) *(10)*.

The enzyme label is linked to antibody or ligand by several means. Glutaraldehyde is often used as a crosslinker to join amino groups of the enzyme and the molecule to be labeled. Maleimide derivaties are also employed to attach the enzyme label.

Biotin-labeled antibodies (or antigens) followed by enzyme-labeled avidin (or streptavidin) are often used in ELISA. However, in most assays, conjugates prepared by covalently coupling enzymes to antibodies (or antigens) by glutaraldehyde, *m*-periodate or maleimide derivatives are used.

Enzyme assays are classified as heterogeneous *(12)* or homogeneous *(6,7,13)* on the basis of whether or not a separation step is necessary. Heterogeneous enzyme immunoassays require a step to separate free from bound ligand physically. In homogeneous assays, on the other hand, no separation step is necessary, as the enzyme activity diminishes when the binding of antibody and ligand occurs. Heterogenous enzyme immunoassays, like all immunologic procedures, always involve various degrees of nonspecific binding, in addition to the specific antigen-antibody binding. This ratio appears to be primarily dependent on the solid phase and on the properties of the enzyme conjugates.

Immobilization of antigen or antibody on a solid phase is obtained either by covalent binding or by adsorption through noncovalent interactions. Paper discs, but also agarose, cellulose, and polyacrylamide particles carrying various active chemical groups, have been used for the covalent immobilization of antigens and antibodies *(14,15)*. However, these types of immunoadsorbent are not often used in ELISA. In principle, covalent binding has the advantages of irreversibly binding ligands and of preparing homogeneous immobilized antigen or antibody solid phases. Various supports have been tested for the immobilization of antigen and antibody by physical adsorption.

Plastic carriers, such as beads, films, plates, and tubes, are the most common and have proved the most successful *(14,15)*. Adsorption to such surfaces, principally polystyrene, occurs mainly by hydrophobic interactions. Because antigen or antibody immobilization on plastic surfaces is very simple and plastic carriers are easy to handle, this type of immobilization has led to the development of enzyme immunoassays suitable for large-scale testing. Of these, a procedure making use of microtitration plates, introduced in ELISA by Voller and colleagues *(16)*, has allowed the design of automatic devices, which are now routinely used.

A few years ago, the major disadvantage of the plastic surface was that the adsorbing capacity varied from one batch of plastic to another. In the plates now commercially available, this serious drawback is only occasionally encountered. Recently, active functional groups were introduced on the surface of the plastic, and proteins were covalently bound or proteins were adsorbed onto surfaces made more charged and hydrophilic after radiation treatment. The results obtained thus far are not conclusive evidence as to whether such procedures can advantageously replace simple physical absorption onto an underivatized plastic support.

1.1. Sandwich or Capture Assays

Sandwich enzyme-multiplied immunoassays, also known as capture assays, are used with antigens having multiple epitopes. Excess antibody attached to solid phase is allowed to combine with the test sample. After an incubation period, enzyme-labeled antibody is added. This second antibody may recognize the same or a different epitope from the solid-phase antibody *(17)*. Enzymatic activity is directly proportional to the amount of antigen in the test sample. This is also considered a noncompetitive assay, as all patient antigen is involved in the reaction.

This technique can be used to detect antigens that are present in very low concentrations, around pg/mL *(18)*. It is suited to antigens that have multiple determinants, such as antibodies, polypeptide hormones, proteins, and microorganisms, especially viruses *(19)*. When used with microorganisms, the epitope must be unique to the organism being tested, and it must be present in all strains of the organisms *(20)*.

Another important use of capture assays is to measure immunoglobulins, especially those of certain classes. For instance, the presence of IgM can be specifically determined, thus indicating an acute infection. Measurement of IgE, which appears in minute quantities in serum, can also be accomplished with this system *(17)*.

In sandwich assays, it is important to have a high-affinity capture antibody on solid phase, as this antibody determines the range of linearity of the titration graph *(17)*. A linear relationship does not exist between optical density and analyte concentration, so the results must be extrapolated from a standard curve. Specificity is another essential antibody quality needed in order for this test system to be effective.

Heterogeneous enzyme assays usually achieve similar sensitivity to that of RIA; however, there may be problems with nonspecific protein binding and crossreactivity. In addition, the test conditions must be carefully controlled, as temperature variations may affect the results *(10)*. Recently, the use of monoclonal antibodies has made this a highly sensitive test system.

Kits are also available for the direct measurements of most cytokines. At present, these kits are for research use only, but Food and Drug Administration

(FDA) approval for diagnostic purposes is expected shortly. Once normal human levels of cytokines are established, this method should prove to be the most sensitive and direct for diagnostic purposes.

In view of these considerations, we have detected the plasma levels of some cytokines interleukin (IL)-4, IL-5, IL-10, and interferon-γ (IFN-γ) by ELISA assay in patients suffering with migraine.

For direct measurement of cytokines in serum, we used ELISA testing in microtiter wells containing monoclonal antibody to individual cytokines. After careful washing, a second anti-IL antibody is added. This one is biotinylated and binds horseradish peroxidase-conjugated streptavidin. These immune complexes are allowed to react, and then a wash step is performed. Substrate is added, and the ensuing color development is read on a spectrophotometer.

2. Materials (*see* Notes 1 and 2)

1. Monoclonal anti-human IFN-γ, IL-4, IL-5, and IL-10 antibodies (PharMingen, San Diego, CA).
2. Biotinylated anti-IFN-γ, -IL-4, -IL-5, and -IL-10 antibodies (PharMingen).
3. Horseradish peroxidase-conjugated streptavidin (GIBCO, Life Technologies, Gaithersburg, MD).
4. 2,2'-Azinobis(3-ethylbenz)thiazoline sulfonic acid (ABTS) (Sigma) substrate.
5. Stop solution: 1 *M* sulfuric acid.
6. Phosphate-buffered saline (PBS) solution: 10 m*M* phosphate buffer, pH 7.4, 150 m*M* NaCl, and 0.1% sodium azide.
7. Washing buffer (PBS-T): 10 m*M* phosphate buffer, pH 7.4, 150 m*M* NaCl, and 0.05% Tween-20 (Sigma).
8. PBS solution containing 1% bovine serum albumin (BSA) (Sigma).

3. Methods
3.1. monoclonal Antibody Coating

1. Prepare an antibody solution of monoclonal anti-human IFN-γ, IL-4, IL-5, and IL-10 at the appropriate concentration.
2. Pipet 0.2 mL of (the above) monoclonal anti-human IFN-γ, IL-4, IL-5, or IL-10 to each well of the microtiter plate (Nunc, Naperville, IL).
3. Incubate at 37°C for 30 min, or incubate (covered) overnight at 4°C.
4. Remove the coating solution. Wash three times with PBS-T (*see* **Notes 3** and **4** for a step to ensure low nonspecific binding).
5. Pipet 0.2 mL of PBS containing 1% BSA. Incubate and wash three times with PBS-T.

3.2. Primary Antigen-Antibody Reaction

1. Dilute serially twofold standard recombinant human cytokines (IFN-γ, IL-4, IL-5, and IL-10) at the appropriate concentrations.

2. Add 0.2 mL of the diluted cytokines in PBS standards and plasma samples to duplicate wells.
3. Incubate overnight at 4°C.
4. Wash as in **Step 4** of **Subheading 3.1.**

3.3. Application of Secondary Monoclonal Antibody

1. Add 0.2 mL of appropriate biotinylated anticytokine antibodies (PharMingen) to each well.
2. Incubate the covered plates overnight at 4°C.
3. Dilute the peroxide-conjugated secondary antibody in PBS-T (*see* **Note 5**).
4. Add 0.2 mL of this solution to each well. The optimal dilution should be predetermined using a titration assay.
5. Incubate at room temperature for 1 h.
6. Wash as in **step 4** of **Subheading 3.1.**

3.4. Substrate Preparation

During the last incubation and immediately *before use*, prepare the ABTS substrate.

3.5. Development

1. Add 0.2 mL of freshly prepared substrate to each well.
2. A color should develop in positive wells within 30 min.
3. Plate may be read directly or by stopping reaction with 50 µL/well of preferred stopping reagent, at 415 nm in a microplate reader.

3.6. Calculations

Calculate the average absorbance for each set of duplicate standards, controls, and samples. Calculate the corrected absorbance by subtracting the absorbance of the zero standard from standard, controls, and samples. A standard curve must be determined each time the assay is performed. Standard curves may be generated with known amounts of appropriate recombinant human cytokines for each plate. The levels of specific cytokines in plasma may be interpolated on standard curves generated by a computer program with appropriate logistic algorithms.

3.7. Statistics

Statistical evaluation was carried out by the Fisher exact test. Data are expressed as the means ± SEM.

3.8. Case Study: Patients

1. Thirty-two patients suffering from migraine without aura (MWA), in the interictal period, were enrolled in our study. Patients ages ranged from 20 to 58 yr (mean 34.2 yr), and the male/female ratio was 9:23. All patients were consecutively

recruited through The Headache Unit-Internal Medicine, DMIL, University of Bari. The diagnosis was made according to The International Headache Society (IHS) criteria *(22)*.

2. All patients affected by allergic disorders or pathologies that could interfere with the study were excluded on the basis of accurate history taking and laboratory investigations (PRIST, RAST, specific IgG). The patients did not take preventative or symptomatic drugs for at least 1 wk before entering the study. Thirty-two donors matched for sex and age were included as healthy controls.

3. Plasma selection: 5 mL of peripheral blood was collected from all participants in heparinized tubes and then centrifuged at 400g for 15 min. Plasma was partitioned into 1-mL aliquots and immediately stored at –80°C for future analyses.

4. Blood eosinophil count: A peripheral blood eosinophil count was performed by VCS Coulter Max M.

5. Discussion: Since conflicting results have been reported on the contribution of cytokines to the pathophysiology of migraine, we undertook this study to investigate the role of cytokines in migraine patients during the interictal period. We compared plasma cytokine levels in 32 MWA patients vs 32 age- and sex-matched healthy controls.

   In healthy controls, plasma levels of all the cytokines tested were undetectable, and for statistical analyses they were considered equal to the detection limit. The detection limits for IFN-γ, IL-4, IL-5, and IL-10 were 3, 6, 1, and 5 pg/mL, respectively.

   Figure 1 shows the cytokine plasma levels in MWA patients. Plasma IFN-γ and IL-10 levels were undetectable in 30 MWA patients (93.7 %). We also measured IL-4 and IL-5 levels in plasma from the same group and found higher IL-4 levels (286 ± 66 pg/mL) in 12 MWA patients (37.5%) ($p = 0.0043$). Interestingly, plasma IL-5 levels in 27 MWA patients (84.3%) were significantly higher (2499 ± 565 pg/mL) than in healthy controls ($p < 0.0001$).

   From a clinical point of view, there was no correlation between increased cytokine levels and such clinical features as attack frequency, headache intensity, duration of illness, and average age of migraine onset. In addition, it is difficult to state the exact role of IL-4 and IL-5 since in our study higher levels of cytokines were not related to increased IgE plasma levels and eosinophil count.

4. Notes

1. Store nonreconstituted reagent undiluted at –20°C. Store all reconstituted reagent at 2–8°C and keep stable at 2–8°C until the expiration date on the label. All reagents should be brought to room temperature for use and returned to proper storage conditions immediately after use.

2. Reagents that contain thimerosal or chloroacetamide may be toxic if ingested, inhaled, or placed in contact with skin. Sulfuric acid is a caustic agent and oxider and is harmful if inhaled or absorbed through the skin. Avoid contact with skin, eyes, or clothing by substrate or stop solution

3. If problems with nonspecific binding occur, an additional blocking step (30 min, 5% BSA-PBS) may be required *(21)*.

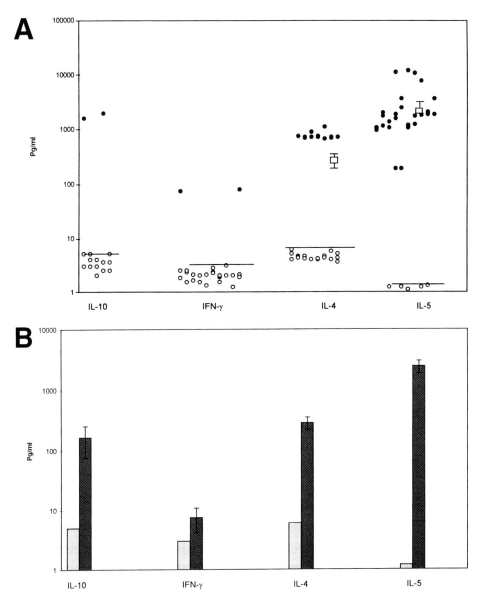

Fig. 1. (**A**) Plasma IL-10, IFN-γ, IL-4, and IL-5, levels (pg/mL) (log scale) in each MWA patient ($n = 32$) assessed during interictal period. The horizontal bars point out the detection limit of each ELISA assay. Filled circles indicate patients who released cytokines. Open circles represent patients whose cytokine levels were undetectable. (**B**) The level (mean ± SEM; log scale) of specific cytokines in MWA patients (■) and healthy controls (▨).

4. In general, in ELISA, nonspecific adsorption can be reduced by including in the medium, during the incubation and washing steps, a nonionic detergent, such as Tween-20, either alone or supplemented with a protein, e.g., BSA or gelatin *(3)*. However, it must be realized that even under the best defined conditions, there will always be nonspecific adsorption of the enzyme conjugate by the coated solid phase.

5. The choice of enzyme label depends essentially on how quickly the results are needed, as well as on the number of samples to be examined. When a large number of samples has to be tested simultaneously, it is preferable to use enzyme for which stable substrates are available and that therefore allows reactions of long duration. Consequently, peroxidase is not well suited to ELISA requiring long-lasting reactions but it is particularly effective in rapid heterogeneous enzyme immunoassays. Comparative assays performed using chromogenic substrates and conjugates of peroxidase, glucose oxidase, alkaline phosphatase, and β-galactosidase have shown that, after the optimal conditions were established, these conjugates had virtually identical sensitivities and were capable of measuring equally small quantities.

References

1. Kiple, K. F. (1993) *The Cambridge World History of Human Disease.* Cambridge University Press, Cambridge, pp. 126–140.
2. Yalow, R. S. and Berson, S. A. (1960) Immunoassay of endogenous plasma insulin in man. *J. Clin. Invest.* **39,** 1157–1175.
3. Avrameas, S., Druet, P., Masseyeff, P., and Feldmann, G., eds. (1983) *Immunoenzymatic Techniques.* Amsterdam, Elsevier.
4. Engvall, E. and Perlmann, P. (1972) ELISA. III. Quantitation of specific antibodies by enzyme-linked immunoglobulin in antigen coated tubes. *J. Immunol.* **109,** 129–135.
5. O'Beirne, A. J. and Cooper, H. R. (1979) Heterogeneous enzyme immmunoassay. *J. Histochem. Cytochem.* **27,** 1148–1162.
6. Miller, L. E., et al. (1991) *Manual of Laboratory Immunology*, 2nd ed., Lea & Febiger, Philadelphia, pp. 61–74.
7. Nakamura, R. M., Turker, E. S., and Carlson, I. H. (1991) Immunoassay in the clinical laboratory, in *Clinical Diagnosis and Management by Laboratory Methods*, 18th ed. (Henry, J. B., ed.), WB Saunders, Philadelphia, PA, pp. 848–884.
8. Ngo, T. T. (1985) Enzyme-mediated imunoassay: an overwiew, in *Enzyme-Mediated Immunoassay* (Ngo, T. T. and Lenhoff, H. M., eds.), Plenum, NY, pp. 3–32.
9. Carpenter, A. B. (1992) Enzyme-linked immunoassays, in *Manual of Clinical Immunology,* 4th ed. (Ngo, T. T. and Lenhoff, H. M., eds.), American Society for Microbiology, Washington, DC, pp. 2–9.
10. Kemeny, D. M. and Chantler, S. (1988) An introduction to ELISA, in *ELISA and Other Solid Phase Immunoassays* (Kemeny, D. M. and Challacombe, S. J., eds.), John Wiley & Sons, Chichester, UK, pp. 1–29.
11. Sheehan, C. (1990) Ligand assays, in *Clinical Immunology: Principles and Laboratory Diagnosis* (Sheehan, C., ed.), JB Lippincott, Philadelphia, PA, pp. 162–178.
12. Standeifer, J. C. (1985) Separation-required (heterogeneous)enzyme immunoassay for haptens and antigens, in *Enzyme-Mediated Immunoassay* (Ngo, T. T. and Lenhoff, H. M., eds.), Plenum Press, NY, pp. 203–222.

13. Maggio, E. T. (1984) Homogeneous enzyme immunoassays, in *Clinical Immunochemistry: Principles of Methods and Applications* (Boguslaski, R. C., Maggio, E. T., and Nakamura, R. M., eds), Little Brown, Boston, MA, pp. 89–97.
14. Baker, T. S., Abbott, S. R., Daniel, S. G., and Wright, J. F. (1985) Immunoradiometric assays, in *Alternative Immunoassays* (Collins, W. P., ed.), John Wiley & Sons, Chichester, UK, pp. 59–76.
15. Barrett, J. T. (1988) *Textbook of Immunology*, 5th ed. CV Mosby, St. Louis, MO.
16. Voller, A., and Bidwell, D. E. (1985) Enzyme immunoassays, in *Alternative Immunoassays* (Collins, W. P., ed.), John Wiley & Sons, Chichester, UK, pp. 77–86.
17. Butler, J. F. (1988) The immunochemistry of sandwich ELISAs: principles and applications for the quantitative determination of immunoglobulins, in *ELISA and Other Solid Phase Immunoassays* (Kemeny , D. M. and Challacombe, S. J., eds.), John Wiley & Sons, Chichester, UK, pp. 155–180.
18. Hemmila, I. (1985) Fluoroimmunoassays and immunofluorometric assays. *Clin. Chem.* **31,** 359.
19. Challacombe, S. J. (1988) Application of ELISA to microbiology, in *ELISA and Other Solid Phase Immunoassays* (Kemeny , D. M. and Challacombe, S. J., eds.), John Wiley & Sons, Chichester, UK, pp. 319–342.
20. Chantler, S. M. and Clayton, A. L. (1988) The use of ELISA for rapid viral antigen detection in clinical specimens, in *ELISA and Other Solid Phase Immunoassays* (Kemeny , D. M. and Challacombe, S. J., eds.), John Wiley & Sons, Chichester, UK, pp. 279–301.
21. Vogt, R. F., Phillips, D. L., Henderson, L. O., Whitfield, W., and Spierto, F. W. (1987) Quantitative differences among various proteins as blocking agents for ELISA microtiter plates. *J. Immunol. Methods* **101,** 43–50.
22. Headache Classification Committee of the International Headache Society (1988) Classification and diagnostic criteria for headache disorders, cranial neuralgias and facial pain. *Cephalalgia* **8,** 1–96.

23

Assaying Interleukins in Plasma in the Course of Acute Myocardial Infarction

Radek Pudil

1. Introduction

Acute myocardial infarction (AMI) is one of the most common diseases in cardiology. Recent studies have shown the important role of an activated immune system and its products (interleukins) in the pathogenesis of AMI in these processes:

1. Ischemia and reperfusion process with immune-mediated myocyte injury and postischemic myocardial inflammation *(1–3)*.
2. Structural and geometric changes in the left ventricle, commonly referred to as remodeling *(4)*.
3. The process of myocyte apoptosis, leading to the loss of myocardial contractile function *(5)*.

Interleukins have also been shown to have hemodynamic properties, which can have a negative effect on formerly impaired cardiac function *(6–9)*. Immune-mediated myocyte injury and postischemic myocardial inflammation dominate in the acute phase of AMI; structural and geometric changes of the myocardium begin later and develop for weeks, months, or years, i.e., in the chronic phase of the disease. The aim of this chapter is to describe the role of the enzyme-linked immunosorbent assay (ELISA) method in assaying of the interleukins in peripheral blood, including problems and troubleshooting in preanalytical and analytical phases.

1.1. Role of Interleukins in the Course of Immune-Mediated Myocyte Injury and Postischemic Myocardial Inflammation

In 1991, Entman et al. *(10)* showed the role of interleukins in the process of ischemia and reperfusion. Activated neutrophils (and their interaction with

From: *Methods in Molecular Medicine, vol. 60: Interleukin Protocols*
Edited by: L. A. J. O'Neill and A. Bowie © Humana Press Inc., Totowa, NJ

endothelial cells and cardiac myocytes) play an important role in the pathology of reperfusion injury by producing free oxygen radicals, arachidonic acid derivatives, and proteolytic enzymes.

This process includes neutrophil activation, their adherence to the endothelium, migration of activated neutrophils into the extravascular space, and interaction of the activated neutrophils with cardiac myocytes and other cells (activated fibroblasts, etc.). An injured myocardial cell initially releases products that promote chemotaxis, neutrophil shape change, and enhanced neutrophil surface expression of CD11/CD18 heterodimers; upon adherence, granular contents are released and free oxygen radicals are produced. The secretory and migratory functions require adherence of CD11/CD18 to intercellular adhesion molecule-1 (ICAM-1) and interaction with other endothelial ligands (E-selectin, VLA-4, etc.) Although all of these are constitutively expressed to some degree, induction of surface expression of ICAM-1 and other ligands is fundamental to the initiation of the inflammatory event. The interactions between activated neutrophils and cardiac myocytes are also dependent on these types of interactions.

The ischemic and reperfusion process in AMI is accompanied by elevation of plasma cytokine interleukin 1-β (IL-1β), IL-6, IL-8, tumor necrosis factor-α (TNF-α), and soluble adhesion molecule levels, as was described in our previous studies *(11,12)*. These interleukins have been shown to play a key role in this process. As was suggested in previous studies, the role of cytokines is to serve as a potent chemotactic factor for leukocytes (IL-8). IL-1β and TNF-α are also potent stimulators of adhesion molecule expression (CD 11/18, ICAM-1, E-selectin) on neutrophils, endothelial cells, and cardiac myocytes.

These interleukins are produced by mononuclear phagocytes and endothelial cells. They are also released by activated platelets and degranulated mast cells and are also produced by cardiac myocytes. Studies in the animal model have shown expression of mRNA for TNF-α, IL-1β, and IL-6 not only in the infarcted but also in the noninfarcted myocardium *(3)*.

Most interleukins are highly pleiotropic in their effects. TNF-α and IL-6 are known to induce myocyte apoptosis, resulting in loss of left ventricular mass as well as the remodeling process, and their overproduction during heart failure has a cardiodepressive effect on myocardial contractility. The association of TNF-α and IL-6 production and activation of the sympathetic nervous system influencing cardiac function is also important. Recent studies have also indicated hemodynamic properties of IL-1β. There is an increasing number of similar observations. Assessment of plasma interleukin levels has a prognostic value.

1.2. Methods of Studying the Role of Interleukins in the Course of AMI

Molecular medicine offers a broad spectrum of methods for the study of these processes, with two methods dominating:

1. Assay of the pro- and anti-inflammatory interleukins, as well as their soluble receptors and receptor antagonists in the blood specimens using the ELISA method.
2. Assessment of mRNA expression for many cytokines and their receptors and cytokine-converting enzymes in the infarcted and noninfarcted myocardium by polymerase chain reaction (PCR) techniques, immunohistochemical analysis, etc. Although these methods are preferably used in vitro or in animal models, their future use for assay of mRNA expression in tissue biopsy specimens is generally suggested.

Only a few data currently exist on the role of interleukins in AMI in humans. The role of interleukins in ischemia and reperfusion in humans is currently studied by peripheral blood sample assay, generally considered to be simple, rapid, reliable, and versatile. Plasma interleukin levels are usually measured with ELISA and related techniques *(13)*.

Although many interleukins were discovered on the basis of their biologic activities, cytokine bioassays preceded immunoassays. In comparison with bioassays, immunoassays provide the measurement of the number of molecules, not the biologic activity. Immunoassays are also characterized by high specificity and sensitivity; with good reproducibility, they offer an international standard and are less time consuming. A broad spectrum of ELISA kits for quantitative determination of the variety of human interleukins is commercially available.

1.3. Testing Strategy

Although the plasma levels of many interleukins change rapidly in the course of AMI, and a sharp peak followed by a decrease, some plasma interleukin levels are only slightly elevated without any significant peak. Recent studies have shown peak plasma IL-1β and IL-6 levels during the first 24 h. Our previous study has demonstrated the nadir plasma IL-6 level at 9 h, and the nadir plasma IL-1β level 15 h after the onset of the symptoms. Similar results have been shown by of Van Lente and Kazmierczak *(14)* and Ikeda et al. *(15)*. Plasma levels of other cytokines, e.g., IL-8 or TNF-α, were elevated throughout the time of observation without any significant peak. This elevation can persist for of 4–6 d after onset of symptoms. Although mRNA expression for TNF-α, IL-1β, IL-6, and IL-8 in the infarcted and noninfarcted myocardium remains significantly higher for 20 wk, after a period of 4–6 d interleukin levels are usually undetectable in peripheral plasma samples.

Thus it is necessary to estimate an optimal blood sample collection schedule. The first blood sample is generally recommended to be taken at the time of admission, i.e., before start of treatment, and then at 3–4-h intervals during the first 48 h and at 6–8-h intervals during the next 48 h. During the next few days there is no need to take blood samples more than once a day.

1.4. Preanalytical Factors and the Measurement of Interleukins in Human Subjects

Interleukin analyses are influenced by a myriad of factors. Factors influencing the outcome of laboratory measurements can be divided into in vivo preanalytical factors (aging, chronobiologic rhythms, diet, effect of treatment, concomitant diseases, especially the effect of serious inflammatory disorders, liver and kidney diseases, and the malignancies), in vitro preanalytical factors (e.g., specimen collection, equipment, transport, storage, etc.), and analytical factors *(16)*. To improve the value of interleukin assessment, factors strongly influencing the results have to be controlled. This can be done using standardized assays and specimen collection procedures. In the course of AMI sufficient attention must be paid to specific preanalytical factors, as described below.

1.4.1. Influence of Heart Failure on Plasma Interleukin Levels in the Course of AMI

The plasma levels of tumor TNF-α and IL-6 in a patient with AMI can be influenced by the presence of previous chronic heart failure, as well as by the development of acute heart failure. Elevation of plasma levels of these cytokines has been described in previous studies and seems to be proportional to the severity of heart failure *(17–20)*. Furthermore, in patients with heart failure the degree of natural variability in circulating interleukin levels increases with time and is greater for IL-6 than for TNF-α, as was shown by Dibbs et al. *(21)*.

1.4.2. Influence of Chronobiologic Rhythm and Hormonal Changes

The influence of circadian rhythms on the measurement of human cytokines is described in Chapter 14. Plasma interleukin levels can also be affected by changes during the menstrual cycle. Although the incidence of AMI in menopausal women is higher, the plasma interleukin levels can also be affected in hormonally active women, e.g., IL-1β secretion is known to be twice as high in the follicular phase as in the luteal phase. Excessive interleukin production during the first few days of AMI is only minimally influenced by these factors but it can be influenced during the following days.

1.4.3. Influence of a Delay in Separation of Plasma From Cells

This delay can decrease or increase in plasma interleukin concentration, e.g., a 50% decrease in plasma TNF-α concentration has been shown by Dugue et al. *(16)*.

Because of the broad spectrum of commercially available ELISA kits for quantitative determination of a variety of human interleukins, and because the differences in performance of ELISA methods depend on both the manufacturer, and the type of interleukin to be assayed, it is impossible to describe each different method step by step.

In the following sections, the use of ELISA to detect plasma IL-6 levels is outlined. Technical problems are then discussed.

2. Materials

2.1. Samples

Peripheral as well as central venous blood, arterial blood, or blood taken from the coronary sinus during invasive procedures may be used for assessment of plasma interleukins in the course of AMI (*see* **Note 1**).

EDTA endotoxin-free tubes are generally recommended for blood collection (*see* **Note 2**).

2.2. Reagents

Quantikine Human IL-6 Immunoassay kit (cat. no. D6050) for the quantitative determination of human IL-6 in tissue culture media, serum, plasma, and other fluids (R&D Systems, Minneapolis, MN). This kit contains:

1. IL-6 microtiter plate (product code D6051): 96-well polystyrene microtiter plate coated with a murine monoclonal antibody against IL-6.
2. IL-6 conjugate (product code 6052): 21 mL of polyclonal antibody against IL-6, conjugated to horseradish peroxidase with preservative.
3. IL-6 standard (product code D6053): 1 vial containing 1.5 ng of recombinant human IL-6 in a buffered protein base with preservative, lyophilized.
4. Assay diluent RD 1A (product code D0011): 12 mL of a buffered protein base with preservative.
5. Calibrator diluent RD 5A (product code D0015): 21 mL of a buffered protein base with preservative.
6. Calibrator diluent RD 6F (product code D0066): 21 mL of animal serum with preservative, for serum/plasma testing. Reconstitution of the IL-6 standard with calibrator diluent (*see* **Note 3**).
7. Wash buffer concentrate (product code D0020): 21 mL of a 25-fold concentrated solution of buffered surfactant with preservative. Preparation of the wash buffer concentrate (*see* **Note 4**).
8. A vial of color reagent A (product code D0030): 12.5 mL of stabilized hydrogen peroxide. Color reagent B (product code D0040): 12.5 mL of stabilized chromogene (tetramethylbenzidine). Preparation of the substrate solutions (*see* **Note 5**).
9. Stop solution (product code D0050): 6 mL of 2 *N* sulfuric acid.
10. Four adhesive strips. **Caution:** *see* **Note 6**.

2.3. Equipment

In addition to standard laboratory equipment, the following are required:

1. Spectrophotometer capable of measurement at 450 nm, preferably configured for microtiter plates, capable of using dual-wave length correction.

2. Pipets: 50, 100, and 200 µL for running assay; adjustable 1, 5, 10, and 25 mL for reagent preparation.
3. Deionized or distilled water.
4. Pipet, squirt bottle, manifold dispenser, or automated microtiter plate washer.
5. Optional equipment: Horizontal microtiter plate orbital shaker with speed range from 400 to 600 rpm.

3. Methods

This protocol is used in our laboratory and was prepared according to the recommendations of the diagnostic kit producer.

3.1. Collection of Blood Samples

1. Put 5 mL of peripheral blood into a sterile EDTA endotoxin-free tube.
2. Pipet 5 mL of blood into a centrifuge tube.
3. Centrifuge at 1000g for 10 min at room temperature (18–24°C).
4. After the centrifuge procedure, immediately perform assessment of the interleukin levels.

If not, pipet the plasma sample aliquots into an Eppendorf tube. Samples should always be stored in closed vessels to avoid evaporation or sublimation (*see* **Note 7**). Samples must be stored at –70°C until assessment (*see* **Note 8**).

3.2. Assay Procedure

Bring all reagents and samples to room temperature before use. It is recommended that all samples and standards be assayed in duplicate (*see* **Notes 9–11**).

1. Open the resealable foil pouch containing the microtiter plate. Remove excess microtiter plate strips from the frame and store in the foil pouch.
2. Pipet 100 µL of assay diluent RD1A into each well.
3. Add 100 µL of standard or sample per well. Cover with the adhesive strip provided and incubate for 2 h at room temperature. (For shaker assay: Incubate for 1 h at room temperature on a horizontal 0.12-inch orbital microtiter plate shaker at 500 ± 100 rpm.)
4. Aspirate each well and wash, repeating the process three times. Wash by filling each well with 400 µL of wash buffer using a squirt bottle, pipet, or manifold dispenser. Complete removal of liquid at each step is essential to good performance. After the last wash, remove any remaining wash buffer by inverting the plate and blotting it against clean paper toweling, or use vacuum aspiration.
5. Add 200 µL of IL-6 conjugate. Cover with a new adhesive strip. Incubate for 2 h at room temperature. (For shaker assay: Incubate 1 h at room temperature on a horizontal 0.12-inch orbital microtiter plate shaker set at 500 ± 100 rpm.)
6. Repeat the aspiration/wash as in **step 4**.
7. Add 200 µL of substrate solution to each well. Incubate for 20 min at room temperature.

8. Add 50 µL of stop solution to each well. If color change does not appear uniform, tap the plate gently to ensure thorough mixing.
9. Determine the optical density of each well within 30 min, using a spectrophotometer set to 450 nm. If wavelength correction is not available, subtract readings at 540 or 570 nm from the readings at 450 nm. This subtraction will correct for optical imperfections in the polystyrene microtiter plate.

3.4. Calculation of Results

Average the duplicate readings. Subtract the average zero standard optical density. Plot the optical density for the standards vs the concentration of the standards and draw the best curve. The data can be linearized by using log/log paper, and regression analysis may be applied to the log transformation.

4. Notes

1. Repeated sampling of the venous blood can be performed by leaving a permanent needle, cannula, or catheter in the peripheral or central vein. Care should be taken to ensure that no clot is formed at the tip or in the lumen of the catheter. Between samples, an anticoagulant (preferably heparin) should be used to flush the cannula. When sampling with a venous catheter, the coagulation tube containing EDTA should be filled after a heparin-containing tube is collected. The first few milliliters of blood, representing 1–2 vol of the catheter, should be discarded to avoid contamination with anticoagulant. Blood should never be collected proximal to the infusion site. Specimens should be collected from the opposite arm.
2. Current research shows that EDTA is the most suitable anticoagulant to avoid spontaneous elevation of interleukin levels after the blood sampling procedure. Heparin could give a false result because of content of contaminating endotoxins.
3. Reconstitute the IL-6 standard with 5 mL of calibrator diluent RRD6F (for serum/ plasma samples), or a diluent that reflects the composition of the samples being assayed. This reconstitution produces a stock solution of 300 pg/mL. Allow the standard to sit for a minimum of 15 min with gentle agitation prior to making dilution. Use this stock solution to produce a dilution series, as described below, within the range of this assay (3.13–300 pg/mL). (A suggested dilution series for standards is 300, 100, 50, 25, 12.5, 6.25, 3.13, and 0 pg/mL. Label six tubes or vials as 100, 50, 25, 12.5, 6.25, or 3.13 pg/mL. Pipet 0.667 mL of appropriate diluent into the 100-pg/mL tube and 0.500 mL diluent into each remaining labeled tube. Pipet 0.333 mL of the 300-pg/mL IL-6 standard into the 100-pg/mL tube and mix thoroughly. Transfer 0.500 mL from the 100-pg/mL tube to the 50-pg/mL tube and mix thoroughly. Repeat this process successively to complete the twofold dilution series. The undiluted IL-6 standard will serve as the high standard (300 pg/mL). Use the appropriate diluent as the zero standard (0 pg/mL). Store the 300-pg/mL IL-6 stock solution frozen (–20°C) for up to 30 d. Avoid freeze-thaw cycles; aliquot if repeated use is expected.
4. To yield 500 mL of wash buffer, dilute 20 mL of this concentrate into deionized (or distilled) water. Store for up to 30 d at 2–8°C. Any precipitate formed during storage will redissolve on dilution. If precipitate has formed, then mix the concentrate well before diluting.

5. Mix the color reagents A and B together in equal volumes within 15 min of use; 200 µL of the resultant mixture is required per well.
6. Wear eye, hand, face, and clothing protection. Some components of the kit contain sodium azide, which may react with lead and copper plumbing to form explosive metallic azides. Flush with large volumes of water during disposal. The stop reagent is an acid solution. Wear eye, hand, and face protection when using this material.
7. The danger of evaporation/sublimation also exists in refrigerators/freezers (condensation of moisture on the cooling elements). Reduce contact with air as much as possible. If this is not done, evaporation/sublimation will result in an apparent increase in the concentration of all nonvolatile components. This is particularly the case when the volume of the sample is relatively small and the surface area is relatively large.
8. The plasma concentration of many interleukins can be decreased by a few hours' storage at room temperature (e.g., TNF-α and IL-4). Recommended temperatures and storage times for plasma specimens are as follows: 4°C, 12 h; –20°C, 1 mo; and –80°C would maintain sample stability for years.
9. It is necessary to fulfil all steps of the procedure according to instructions provided by the manufacturer. Each commercially available ELISA kit requires its own procedure, which is usually different from that of another. All kits are provided with standards calibrated against WHO international standards. A standard curve of absorbency vs log10 antigen concentration is constructed, and the concentration of the antigen in the test sample is read off the standard curve. Some of these procedures are one-step immunoreactions; others include the immunologic step(s), enzymatic step and reading phase.
10. In all these procedures, the manufacturers' recommendations must be followed as to incubation time (appropriate temperature and conditions—shaking, etc.) and washing procedures.
11. We have tested a number of commercially available assay kits and reagents and have found the RD Quantikine (Minneapolis, MN), and Immunotech (Marseilles, France) to be fast and reliable. All these kits were intended for research use only, not for use in diagnostic procedures.

References

1. Irwin, M. W., Mak, S., Mann, D. L., Qu, R., Penninger, J. M., Yan, A., et al. (1999) Tissue expression and immunolocalization of tumor necrosis factor-alpha in postinfarction dysfunctional myocardium. *Circulation* **99,** 1492–1498.
2. Marx, N., Neumann, F. J., Ott, I., Gawaz, M., Koch, W., Pinkau, T., et al. (1998) Induction of cytokine expression in leukocytes in acute myocardial infarction. *J. Am. Coll. Cardiol.* **30,** 165–170.
3. Gwechenberger, M., Mendoza, L.-H., Youker, K. A., Frangogiannis, N. G., Smith, C. W., Michael, L. H., et al. (1999) Cardiac myocyte produce interelukin-6 in culture and in viable border zone of reperfused infarctions. *Circulation* **99,** 546–551.

4. Ono, K., Matsumori, A., Shioi, T., Furukawa, Y., and Sasayama, S. (1998) Cytokine gene expression after myocardial infarction in rat hearts: possible implication in left ventricular remodeling. *Circulation* **98,** 149–156.

5. Pulkki, K. J. (1997) Cytokines and cardiomyocyte death. *Ann. Med.* **29,** 339–343.

6. Francis, S. G. (1999) TNF alpha and heart failure. The difference between proof of principle and hypothesis testing. *Circulation* **99,** 3213–3214.

7. Ferrari, R. (1998) Tumor necrosis factor in CHF: a double facet cytokine. *Cardiovasc. Res.* **37,** 554–559.

8. Cecconi, C., Curello, S., Bachetti, T., Corti, A., and Ferrari, R. (1998) Tumor necrosis factor in congestive heart failure: a mechanism of disease for the new millenium? *Prog. Cardiovasc. Dis.* **48(Suppl. 1),** 25–30.

9. Piano, M. R., Bondmass, M., and Schwertz, D. W. (1998) The molecular and cellular pathophysiology of heart failure. *Heart Lung* **27,** 3–19.

10. Entman, M. L., Michael, L., Rossen, R. D., Dreyer, W. J., Anderson, D. C., Taylor, A. A., et al. (1991) Inflammation in the course of early myocardial ischemia. *FASEB J.* **5,** 2529–2537.

11. Pudil, R., Pidrman, V., Krejsek, J., Gregor, J., Tichy, M., Andrys, C., et al. (1999) Cytokines and adhesion molecules in the course of acute myocardial infarction. *Clin. Chim. Acta* **280,** 127–134.

12. Pudil, R., Pidrman, V., Krejsek, J., Gregor, J., Tichy, M., Andrys, C., et al. (1998) Effect of reperfusion on plasma cytokine and adhesion molecule levels in the course of acute myocardial infarction. *Cor Vasa* **40,** 166–172.

13. Reen, D. J. (1994) Enzyme-linked immunosorbent assay (ELISA), in *Methods in Molecular Biology* (Walker, J. M., ed.), Humana, Totowa, NJ, pp. 461–467.

14. Van Lente, F. and Kazmierczak, S. C. (1995) Interleukin 6 as a first indicator of acute myocardial infarction. *Clin. Chem.* **41,** 1189–1190.

15. Ikeda, U., Ikeda M., Kano, S., and Shimada, K. (1993) Neutrophil adherence to rat cardiac myocyte by proinflammatory cytokines. *J. Cardiovasc. Pharmacol.* **23,** 647–652.

16. Dugue, B., Lepanen, E., and Grasbeck, R. (1996) Preanalytical factors and the measurement of cytokines in human subjects. *Int. J. Clin. Lab. Res.* **26,** 99–105.

17. Koller-Strametz, J., Pacher, R., Frey, B., Kos, T., Woloszuk, W., and Stanek, B. (1998) Circulating tumor necrosis factor-alpha in chronic heart failure: relation to its soluble receptor II, interelukin-6, and neurohumoral variables. *J. Heart Lung Transplant.* **17,** 356–362.

18. Satoh, M., Nakamura, M., Saitoh, H., Satoh, H., Maesawa, C., Segawa, I., et al. (1999) Tumor necrosis factor alpha converting enzyme and tumor necrosis factor alpha in human dilated cardiomyopathy. *Circulation* **99,** 3260–3265.

19. Colucci, W. S. (1997) Molecular and cellular mechanisms of myocardial failure. *Am. J. Cardiol.* **80,** 15–25.

20. Meldrum, D. R. (1998) Tumor necrosis factor in the heart. *Am. J. Physiol.* **274,** 557–195.

21. Dibbs, Z., Thornby, J., White, B. G., and Mann, D. L. (1999) Natural variability of circulating levels of cytokines and cytokine receptors in patients with heart failure: implications for clinical trials. *J. Am. Coll. Cardiol.* **33,** 1935–1942.

IV

ASSAYING INTERLEUKINS IN PARTICULAR BIOLOGICAL FLUIDS

24

Measurement of Cytokines in Peritoneal Fluids

Reijo Punnonen and Juha Punnonen

1. Introduction

Cytokines are small-molecular-weight proteins that mainly function in soluble, secreted form. Cytokines regulate a wide variety of cellular functions, such as immune responses and the growth and differentiation of hemopoietic, epithelial, and mesenchymal cells *(1,2)*. Typical features of cytokines are pleiotropy and redundancy, that is, each cytokine has numerous functions, and one function is often mediated by several different cytokines. Based on their functional or structural similarities, cytokines can be roughly divided into interleukins (IL), tumor necrosis factors (TNFs), interferons (IFNs), hemopoietic growth factors, and chemokines. Practically all nucleated cells produce certain cytokines at moderate levels, but a high level of cytokine production is typically a characteristic of the cells of the immune system, particularly of activated monocytes/macrophages and T-lymphocytes.

T helper (Th) cells are divided into at least three subsets based on their cytokine synthesis profiles, and the pattern of cytokine production by antigen-specific T cells has been suggested to affect the outcome of several diseases profoundly, including infectious diseases, allergy, autoimmune diseases, and malignancies *(3–5)*. Th1 cells produce high levels of IL-2 and IFN-γ and no or minimal levels of IL-4, IL-5, and IL-13. In contrast, Th2 cells produce high levels of IL-4, IL-5, and IL-13, whereas IL-2 and IFN-γ production is minimal or absent *(3–5)*. Th1 cells activate macrophages and dendritic cells, and they also augment the cytolytic activity of CD8+ cytotoxic T-lymphocytes and natural killer cells. Th2 cells provide efficient help for B cells, and they mediate allergic responses due to the capacity of Th2 cells to induce IgE isotype switching and differentiation of B cells into IgE-secreting cells *(6)*. Th0 cells produce high levels of IL-2 and typically low levels of both IL-4 and IFN-γ. More

From: *Methods in Molecular Medicine, vol. 60: Interleukin Protocols*
Edited by: L. A. J. O'Neill and A. Bowie © Humana Press Inc., Totowa, NJ

recently, two additional T-cell subsets have been demonstrated. Th3 cells are characterized by production of high levels of transforming growth factor (TGF)-β, and T-regulatory cells were identified as cells producing high levels of IL-10 *(7,8)*. Identification of different T-cell subsets generally requires analysis of cytokine production at the single cell level, because T-cell populations are typically mixtures of different T-cell subsets.

Peritoneal fluid (PF) cytokine measurements provide the opportunity to study cytokine production at sites of disease processes such as cancer, endometriosis, fibrosis, abdominal infections, and inflammatory diseases of the gastrointestinal tract *(9–14)*. Analysis of cytokine production in PF provides information of the disease mechanisms and activity. Moreover, the cytokine profile of PF gives an insight into the types of cells that are present in the peritoneal cavity and to the activation and differentiation status of the different T-helper cell subsets.

In the present chapter we describe methods for measurement of cytokine production with special emphasis on PF. Cytokines often have additive and/or synergistic effects on responses induced by other cytokines, and one cytokine may stimulate or prevent the expression of another cytokine or its receptor. Therefore, it is important to study simultaneous expression of several cytokines that may crossregulate each other's functions. We describe the means to measure total cytokine levels present in PF and the means to analyze cytokine production by individual cells.

2. Materials
2.1. PF Samples

PF can be obtained as an ascites puncture, or during laparoscopy or surgery *(9–15)*. PF is typically aspirated in the beginning of the operations from the cul-de-sac. In patients with malignancies, the quantity of PF may dramatically increase, resulting in ascites formation. In these cases the volume of PF typically exceeds 0.5 L, and therefore ascites puncture is a convenient means of obtaining samples of PF. In addition, PF samples may be obtained by intravaginal puncture of the fossa Douglas. Although exact measurements are often difficult to obtain, it is always useful to obtain information on the total volume of PF, because this will allow estimations of the total amounts of cytokines present in PF. Cases with bleeding from the abdominal wall should be discarded (*see* **Note 1**). The samples should be immediately put on ice and delivered to the laboratory. The samples should be centrifuged at 400*g* for 10 min to remove any cells or cell debris. The supernatants should then be stored at –70°C until the cytokine levels are determined (*see* **Note 2**). Storage at –20°C for short periods is often acceptable, but the longer the samples are stored the higher the probability of altered ratios of cytokines in each sample is (*see* **Note 3**).

2.2. Reagents
2.2.1. ELISA

1. Immulon microtiter plates for enzyme-linked immunosorbent assay (ELISA) were obtained from Dynex Technologies (Chantilly, VI).
2. Purified recombinant human cytokines and cytokine-specific ELISA kits were obtained from R&D Systems (Minneapolis, MN).
3. PBS was obtained from Gibco BRL (Paisley, Scotland).
4. Washing buffer: Phosphate-buffered saline (PBS) supplemented with 0.05% (v/v) Tween-20, pH 7.4.
5. Blocking buffer: PBS supplemented with 1% (w/v) bovine-serum albumin (BSA; Sigma, St. Louis, MO) or 1% (v/v) fetal calf serum (FCS; Bioproducts for Science, Indianapolis, IN).
6. ELISA substrate: 1 mg/mL 2,2'-azinobis(3-ethylbenzothiazoline-6-sulfonic acid) in 0.1 M citrate/0.1 M phosphate buffer, containing 0.003% (v/v) H_2O_2, pH 4.5.

2.2.2. Flow Cytometry

1. Wash buffer: PBS supplemented with 0.5% (w/v) BSA and 0.01% (w/v) NaN_3.
2. Fluorescein isothiocyanate (FITC)- and phycoerythrin (PE)-conjugated human surface antigen-specific and cytokine monoclonal antibodies were purchased from Becton Dickinson (San Jose, CA).
3. 2% (v/v) Formaldehyde.
4. Permeabilization buffer: PBS supplemented with 0.5% (w/v) BSA, 0.01% (w/v) NaN_3, and 0.1% (w/v) saponin.
5. FITC-, PE- and PerCP-conjugated IgG1 isotype controls.

3. Methods
3.1. Cytokine Measurements Using ELISA

The recommended, but by no means the only, method for the measurement of total cytokine levels in PF is cytokine-specific ELISA. Several commercially available kits for cytokine measurements are available (e.g., from R&D Systems, Endogen, PeproTech, and Genzyme), but their high cost often prevents their usage in large studies. Establishment of specific ELISAs in the laboratory is quite feasible and cost-effective and provides the same quality of results as commercially available kits. Even when the required antibodies (Abs) are purchased commercially, the cost of the analysis per sample is only a fraction of that when complete kits are used. Cytokine-specific Abs are typically available through the same companies that provide ELISA kits, and many of them have been pretested for use in ELISA. Although much more work is required, the cytokine-specific Abs can be generated in the laboratory, and several sensitive ELISA protocols have been successfully established using such Abs *(16–19)*.

A typical protocol for cytokine-specific ELISA is described below. Minor modifications are often required depending on the quality of the Abs, buffers, and plates. In addition, several different substrates can be used. In the present example, horseradish peroxidase (HRP) is used. Samples from different study groups should be measured in parallel in each assay to avoid differences due to possible interassay variance.

1. Coat the wells of 96-well plates with 100 µL of capture Ab specific for the cytokine of interest, diluted in PBS (*see* **Note 4**). Incubate overnight at room temperature (RT). Some plates may be more efficiently coated at 4°C.
2. Wash the plates three times with at least 200 µL/well of washing buffer.
3. Block nonspecific binding by adding 200 µL/well of blocking buffer and incubate for at least 1 h at RT. Subsequently, wash the plates as in **step 2**.
4. Add 100 µL of samples and standards to the plates. Duplicate or triplicate measurements are recommended. Incubate for 2–3 h at RT and wash the plates three times.
5. Add detection Ab specific for the cytokine of interest (*see* **Notes 4** and **5**).
6. Incubate for approx 2 h, and wash plates three times as in **step 2**. If detection antibody is HRP-conjugated, proceed directly to **step 8**.
7. When using biotinylated secondary Ab, add 100 µL of streptavidin-HRP to each well, and incubate 20–30 min.
8. Add ELISA substrate and incubate 20–30 min. Keep direct light away from the plate.
9. Determine the optical density (OD) at a wavelength of 450 nm using a microplate reader.

3.2. Analysis of Cytokine Synthesis at the Single Cell Level Using Flow Cytometry

In several applications, information on the cytokine synthesis profiles of individual cells provides information on the types of active immune responses. Such information is crucial when evaluating the possibility of treating diseases by altering the Th1/Th2 balance in vivo. As an example, Th2 responses are generally considered to favor allergic responses, whereas Th1 cells contribute to several autoimmune diseases, reversal of the skewed Th cell differentiation may provide potential opportunities to treat these diseases. The ratios of Th1 and Th2 cytokines in PF can be measured by ELISA, but analysis of cytokine production at the single cell level generally provides more detailed information. Flow cytometry can analyze thousands of cells per second, and permeabilization of cell membranes allows staining of intracellular cytokines *(20)*. Moreover, flow cytometry allows simultaneously staining with MAbs that recognize cell surface antigens, providing the means to analyze cytokine production in various lymphocyte subpopulations. PF lymphocytes at 10^6 are sufficient for analysis of Th1/Th2 ratios, but somewhat higher numbers of cells are typically useful for more detailed analysis of the lymphocyte subsets.

To measure intracellular cytokines in T helper cells, in vitro T-cell activation is typically required. Several mitogens, such as phytohemagglutinin (PHA) or phorbol myristate acetate (PMA), can be used, or T cells can be stimulated by anti-CD3 + anti-CD28 MAbs *(21)*. The activated cells are then harvested, washed, permeabilized, and stained with MAbs specific for the cytokines of interest. The following is a typical protocol for intracellular cytokine staining to measure cytokine production at single cell level by flow cytometry.

1. The cells are washed twice with wash buffer (*see* **Subheading 2.2.2.**).
2. When desired, the cells are stained with MAbs specific for cell surface antigens to allow identification of cytokine-secreting cells, for example, staining with anti-CD4 and anti-CD8 MAbs for 30 min, after which the cells are washed twice.
3. The cells are fixed with 2% formaldehyde for 20 min at RT.
4. The cells are subsequently permeabilized in permeabilization buffer for 10 min at RT.
5. The permeabilized cells are stained with FITC- and PE-conjugated anticytokine MAbs diluted in permeabilization buffer for 30 min on ice and then washed twice with permeabilization buffer and once with wash buffer.
6. FITC-, PE-, and PerCP-conjugated IgG1 isotype controls can be used as negative controls to differentiate between positive and negative cells. Labeled cells are analyzed by FACSCalibur flow cytometer and CellQuest software (Becton-Dickinson), for example. Cells with light scatter characteristics of lymphocytes should be gated, and it is recommended that at least 5000–10,000 cells of each sample be analyzed. Fluorescence is measured using detectors specific for each wavelength, and data can be presented as either histograms or dot plots.

Flow cytometry is by far the most efficient technology for analyzing the phenotypes of single cells. The major advantages include high sensitivity and rapid analysis of large numbers of cells *(20)*. Thousands of cells can be analyzed per second compared with some hundreds per slide using immunohistochemistry. In addition, flow cytometry can easily and rapidly analyze several cytokines simultaneously. An alternative method for detection of cellular cytokines is reverse transcriptase-polymerase chain reaction, which is also very sensitive *(22)*, but the technique is not feasible for analysis of individual cells. The disadvantages of flow cytometry include high price of instrumentation and relatively difficult sample preparation. In addition, flow cytometry provides information on only one single time point. Theoretically, it is possible that some cytokines are induced in the PF cells during the surgery, and positive results can be obtained, although the given cytokine may not have been produced before the surgery. In contrast, ELISA provides data on the accumulated amounts of cytokines, and therefore, the risk of artifacts because of sample preparation is reduced.

4. Notes

1. It is also important to obtain full clinical histories of the patients, because they may be undergoing therapies that have profound effects on the cells of the

immune system. Such therapies include, but are not limited to, immunosuppressive drugs and ongoing chemo- or radiotherapy. Furthermore, active infections typically alter the production levels of many cytokines.

2. Sample preparation and storage are crucial for the quality of the results. The samples should be stored at 4°C until they reach the laboratory and they should be centrifuged as soon as they arrive. Immediate processing of the samples reduces interference caused by lysis of cells present in the PF or by any proteases that may be present. In addition, if lymphocytes or macrophages are present in the PF samples, activation of these cells ex vivo may result in false-positive results.

3. Repeated freezing and thawing is common when testing clinical samples in several different tests. However, for cytokine assays this is not recommended, because the activity and biochemical properties of several cytokines may be altered, and different cytokines may be differently affected.

4. Coating of the plates using the right amount of the Abs specific for the given cytokine is essential for the quality of the measurements. When the background given by control samples is high, it is often an indication of too much coating Ab, but it can also be caused by excessive secondary Ab. Generally, the best approach is to titrate the amounts of both coating and secondary Abs.

5. Commercially available biotinylated and HRP-conjugated Abs are available. However, nonconjugated Abs can be used followed, for example, by biotinylated or HRP-conjugated secondary antibody.

References

1. Paul, W. E. and Seder, R. A. (1994) Lymphocyte responses and cytokines. *Cell* **76,** 241–251.
2. Oppenheim, J. J., Murphy, W. J., Chertox, O., Schirrmacher, V., and Wang, J. M. (1997) Prospects for cytokine and chemokine biotherapy. *Clin. Cancer Res.* **3,** 2682–2686.
3. Mosmann, T. R. and Coffman, R. L. (1989) TH1 and TH2 cells: different patterns of lymphokine secretion lead to different functional properties. *Annu. Rev. Immunol.* **7,** 145–173.
4. Lucey, D. R., Clerici, M., and Shearer, G. M. (1996) Type 1 and type 2 cytokine dysregulation in human infectious, neoplastic, and inflammatory diseases. *Clin. Microbiol. Rev.* **9,** 532–562.
5. Coffman, R. L., Mocci, S., and O'Garra A. (1999) The stability and reversibility of Th1 and Th2 populations. *Curr. Top. Microbiol. Immunol.* **238,** 1–12.
6. De Vries, J. E. and Punnonen, J. (1996) Interleukin-4 and interleukin-13, in *Cytokine Regulation of Humoral Immunity: Basic and Clinical Aspects* (Snapper, C. M., ed.), John Wiley & Sons, West Sussex, UK, pp. 195–215.
7. Chen, Y., Kuchroo, V. K., Inobe, J., Hafler, D. A., and Weiner, H. L. (1994) Regulatory T cell clones induced by oral tolerance: suppression of autoimmune encephalomyelitis. *Science* **265,** 1237–1240.
8. Groux, H., O'Garra, A., Bigler, M., Rouleau, M., Antonenko, S., de Vries, J. E., et al. (1997) A CD4+ T-cell subset inhibits antigen-specific T-cell responses and prevents colitis. *Nature* **389,** 737–742.

9. Price, F. V., Chambers, S. K., Chambers, J. T., Carcangiu, M. L., Schwartz, P. E., Kohorn, E. I., et al. (1993) Colony-stimulating factor-1 in primary ascites of ovarian cancer is a significant predictor of survival. *Am. J. Obstet. Gynecol.* **168,** 520–527.

10. Moradi, M. M., Carson, L. F., Weinberg, B., Haney, A. F., Twiggs, L. B., and Ramakrishnan, S. (1993) Serum and ascitic fluid levels of interleukin-1, interleukin-6, and tumor necrosis factor-alpha in patients with ovarian epithelial cancer. *Cancer* **72,** 2433–2440.

11. Punnonen, J., Teisala, K., Ranta, H., Bennett, B., and Punnonen, R. (1996) Increased levels of interleukin-6 and interleukin-10 in the peritoneal fluid of patients with endometriosis. *Am. J. Obstet. Gynecol.* **174,** 1522–1526.

12. Punnonen, R., Teisala, K., Kuoppala, T., Bennett, B., and Punnonen, J. (1998) Cytokine production profiles in the peritoneal fluids of patients with malignant or benign gynecologic tumor. *Cancer* **83,** 788–796.

13. Zeyneloglu, H. B., Senturk, L. M., Seli, E., Oral, E., Olive, D. L., and Arici, A. (1998) The role of monocyte chemotactic protein-1 in intraperitoneal adhesion formation. *Hum. Reprod.* **13,** 1194–1199.

14. Brauner, A., Hylander, B., and Lu, Y. (1998) Granulocyte stimulating factor in patients on peritoneal dialysis and LPS stimulated peripheral blood mononuclear cells. *Inflammation* **22,** 393–401.

15. Punnonen, R., Seppälä, E., Punnonen, K., and Heinonen, P. K. (1986) Fatty acid composition and arachidonic acid metabolites in ascitic fluid of patients with ovarian cancer. *Prostaglandins Leukot. Med.* **22,** 153–158.

16. Chretien, I., Van Kimmenade, A., Pearce, M., Banchereau, J., and Abrams, J. S. (1989) Development of polyclonal and monoclonal antibodies for immunoassay and neutralization of human interleukin-4. *J. Immunol. Methods* **117,** 67–73.

17. Bacchetta, R., de Waal Malefijt, R., Yssel, H., Abrams, J., de Vries, J. E., Spits, H., et al. (1990) Host-reactive CD4$^+$ and CD8$^+$ T cell clones isolated from a human chimera produce IL-5, IL-2, IFN-gamma and granulocyte/macrophage-colony-stimulating factor but not IL-4. *J. Immunol.* **144,** 902–908.

18. Yssel, H., Johnson, K. E., Schneider, P. V., Wideman, J., Terr, A., Kastelein, R., et al. (1992) T cell activation-inducing epitopes of the house dust mite allergen Der p I. Proliferation and lymphokine production patterns by Der p I-specific CD4$^+$ T cell clones. *J. Immunol.* **148,** 738–745.

19. Wahlgren, M., Abrams, J. S., Fernandez, V., Bejarano, M. T., Azuma, M., Torii, M., et al. (1995) Adhesion of *Plasmodium falciparum*-infected erythrocytes to human cells and secretion of cytokines (IL-1-beta, IL-1RA, IL-6, IL-8, IL-10, TGF beta, TNF alpha, G-CSF, GM-CSF). *Scand. J. Immunol.* **42,** 626–636.

20. Maino, V. C. and Picker, L. J. (1998) Identification of functional subsets by flow cytometry: intracellular detection of cytokine expression. *Cytometry* **34,** 207–215.

21. Isomäki, P., Luukkainen, R., Lassila, O., Toivanen, P., and Punnonen, J. (1999) Synovial fluid T cells from patients with rheumatoid arthritis are refractory to the T helper type 2 differentiation-inducing effects of interleukin-4. *Immunology* **96,** 358–364.

25

Measurement of Cytokines in Seminal Plasma

Marek Glezerman, Eitan Lunenfeld, and Mahmoud Huleihel

1. Introduction

Cytokines are a family of immunoregulatory peptide growth factors. They are produced mainly by immune cells after immune challenge (infection/inflammation). Various cells of nonimmune cell origin such as epithelial, muscle, endothelial, fibroblast, and mesangial, and also sperm cells are capable of producing cytokines. Cytokines are pleiotropic factors with autocrine and paracrine effects and may therefore play an important role in the testicular microenvironment. The main proinflammatory cytokines are tumor necrosis factor-α (TNF-α), interleukin (IL)-1, and IL-6. The first cytokine produced after immunologic challenge is TNF-α, which induces the production of IL-1 followed by IL-6. The amplitude of the immune response is controlled by feedback inhibition of the proinflammatory cytokines and also by downregulator cytokines such as IL-4, IL-10, IL-12, and/or cytokine-soluble receptors and IL-1 receptor antagonist. Ample evidence has accumulated indicating the involvement of cytokines in the physiology and pathophysiology of reproduction (1).

1.1. Male Genital Infection

The male (and the female) genital system is exposed to microbial and viral infections. Inflammatory processes may affect either the prostate or the seminal vesicles, or both secondary sex glands. In 40% of infertile couples, a male factor is implicated for which the etiology is often unknown. Acute and chronic infections of the genitourinary tract may play a contributing role in male-factor infertility. An infectious process may impair fertility by a variety of mechanisms. In the extreme, obstruction of the genital may ensue, but the infective process may also affect the spermatogenetic system and/or sperm functions via mediators. Cytokines have been implicated in this realm (1–4).

From: Methods in Molecular Medicine, vol. 60: Interleukin Protocols
Edited by: L. A. J. O'Neill and A. Bowie © Humana Press Inc., Totowa, NJ

1.2. Cytokines and Their Soluble Receptors in Seminal Plasma

Semen is composed of cells (sperm cells, leukocytes, and epithelial cells) and plasma (peptide and nonpeptide soluble factors). Seminal plasma is derived from various glands along the male reproductive tract, mainly epididymis, seminal vesicles, prostate, and bulbourethral glands, but also Sertoli cells in the testis. Lymphocytes and monocytes are present in the human male genital tract even in the apparent absence of genital tract infection. Large numbers of leukocytes have been detected in some semen samples in the presence of male genital infection and infertility *(3,4)*. Seminal plasma contains various cytokines and anti-inflammatory and immunosuppressive factors that are assumed to protect sperm from immunologic damage and prevent sensitization of the female genital system to sperm antigens after coitus *(5)*. Although cells of the immune system are the major source of cytokines, other cells in the reproductive tract apparently also produce cytokines.

1.3. Inhibitory Cytokines in Semen

TNF-α is present in seminal plasma of fertile and infertile patients in similar amounts *(6)*. We have recently shown that the levels of soluble TNF receptor type I were significantly lower in semen with oligoteratozoospermia in the presence of leukospermia compared with normal, azoospermic, and oligoteratozoospermic semen samples with no evidence of infection *(7)*. IL-8 possesses specific chemotactic activity for accumulation and activation of neutrophils at an inflammatory site *(8)*. Shimoya et al. *(9)* have demonstrated the presence of IL-8 in semen of normal fertile men. They have further demonstrated an increase in IL-8 in semen of infertile men with leukospermia and a high degree of correlation between IL-8 concentration in seminal plasma and polymorphonuclear cell (PMN) elastase level in seminal plasma. Interferon-γ (IFN-γ) is a product of T cells and natural killer cells and has distinct biologic effects on cell growth and differentiation in a variety of cell systems. Naz and Kaplan *(10)* detected IFN-γ in seminal plasma of fertile and infertile men. They claimed that IFN-γ levels correlated significantly with the sperm number in semen and some sperm motility characteristics, namely, linearity and beat frequency *(10)*. IL-10 exhibits an important regulatory function during the initiation and maintenance of inflammation and is capable of blocking the expression of proinflammatory cytokines, including IL-8. IL-10 is constitutively detectable in seminal plasma *(11)*.

1.4. Growth Cytokines in Semen

Measuring the concentration of IL-1β in seminal plasma of men with accessory sex gland infection and an increased number of PMNs, Comhaire et al. *(12)* found significantly higher IL-1β levels compared with those of controls. In addition, there was a significant correlation between the concentration of PMNs and that of IL-1β. We have recently, demonstrated that IL-1β is present in similar amounts in seminal plasma of fertile and infertile men; IL-1 receptor antagonists were expressed at variable magnitudes in different groups of patients. IL-1 receptor antagonists were present in low amounts in seminal plasma of fertile men, and their levels were increased in azoospermia, oligoteratozoospermia, and, more significantly, oligoteratozoospermia in the presence of leukospermia *(7)*.

IL-2 concentrations in seminal fluids with identified bacterial agents were lower than in control groups *(6)* and are present in significantly higher levels in the seminal plasma of infertile men compared with fertile men *(13)*. Furthermore, higher seminal plasma concentrations of soluble IL-2 receptor were detected in ejaculates with high levels of PMNs or elastase *(14)* or low sperm motility *(15)*. Paradisi et al. *(16)* were not able to demonstrate significant differences in total soluble IL-2 receptor in the seminal plasma of fertile and infertile men. Furthermore, no specific relationship seems to exist between the concentration of IL-2 and its soluble receptor in semen. Naz and Kaplan *(10)* noted that the levels of IL-6 in seminal plasma of fertile men were significantly lower when compared with those of infertile men and IL-6 levels in seminal plasma and cover a wide range in men with normal and abnormal spermiograms *(17)*. Comhaire et al. *(12)* observed that the concentration of IL-6 in seminal plasma of men with male accessory gland infection and an increased number of PMNs was significantly higher than that of controls. In addition, there was a significant correlation between the concentration of PMNs and that of IL-6. This group suggested that IL-6 and IL-1β in semen could be used as markers of an inflammatory state of the accessory sex glands. IL-6 at a criterion value of 45 pg/mL was reported to have a specificity of 80% and a sensitivity of 92%. The same group also reported that IL-6 concentrations were significantly higher in men with varicocele without white blood cells in the semen compared with matched controls without varicocele *(18)*.

The endocrine system and the paracrine/autocrine system, both mediated by cytokines, are probably interactive: A study carried out in rats demonstrated that Sertoli cells secrete bioactive IL-6 when cultured in vitro *(19)*. It was further found that follicle-stimulating hormone (FSH) augments Sertoli cell IL-6 secretion in a dose-dependent manner. Thus, hormonal imbalance, especially related to FSH, may affect the levels of IL-6. The concentration in semen of IL-6-soluble receptor is unrelated to that of IL-6 and IL-1β and was not influenced by accessory gland infection *(20)*.

1.5. Immune Response Inhibitory Effect of Seminal Plasma

Seminal plasma is involved in the inhibition of immune responses in vitro as well as in vivo. These include suppression of B-cell function and proliferation, natural cell killing, T-cell proliferation in response to phytohemagglutinin (PHA) and concanavalin A, mixed lymphocyte response, primary and secondary humoral responses, inhibition of macrophages and granulocytes, phagocytosis, and the production of reactive oxygen species *(5,21,22)*. Cytokines, cytokine inhibitors, and/or their soluble receptors in addition to other mechanisms control immune response amplitude. The physiologic role of the inhibitory effect of seminal plasma probably acts mainly to protect the sperm cells in the male genital tract and to prevent immunologic damage of sperm in the female genital tract by decreasing the sensitization of leukocyte responses. We have recently demonstrated that seminal plasma from infertile men with and without leukospermia is less inhibitory for spleen cell proliferation than seminal plasma of fertile men *(23)*. IL-12 plays a central role in the regulation of immune responses, as documented by a variety of actions, such as its ability to activate natural killer cells and cytotoxic T-lymphocytes and to enhance IFN-γ production. IL-12 has been detected in seminal plasma of both fertile and infertile men *(24,25)*, with the infertile group having lower levels *(25)*.

1.6. The Effect of Cytokines on Sperm Function

TNF-α has been implicated in a dose-dependent reduction of sperm motility and in reduction of the fertilizing capacity of human sperm in sperm penetration assays *(26,27)*. Others *(28,29)* reported that recombinant TNF affected neither sperm motility nor penetration of bovine cervical mucus or hamster ova, mouse in vitro fertilization, or preimplantation development. Incubation of human spermatozoa with a combination of TNF-α and IFN-γ significantly reduces human sperm viability and sperm integrity, as demonstrated by the use of the hypoosmotic swelling test and percentage of motility *(30)*. IL-6 increases the fertilizing capacity of human sperm cells by affecting capacitation and/or acrosome reaction *(31)*.

2. Materials
2.1. Cytokine Immunoassay

1. Coating buffer: 0.1 M carbonate, pH 9.5. For some cytokines phosphate-buffered saline (PBS) may also be used (*see* **Note 1**).
2. PBS, pH 7.4: Dissolve 80 g NaCl, 2.0 g KCl, 11.5 g Na_2HPO_4, and 2.0 g KH_2PO_4 in 900 mL distilled water. Adjust pH to 7.4 with 1 M NaOH if necessary. Make volume up to 1 L with distilled water. Store at room temperature. Dilute 1 in 10 with distilled water for use.
3. Washing buffer: PBS + 0.05% (v/v) Tween-20.
4. Blocking buffer: PBS + 10% (v/v) fetal calf serum (FCS) or 2% (w/v) bovine serum albumin (BSA).
5. Standard diluent: Cell culture medium or serum (depending on the samples examined).

6. Dilutions for second antibody and horseradish peroxidase (HRP): PBS + 0.05% (v/v) Tween-20 + 2% (w/v) BSA or 10% (v/v) FCS.
7. Primary and secondary antibodies for ELISA.
8. Appropriate ELISA detection system.
9. Stop solution: 2 N H$_2$SO$_4$.
10. 96-well ELISA plates.

2.2. Cytokine Bioassays

1. Cells for bioassays: 1A-5 helper T-cell line (IL-1), CTLD cell line (IL-1, IL-2), cell line FDC-P2 (IL-3), B9 cell line (IL-6), L-929 fibroblasts (TNF), and murine bone marrow cells (colony-stimulating factors [CSFs]).
2. Recombinant cytokines for standards: IL-1, IL-2, IL-3, IL-6, human TNF, and CSF-1.
3. 1 mg/mL MTT.
4. Isopropanol in 0.04 N hydrochloric acid.
5. Ham F-10 medium containing serum (membrane IL-1 bioassay).
6. 1% Formaldehyde.
7. Cyclohexamide.
8. Media for cell culture (*see* **Notes 2–5**) and FCS.
9. Agar.
10. Neutral red stain.
11. Orcein stain.

3. Methods

When assessing cytokine levels in semen, it should be kept in mind that cytokines in seminal plasma may be adsorbed to sperm cells or to other cells and may be biologically inactivated by various mechanisms, including inhibitory factors (specific and/or nonspecific) and/or proteases. Their specific soluble receptors or other nonspecific inhibitors affect the levels of bioactive cytokines in seminal plasma. Prostaglandins, inhibin, and other inhibitory factors may affect cytokine activity. Therefore, the total biologic effect of cytokines should be viewed in light of a balance between the levels of cytokine and their inhibitors. A reasonable approach to examine the actual active levels of cytokines in seminal plasma is to assess the samples after liquefaction and separation of seminal plasma from the cells by centrifugation (300g, 10 min). Subsequently, seminal plasma is separated into aliquots of small volumes needed for cytokine immunoassays (200 µL/patient/cytokine). The samples are then frozen at –70°C until processed. Each vial should be used only for one experiment, since thawing and freezing of the samples will destroy cytokines or their bioactivity. The levels of cytokines can be evaluated by immunoassay (by using a specific ELISA) and by bioassays (by using cell systems specific for each cytokine). Some bioassays for cytokines such as IL-1, IL-2, IL-3, IL-6, TNF-α, and CSFs are discussed below.

3.1. Cytokine Immunoassay

This method is a sandwich enzyme immunoassay, which is used to evaluate the quantities of the cytokines examined in conditioned media of tissues/cells, plasma, or body fluids. Usually the primary (coated) anticytokine antibodies used are monoclonal antibodies specific for the cytokines examined. Therefore, the quantities from the immunoassay indicate the real values of the cytokines examined.

1. Primary anticytokine monoclonal antibody (diluted to the optimal concentration; *see* **Note 6**) is coated by coating buffer to ELISA plates (100 µL/well) overnight at 2–8°C. Plates are covered to prevent drying and contamination.
2. After overnight incubation the coated antibody is aspirated from the wells and the wells are washed five times with washing buffer (*see* **Note 7**).
3. Thereafter, the wells are blocked with blocking buffer (200 µL/well), and the plates are covered and incubated for 2 h at 37°C.
4. After incubation the wells are aspirated and 100 µL/well (in duplicate) of various concentrations of cytokine the standard to be used for standard curve (*see* **Note 8**), or samples, are added to the plates. The plates are covered and incubated for 1 h at 37°C.
5. The plates are washed five times with washing buffer, and 100 µL/well of the diluted second antibody (biotinylated rabbit anticytokine antibody in optimal concentration) is added to the plates. The plates are covered and incubated for 1 h at 37°C.
6. The plates are again washed five times with washing buffer, and 100 µL/well of HRP-conjugated streptavidin goat anti-rabbit antibody (detection reagent) is added. The plates are covered and incubated for 15 min at 37°C.
7. After incubation, the plates are washed five times with washing buffer, 100 µL/well of substrate solution (tetramethylbenzidine [TMB]) is added for 10 min, and the plates are again incubated at room temperature (20–26°C). Positive samples will show blue color in the wells.
8. At the end of the incubation period one should add 100 µL/well of the stop solution (the pale blue color will turn yellow) and read the plates at 450 nm as soon as possible, but within a maximum of 60 min. The quantities of the samples examined are calculated from the standard curve values.

3.2. Cytokine Bioassay

These methods will give the net value of bioactive levels of the cytokine examined, and the results do not necessarily correlate with the quantitative amounts of the cytokines examined. The reason for this apparent discrepancy is based on the presence or absence of specific or nonspecific inhibitory factors of the cytokines examined in the samples. Moreover, since in this method cell proliferation or cell lysis is observed, other factors that may be present in the sample examined, such as other undetermined cytokines, may affect the proliferation or lysis of these cells. This is an inherent problem of any bioassay that must be taken into account. To examine the bioactivity of a cytokine in the seminal plasma, low concentrations of the plasma are needed (0.1–5% v/v). It should be kept in mind that some sera, such as FCS may be toxic to the cells used in the bioassay. To remove prostaglandins, some of which (such as PGE) are known to decrease cytokine bioactivity, the semen sample should be dialyzed prior to processing.

Samples should always be assessed in triplicates and for at least two dilutions of the plasma examined. Samples of blood plasma are recommended as a reference to cytokine levels in the seminal plasma. Seminal plasma from men with genital infection should be filtered through 0.45-μm filters prior to examination. However, this process may cause the loss of some factors/molecules, which may affect the bioactivity of the cytokines.

3.2.1. IL-1 Bioassay

To examine the levels of IL-1 bioactivity in seminal plasma (SP) of fertile and infertile men, the 1A-5 helper T-cell line and the CTLD cell line may be used. 1A-5 helper T-cell line produces IL-2 in the presence of IL-1 and PHA *(32)*. This IL-2 activity can be detected using a CTLD cell line, which proliferates in the presence of IL-2 *(33)*.

1. SP (0.1–5% v/v) is added to 1A-5 cells (5×10^4 cells/well, 100 μL) in 96-well plates (*see* **Note 9**). Recombinant IL-1 is used as positive control of the bioassay. The range of rIL-1 concentrations for a standard curve is 0.01–50 U/mL. Usually the optimal concentration obtained is 0.1 or 1 U/mL.
2. At 24 h after incubation, plates are frozen and thawed three times, and CTLD cells (5×10^3 cells/well, 20 μL) are added to the plates (*see* **Note 2**). Recombinant IL-2 is used as a positive control for the bioassay (*see* **Note 10**). The range of rIL-2 concentrations is 0.01–10 U/mL. Usually the optimal concentration obtained is 1 U/mL.
3. At 48–72 h later, cell proliferation is determined by addition of 1 mg/mL MTT, followed 3 h later by isopropanol in 0.04 *N* hydrochloric acid, at room temperature.
4. Optical density of cleaved MTT molecules (brown color) are measured by spectrophotometry. Results are expressed as the net absorbance values at 450 and 630 nm *(34)*.

3.2.2. Membrane IL-1 Bioassay

Fixation, as described by Kurt-Jones et al. *(35)*, of the swim-up sperm cells ($3–5 \times 10^4$ cells/well) is performed in 96-well plates after 24 h of culture. Swim-up sperm cells are centrifuged at 300*g* for 10 min, and the medium is removed. Cells are washed three times with Ham F-10-containing serum, fixed for 15 min at room temperature with 1% formaldehyde in culture medium, washed four times, and incubated overnight in culture medium to allow the release of soluble materials from the cells. Thereafter, the medium is discarded and cells are assayed for membrane-associated IL-1 by addition of 1A-5 cells + PHA, and later the CTLD cell line, onto the fixed swim-up sperm cells, as in **Subheading 3.2.1.**

3.2.3. IL-2 Bioassay

Supernatants or fluids to be examined for IL-2 bioactivity are divided (10–50%) in triplicate into 96-well plates. CTLD cells (5×10^3 cells/well, completing the well volume to 100 μL) are added to the plates. Positive control and proliferation evaluation by MTT is performed as described above for the IL-1 bioassay (*see* **Subheading 2.2.1.**).

3.2.4. IL-3 Bioassay

The proliferation assay of the IL-3-dependent cell line FDC-P2 is used *(36)*.

1. Supernatant or fluids to be examined for IL-3 bioactivity (10–50% v/v) are divided into 96-well plates in triplicate.
2. FDC-P2 cells (5×10^3 cells/well, completing the wells to 100 μL final volume) should be added to 96-well plates (*see* **Note 3**). Recombinant IL-3 is used as a positive control for the bioassay. The range of rIL-3 concentrations is 0.01–10 U/mL. Usually the optimal concentration obtained is 1 U/mL.
3. At 48–72 h later, cell proliferation is determined by addition of 1 mg/mL MTT, followed 3 h later by isopropanol in 0.04 N hydrochloric acid, at room temperature.
4. Optical density of cleaved MTT molecules (brown color) is measured by spectrophotometry. Results are expressed as the net absorbance values at 450 nm and 630 nm *(34)*.

3.2.5. IL-6 Bioassay

IL-6 activity in seminal plasma of fertile and infertile men is determined by the B9 cell proliferation assay *(37)*. The B9 cell line (5×10^3 cells/well, 100 μL) is added to 0.1–1% (v/v) conditioned media in 96-well plates (*see* **Note 4**). Human recombinant IL-6 is used as a positive control. The range of rIL-6 concentrations for standard curves is 0.01–50 U/mL. Usually the optimal concentration obtained is 0.1 or 1 U/mL. After incubation for 72–96 h, cell proliferation is determined by MTT staining as described above.

3.2.6. TNF Bioassay

TNF levels in SP are determined using a cytotoxicity assay of TNF-susceptible L-929 fibroblasts *(38)*. Twenty-four hours after seeding (5×10^4 cells/well) in 96-well plates, plates are washed and SP is applied to L-cells in serial dilutions (10–60% v/v) in the presence of 40 mg/mL cyclohexamide (*see* **Note 5**). Sixteen hours later, cytotoxicity is quantified by measuring the uptake of neutral red by ELISA reader at 530 nm. Human recombinant TNF is used as a positive control. The range of rTNF-α concentrations for a standard curve is 0.001–10 ng/mL. Usually the optimal concentration obtained is 1 ng/mL.

3.2.7. Colony-Stimulating Factors

CSF activity is evaluated in the examined samples by their ability to stimulate colony formation from murine bone marrow cells (BMC) in soft agar cultures according to Pluznik and Sachs *(39)*. BMCs (4×10^6 cells/plate/ 20 µL) are cloned in soft agar medium (0.37%) on a harder agar base (0.5%) and supplemented with 25% of supernatants/fluids and 20% FCS in 96-well plates (80 µL/well). L-cell conditioned medium (LCM; 10, 20, and 30% v/v) and/or recombinant CSF-1 (0.01–10 U/mL) are used as positive control. Plates are left at room temperature to harden the agar. BMCs (4×10^4/well) are added in the second soft agar layer (0.37% supplemented with 25% FCS) at 100 µL/well. The second soft agar layer should be warmed in 50°C water and be cooled when the BMCs are mixed. Colonies, containing more than 50 cells, are counted microscopically after 7 d of incubation. For identification of the cell morphology within colonies, plates are stained with orcein *(40)*.

These assays are performed in 96-well plates, and each sample examined in triplicate. The final evaluation is usually expressed as pg or ng cytokine/mL SP. One should compare the levels of cytokine not only with the concentration but also with the protein content of the SP (pg cytokine/mL SP/mg·protein in mL SP).

4. Notes

1. Care should be taken to avoid any possibility of microbial contamination of the reagents and buffers. This may affect the sensitivity of the immunoassay..
2. CTLD cells are cultured in RPMI medium containing 5% FCS, 1% combined antibiotics, 1% glutamine, 10^{-5} *M* mercaptoethanol, and recombinant IL-2 (10 U/mL).
3. FDC-P2 cells are cultured in RPMI medium containing 5% FCS, 1% combined antibiotics, 1% glutamine, 10^{-5} *M* mercaptoethanol, and recombinant IL-3 (10 U/mL). This cell line also proliferates in the presence of granulocyte-macrophage colony-stimulating factor. Therefore anti-IL-3 antibodies are recommended to neutralize the IL-3 activity in the examined fluids.
4. B9 cells are cultured in RPMI medium containing 5% FCS, 1% combined antibiotics, 1% glutamine, 10^{-5} *M* mercaptoethanol, and recombinant IL-6 (10 U/mL).
5. L-cells are cultured in Dulbecco's modified Eagle's medium containing 5% FCS, 1% combined antibiotics, and 1% glutamine.
6. To get an optimal concentration for the first anticytokine antibody (coated antibody) and the second antibody, a standard curve with different concentrations of recombinant cytokines (4–1000 pg/mL) with various concentrations of the first antibody (0.5, 1, and 5 µg/mL; usually the optimal is 1 µg/mL) and secondary antibody should be prepared.
7. Proper washing is important to reduce background staining. Wells should be filled with washing buffer, and after aspiration one needs to blot the plate on a dry absorbent pad or paper towels to remove all liquid from the wells.
8. Standard curves of most cytokines should be in the range of 4–1000 pg/mL.

9. 1A-5 helper T cells are cultured in RPMI medium containing 5% FCS, 1% combined antibiotics, 1% glutamine, and 10^{-5} M mercaptoethanol.
10. In case the IL-1 system bioassay did not succeed, the positive control for CTLD will be helpful to determine whether the problem relates to the 1A-5 or CTLD cells.

References

1. Simon, C. and Polan, M. L. (1994) Cytokines and reproduction. *West. J. Med.* **60,** 425–429.
2. Naz, R. K., Chaturvedi, M. M., and Aggarwal, B. B. (1994) Role of cytokines and protooncogenes in sperm cell function: Relevance to immunologic infertility. *Am. J. Reprod. Immunol.* **32,** 26–37.
3. Litvin, Y. S. and Nagler, H. (1992) Infertility and genitourinary infections. *Infect. Urol.* **5,** 104–107.
4. Bar-Chama, N. and Fisch, H. (1993). Infection and pyospermia in male infertility. *World. J. Urol.* **11,** 76–81.
5. James, K. and Hargreave, T. B. (1984) Immunosupression by seminal plasma and its possible clinical significance. *Immunol. Today.* **5,** 357–363.
6. Hussenet, F., Dousset, B., Cordonnier, J. L., Jacob, C., Foliguet, B., Grignon, G., and Nabet, P. (1993) Tumor necrosis factor alpha and interleukin 2 in normal and infected human seminal plasma. *Hum. Reprod.* **8,** 409–411.
7. Huleihel, M., Lunenfeld, E., Levy, A., Potashnik, G., and Glezerman, M. (1996). Distinct expression levels of cytokines and soluble cytokine receptors in seminal plasma of fertile and infertile men. *Fertil. Steril.* **66,** 135–139.
8. Yoshimura, T., Matsushima, K., Oppenheim, J. J., and Leonard, E. J. (1987) Neutrophil chemotactic factor produced by lipopolysacharide (LPS)–stimulated human blood mononuclear leukocytes: partial characterization and separation from interleukin-1 (IL-1). *J. Immunol.* **139,** 788–793.
9. Shimoya, K., Matsuzaki, N., Tsutsui, T., Taniguchi, T., Saji, F., and Tanizawa, O. (1993) Detection of intreleukin-8 (IL-8) in seminal plasma of infertile patients with leukospermia. *Fertil. Steril.* **59,** 885–888.
10. Naz, R. K. and Kaplan, P. (1994) Increased levels of interleukin-6 in seminal plasma of infertile men. *J. Androl.* **15,** 220–227.
11. Rajasekaran, M., Hellstrom, W., and Sikka, S. (1996) Quantitative assessment of cytokines (Groa and IL-10) in human seminal plasma during genitourinary inflammation. *Am. J. Reprod. Immunol.* **36,** 90–95.
12. Comhaire, F., Bosmans, E., Ombelet, W., Punjabi, U., and Schoonjans, F. (1994) Cytokines in semen of normal men and of patients with andrological diseases. *Am. J. Reprod. Immunol.* **31,** 99–103.
13. Paradisi, R., Capelli, M., Mandini, M., Bellavia, E., Focacci, M., and Flamigni, C. (1995) Interleukin–2 in seminal plasma of fertile and infertile men. *Arch. Androl.* **35,** 35–41.
14. Miska, W. and Mahamoud, M. (1993) Determination of soluble interleukin–2 receptor in human seminal. *Arch. Androl.* **30,** 23–28.

15. Shimonovitz, S., Barak, V., Zacut, D., Ever-Hadani, P., Ben Chetrit, A., and Ron, M. (1994) High concentration of soluble interleukin–2 receptors in ejaculate with low sperm motility. *Hum. Reprod.* **9,** 653–655.
16. Paradisi, R., Mancini, R., Bellavia, E., Beltrandi, E., Pession, A., Venturoli, S., and Flamigni, C. (1997) T-helper 2 type cytokine and soluble interleukin–2 receptor levels in seminal plasma of infertile men. *Am. J. Reprod. Immunol.* **38,** 94–99.
17. Matalliotakis, I., Kiriakou, D., Fragouli, I., Sifakis, S., Eliopoulos, G., and Koumantakis, E. (1998) Interleukin-6 in seminal plasma of fertile and infertile men. *Arch. Androl.* **41,** 43–50.
18. Zalata, A., Hafetz, T., Van Hoecke, M. J., and Comhaire, F. (1995) Evaluation of endorphin and interleukin–6 in seminal plasma of patients with certain andrological diseases. *Hum. Reprod.* **10,** 3161–3165.
19. Syed, V., Gerard, N., Kaipia, A., Bardin, C. W., Parvinen, M., and Jegou, B. (1993) Identification, Ontogeny, and regulation of an interleukin-6-like factor in the rat seminiferous tubule. *Endocrinology* **132,** 293–299.
20. Dousset, B., Hussenet, F., Daudin, M., Bujan, L., Foliguet, B., and Nabet, P. (1997) Seminal cytokine concentrations (IL-1β, IL-2, IL-6, sIL-2R, sIL-6R), semen parameters and blood hormonal status in male infertility. *Hum. Reprod.* **12,** 1476–1479.
21. Lee, H. K., Lee, H. H., Park, Y. M., Lee, J. H., and Ha, T. Y. (1991) Regulation of human B cell proliferation and differentiation by seminal plasma. *Clin. Exp. Immunol.* **85,** 174–179.
22. Valley, P. J. and Ress, R. C. (1986) Seminal plasma supression of human lymphocyte response in vitro requires the presence of bovine serum factors. *Clin. Exp. Immunol.* **86,** 181–187.
23. Huleihel, M., Levy, A., Lunenfeld, E., Horowitz, S., Potashnik, G., and Glezerman, M. (1997) Distinct expression of cytokines and mitogenic inhibitory factors in semen of fertile and infertile men. *Am. J. Reprod. Immunol.* **37,** 304–309.
24. Huleihel, M., Lunenfeld, E., Horowitz, S., Levy, A., Potashnik, G., Mazor, M. and Glezerman, M. (1999) Expression of IL-12, IL-10, PGE2, sIL-2R and sIL-6R in seminal plasma of fertile and infertile men. *Andrologia* **31,** 283–288.
25. Naz, R. K. and Evans, L. (1998) Presence and modulation of interleukin-12 in seminal plasma of fertile and infertile men. *J. Androl.* **19,** 302–307.
26. Anderson, D. J. and Hill, J. A. (1988) Cell mediated immunity in infertility. *Am. J. Reprod. Immunol.* **17,** 22–30.
27. Naz, R. K. and Kumar, R. (1991) Transforming growth factor-β enhances expression of 50 kDa protein related to 2–5 oligoadenylate synthetase in human sperm cells. *J. Cell. Physiol.* **146,** 156–163.
28. Wincek, T. J., Meyer, T. K., Meyer, M. R., and Kuehl, T. J. (1991) Absence of a direct effect of recombinant tumor necrosis factor-alpha on human sperm function and murine preimplantation development. *Fertil. Steril.* **56,** 332–339.
29. Haney, A. F., Hughes, S. F., and Weinberg, J. B. (1992) The lack of effect of tumor-necrosis-factor alpha, interleukin-1a and interferon-gamma on human sperm motility in vitro. *J. Androl.* **13,** 249–253.

30. Estrada, L. S., Champion, H. C., Wang, R., Rajasekaran, M., Hellstrom, W. J., Aggarwal, B., and Sikka, S. C. (1997) Effect of tumor necrosis factor-alpha and interferon-gamma on human sperm motility, viability and motion. *Int. J. Androl.* **20,** 237–242.

31. Naz, R. K. and Kaplan, P. (1994) Interleukin-6 enhances the fertilizing capacity of human sperm by increasing capacitation and acrosome reaction. *J. Androl.* **5,** 228–233.

32. Gillis, S. M. M. and Mizel, S. B. (1981) T cell lymphoma model for the analysis of interleukin 1 mediated T cell activation. *Proc. Natl. Acad. Sci. USA* **78,** 1133–1137.

33. Gillis, S. M. M., Ferm, W. O., and Smith, K. A. (1978) T cell growth factor: parameters of production and quantitative microassay for activity. *J. Immunol.* **120,** 2027–2032.

34. Mosman, T. (1983) Rapid colorimetric assay for cellular growth and survival: application to proliferation and cytotoxicity assays. *J. Immunol. Methods* **65,** 55–60.

35. Kurt-Jones, E. A., Beller, D. I., Mizel, S. B., and Unanue, E. R. (1985) Identification of a membrane-associated interleukin 1 in macrophages. *Proc. Natl. Acad. Sci. USA* **82,** 1204–1208.

36. Prestidge, R. L., Watson, J. D., Urdal, D. L., Mochizuki, D., Conlon, P., and Gillis, S. (1984) Biochemical comparison of murine colony-stimulating factors secreted by a T cell lymphoma and a myelomonocytic leukemia. *J. Immunol.* **133,** 293–298.

37. Aarden, L. A., De-Groot, E. R., Schaap, O. L., and Lansdorp, P. M. (1987) Production of hybridoma growth factor by human monocytes. *Eur. J. Immunol.* **17,** 1411–1416.

38. Flick, D. A. and Gifford, G. E. (1984) Comparison of in vitro cell cytotoxic assays for tumor necrosis factor. *J. Immunol. Methods.* **68,** 167–175.

39. Pluznik, D. H. and Sachs, L. (1965) The cloning of normal "mast" cell tissue culture. *J. Cell. Comp. Physiol.* **66,** 319–324.

40. Shazan, A. and Goldman, R. (1985) 1,25 dihydroxy vit-D_3 in the regulation and differentiation of macrophages and granulocytes. *Int. J. Cell. Clon.* **3,** 65–71.

26

Measurement of Cytokines in Induced Sputum

Application to the Investigation of Asthma and COPD

Peter G. Gibson and Jodie L. Simpson

1. Introduction

Cytokines are important mediators of the persistent cycle of inflammation and repair that characterizes chronic airway diseases such as asthma, chronic obstructive pulmonary disease (COPD), and cystic fibrosis (CF). Interleukin (IL)-5 is a key mediator of the eosinophil infiltrate that characterizes asthma, whereas IL-8 is a potent chemoattractant for neutrophils in COPD and CF. IL-5 and IL-8 can be measured in airway samples obtained by the relatively noninvasive technique of sputum induction. Procedures for sputum induction have recently been standardized, and samples of airway secretions can now be obtained from most adults and children over 7 years of age. Sputum is induced via inhalation of hypertonic saline (4.5%) and assisted expectoration *(1)*. The measurement of cytokines in induced sputum allows a direct estimation of the airway levels of these mediators in health and disease. This chapter details methods that have successfully been applied to the immunochemical assay of IL-5 and IL-8 in induced sputum.

1.1. Sputum Processing

The aim of sputum processing is to obtain a cell-free fluid sample for measurement of fluid-phase cytokines as well as cellular preparations (single cell suspensions, cytospin slides) to assess cell numbers and function. Induced sputum is a mixture of lower respiratory secretions, saliva, and saline. Lower respiratory secretions consist of cells and fluid-phase mediators enmeshed in a network of mucoproteins and, in some cases, extracellular DNA and actin fibers *(2)*. The purpose of initial sputum processing is to select lower respiratory portions from the sputum sample and to separate these into a cell-free fluid

From: *Methods in Molecular Medicine, vol. 60: Interleukin Protocols*
Edited by: L. A. J. O'Neill and A. Bowie © Humana Press Inc., Totowa, NJ

phase and a single cell suspension of viable lower respiratory cells with minimal squamous contamination. Soluble cytokines are assayed in the fluid phase, and cell-associated cytokines are assayed in cell suspension.

1.2. Slide Fixation and Storage

The aim is to fix and store cells on cytospin slides without loss of cytokine immunoreactivity. The immunoreactive determinants of intracellular cytokines need to be fixed, preserved without degradation, and made accessible to the monoclonal antibodies for detection. Formaldehyde and paraformaldehyde fixatives crosslink proteins with methylene bridges formed by condensation reactions. Maximum crosslinking occurs in the pH range of 7.5–8.0; at lower pH, crosslinking is not favored (3). Permeabilization is required to allow the free transfer of antibodies into the cells. Saponins are used for permeabilization as they interact with cholesterol, phospholipid, and proteins to cause small pore openings in the membrane, some of which are permanent. Because only some of the membrane pores created by the action of saponin are permanent, using saponin in all wash solutions and diluents means that permeabilization is active at each stage of immunoassay. The addition of high-concentration sucrose preserves carbohydrate moieties of cytokines, many of which contain the antigenic determinants targeted by detecting antibodies. A combination of paraformaldehyde, saponin, and sucrose gives satisfactory results for the detection of intracellular cytokines in induced sputum samples.

1.3. Immunocytochemical Detection of Cell-Associated Cytokines

The alkaline phosphatase anti-alkaline phosphatase (APAAP) technique is a useful means to assay cell-associated cytokines in induced sputum. This indirect antibody technique involves labeling of a secondary antibody (raised against an immunoglobulin of the same species as the primary antibody) with the enzyme (alkaline phosphatase) and then detection of the primary antibody without the need for the enzyme to be directly conjugated to the primary antibody. The indirect technique allows increased sensitivity compared with the direct technique, although it involves increased assay time. Alkaline phosphatase is often preferred to peroxidase for its increased sensitivity, achieved by production of more color molecules per enzyme molecule (4). Chromogenic substrates are used to create different coloured reaction products in conjunction with the enzyme systems. Alkaline phosphatase substrates include BCIP/NBT, which creates a permanent blue precipitate at the site of alkaline phosphatase localization, or Fast Red TR/naphthol, which precipitates to a red color. Fast Red substrate is recommended for cell smears and cytospins when using alkaline phosphatase (4). Levamisole may be added directly to the substrate solution to quench endogenous alkaline phosphatase activity, which may be present in epithelial cells (5).

1.4. Measurement of Cytokines in Sputum Fluid Phase by ELISA

IL-5 is an important cytokine that mediates the eosinophilic airway inflammation characteristic of asthma *(6)*. IL-5 is synthesized by T-lymphocytes, eosinophils, and mast cells as a 40–45-kDa glycoprotein and plays an important role in the differentiation of eosinophils in bone marrow and their activation in tissue. It is also a chemoattractant for eosinophils and promotes eosinophil survival, by inhibition of eosinophil apoptosis *(7)*. Inhalation of IL-5 by asthmatics causes airway eosinophilia and increased airway responsiveness *(8)*, whereas a humanized anti IL-5 antibody reduced airway eosinophil levels *(9)*.

IL-8 is a dimeric CXC chemokine produced by a variety of cell types including monocytes, macrophages, neutrophils, and lymphocytes *(10)*. It is one of the mediators responsible for the attraction and activation of neutrophils, is resistant to many denaturing treatments such as oxidation or hydrolysis, and can persist in its active form for long periods *(11)*. IL-8 causes neutrophil transendothelial migration, chemoattraction, degranulation, and stimulation of the respiratory burst. IL-8 is the major chemoattractant responsible for neutrophil accumulation in the lung. It is a relevant mediator in acute virus-induced asthma, CF, and COPD.

1.5. Use of Protease Inhibitors to Improve IL-5 Recovery

Sputum samples contain proteases, which can degrade proteins and influence enzyme-linked immunosorbent assay (ELISA) for IL-5. The addition of a protease inhibitor cocktail can improve recovery of spiked IL-5 from 33 to 80%. Sputum samples vary greatly in the extent to which they degrade IL-5. The addition of protease inhibitors is recommended for sputum IL-5 assay.

2. Materials
2.1. Sputum Processing

1. Sputolysin: 9.23 mg/mL dithiothreitol (DTT). A 1:10 working solution of DTT is prepared in distilled water. Trypan blue and phosphate-buffered saline (PBS).
2. Petri dish, glass slides; disposable pipets; polypropylene tubes (15 mL); 5-mL syringes; mixing cannula; 1.5-mL Eppendorf tubes; forceps.
3. Positive displacement pipet, filter nylon (60-μm pore size), and filter holder (Swinnex 25 mm).
4. Hemocytometer and microscope.

2.2. Slide Fixation and Storage

1. PLP fixative: 3% (w/v) paraformaldehyde, 0.1 M disodium hydrogen orthophosphate, 0.9 g L-lysine monohydrate, 0.15 g sodium *m*-periodate, pH 7.4. Solution can be stored for 1 mo in dark glass at room temperature.
2. 15% (w/v) Sucrose (stored at 4°C).

2.3. Immunocytochemical Detection of Cell-Associated Cytokines

1. Control slides: Lipopolysaccharide-activated granulocytes or monocytes.
2. Reagents: 20% normal rabbit serum (DAKO, cat. no. X0902); TBS (H+S): Weigh out: 6.05 g Tris base, 8.77 g NaCl. Dissolve in 1000 mL distilled water and adjust to pH 7.6. Add 2.38 g HEPES and 0.10 g saponin. Remove 100 mL of this solution and add to a clean 100-mL bottle. Add 1.0 g bovine serum albumin (BSA; Sigma A8022) to the 100 mL. Store both solutions at 4°C until required.
3. Immunochemicals: Primary antibody—monoclonal anti-IL-8 (PharMingen), anti-IL-5, anti-granulocyte macrophage-colony (GM-CSF) and anti-eotaxin (R&D) diluted to 10 µg/mL have been used successfully with these methods; link–rabbit anti-mouse immunoglobulin (DAKO, cat. no. Z0259); APAAP— complex of alkaline phosphatase and mouse monoclonal anti-alkaline phosphatase (DAKO D0651) and Fast Red substrate (DAKO K597).
4. Mouse monoclonal $IgG_{1/2}$ antibody negative control (DAKO X0931).
5. Hematoxylin (Carrazi, from Fronine, Riverstone, NSW, Australia) and Faramount (DAKO cat. no. S3025).

2.4. Measurement of Cytokines in Sputum Fluid Phase by ELISA

1. Nunc Maxisorb microtiter plates.
2. Assorted chemicals: NaCl, KCl, NaN_3, KH_2PO_4, Na_2HPO_4.
3. pH standards 4, 7, and 10 (Sigma B5020, B4770, and B4895) and pH adjustment solutions (1 M NaOH and 1 M HCl).
4. Sucrose, Tris base, BSA, fatty acid free (Sigma A6003), PBS, pH 7.3, Tween-20 (Sigma P1379), TMB Sigma one-step (Sigma T8665), H_2SO_4 (Sigma 25810-5).
5. R&D Human IL-8 Duo Set consisting of R&D Human IL-8 Capture antibody, detection antibody, horseradish peroxidase (HRP)-streptavidin, human IL-8 standard.
6. PharMingen Human IL-5 OptEIA Set (2633KI), comprising anti-human IL-5 capture antibody, biotinylated anti-human IL-5 detection antibody, HRP-conjugated avidin, recombinant human IL-5 standard, and assay diluent (26411E).

2.5. Use of Protease Inhibitors to Improve IL-5 Recovery

A protease inhibitor cocktail (ICN Biomedicals) consisting of EDTA sodium salt, 4-2-aminoethyl-benzenesulfonyl fluoride (AEBSF), leupeptin, and pepstatin is used. A stock solution combining each of the four protease inhibitors (2 mg/mL, 40 mg/mL, 10 µg/mL, and 10 µg/mL respectively) is prepared and stored at –20°C.

3. Methods
3.1. Sputum Processing (see *Fig. 1*)

1. Use clean forceps to separate out the mucus clumps, using inverted microscopy to inspect the sample if it is uncertain whether the sample contains mucus plugs.
2. Pipet all suitable mucus clumps (minimum of 300 µL and not more than 1 mL) into a labeled 15-mL polypropylene tube using positive a displacement pipet.

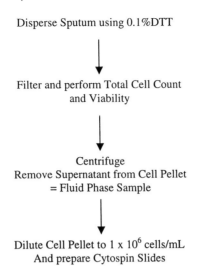

Disperse Sputum using 0.1%DTT

↓

Filter and perform Total Cell Count
and Viability

↓

Centrifuge
Remove Supernatant from Cell Pellet
= Fluid Phase Sample

↓

Dilute Cell Pellet to 1 x 10^6 cells/mL
And prepare Cytospin Slides

Fig. 1. Flowchart summarizing the sputum processing method.

3. Add four times the volume of working sputolysin to the sample and mix. Protease inhibitors can be added for IL-5 assay at this stage (*see* **Subheading 3.5.**). Place sample in a shaking water bath at 37°C for 30 min to disperse mucus.
4. Add PBS (same volume as working sputolysin from **step 3**), and filter the sputum and sputolysin mixture through the 60-μm nylon filter apparatus. Perform a total cell count and viability assay using a Neubauer hemocytometer and Trypan blue stain.
5. Centrifuge the remaining cell suspension at 200g for 10 min, remove the supernatant into labeled Eppendorf tubes, and freeze. This is the *fluid phase sample*.
6. Resuspend the pellet in PBS to 1×10^6 cells/mL and prepare cytospin slides.

3.2. Slide Fixation and Storage

1. Immerse slides in PLP fixative for 30 min at room temperature, and then air-dry.
2. When dry, place slides into a second coplin jar and Cover with 15% sucrose for a further 30 min. Then remove, air-dry, and freeze.

3.3. Immunocytochemical Detection of Cell-Associated Cytokines (see *Fig. 2*)

1. Place sample and three control slides (positive, negative, substrate) into Coplin jars containing TBS (H + S). *Be sure to separate the negative and substrate controls into separate jars at all times* to avoid cross-contamination of the negative control (*see* **Note 1**).
2. Prepare the Ig negative control by adding 50 μL of Ig to 450 μL of TBS (H + S) BSA.
3. Wipe each slide around the cell circle with a Kimwipe to remove excess wash fluid.
4. Using a Pasteur pipet, add 1 drop of NRS to the cell circle on each slide except for the substrate (SUB) control. The SUB control has a drop of TBS (H + S)

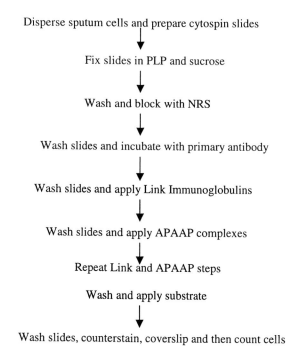

Fig. 2. Flowchart summarizing the APAAP detection method. PLP, periodate lysine paraformaldehyde; NRS, normal rabbit serum; APAAP, APAAP, alkaline phosphatase anti-alkaline phosphatase.

added. Cover the containers with the appropriate lid and incubate the slides at room temperature for 20 min. Do not pipet solutions directly onto cells, but add at the edge of the cell circle.

5. Remove slides from container, and allow the NRS to drain off by placing slides on their end on some absorbent towel. Do not allow cells to dry at any step.

6. Transfer the slides back into the container and add 1 drop of antibody to each slide with the exception of the SUB control, which again has only TBS (H + S); the negative (NEG) control has 1 drop of mouse IgG added. Refrigerate overnight at 4°C.

7. Remove slides from container and place in coplin jars filled with TBS (H + S) for 5 min. Wash NEG and SUB in separate jars. We use Coplin jars for washing in preference to a wash bottle to minimize cell loss.

8. Prepare the LINK, add 1 drop of it to each, slide, with the exception of the SUB control, and incubate for 30 min at room temperature; then wash.

9. Prepare the APAAP, add 1 drop of it to each slide, with the exception of the SUB control, and incubate for 30 min at room temperature.

10. Wash slides, add 1 drop of LINK to each slide, with the exception of the SUB control, and incubate for 10 min at room temperature.

11. Wash slides, add 1 drop of APAAP to each slide, with the exception of the SUB control, and incubate for 10 min at room temperature.
12. Prepare the substrate, wash slides, and add 1 drop of substrate to every slide including the SUB control. The reaction should be stopped when the positive control cells show an intense red coloring in the cell granules. To do this, place slides in a slide holder and wash the slides in distilled water (1 min).
13. Counterstain with hematoxylin and coverslip using Faramount Aqueous mountant.

3.4. Measurement of Cytokines in Sputum Fluid Phase by ELISA

Detailed instructions are provided with the kit. Briefly, the plates are coated with diluted antibody made up to the manufacturer's instructions. Coated plates are incubated overnight at 4°C. Blocking buffer is then added and the plate washed. Standards and samples are applied, followed by washing and application of diluted conjugate, then washing and substrate solutions. The plates are read and a standard curve prepared, which is used to calculate values for samples tested (*see* **Note 2**).

3.5. Effects of Protease Inhibitors

1. The sputum is processed according to **Subheading 3.1.** with the following changes to **step 3**: To the sputum sample add 1/4 of the volume of protease inhibitor cocktail (e.g., a 400-µL sputum sample will have 100 µL added), and make up the remaining volume with 0.1% sputolysin (for the same 400-µL sample, you need to add 1.5 mL of sputolysin).
2. Place in shaking water bath at 37°C for 30 min to disperse mucus. Continue as per **Subheading 3.1., step 4**.

4. Notes

1. Immunocytochemical detection of cell-associated cytokines: Thorough washing is important. Insufficient washing will result in background staining. Reagent and procedure controls are necessary for the validation of the procedure. Procedure controls determine whether the assay and reagents are working correctly. The primary antibody is the most critical of all reagents. To check its specificity on each run, it is replaced on one slide with either affinity-absorbed antiserum, another irrelevant antibody, or preimmune or nonimmune serum from the same species that produced the antibody; the latter is usually used. If the negative control has worked and there are still staining difficulties, then each reagent can be replaced by an alternative one at a time to determine the cause. For example, use a different lot number of APAAP reagent to determine whether the APAAP reagent is generating the problem.
2. Measurement of cytokines in sputum fluid phase by ELISA: Assay sensitivity may be adjusted by modifying reagent concentrations, sample volumes, and incubation times. A poor standard curve can be because of a number of factors,

such as not enough HRP-strepavidin added, not enough secondary antibody, insufficient binding of primary antibody, or improper calculation of the standard dilutions. Each step must be investigated individually. Poor duplicates may be the result of insufficient washing, buffer contamination, contaminated plate sealers, or poor pipet technique. If a signal is expected and the standard curve is correct, then the sample matrix may be masking the detection. Dilute samples 1:2 in an appropriate diluent and repeat or perform a series of dilutions to test sample recovery. Dithiothreitol does not alter ELISA for IL-5 or IL-8. IL-5 recovery is improved by the addition of protease inhibitors, whereas this has no effect on IL-8 assay.

References

1. Gibson, P. G. (1998) Use of induced sputum to examine airway inflammation in childhood asthma. *J. Allergy Clin. Immunol.* **102,** S100–101.
2. Shiels, C. A., Kas, J., Travassos, W., Allen, P. G., Janmey, P. A., Wohl, M. E., et al. (1996) Actin filaments mediate DNA fiber formation in chronic inflammatory airway disease. *Am. J. Pathol.* **148,** 919–927.
3. Melan, M. A. (1994) Overview of cell fixation and permabilisation, in *Immunocytochemical Methods and Protocols* (Javois, L. C., ed.), Humana, Totowa, NJ, pp. 55–65.
4. Bratthauer, G. L. (1994) Overview of antigen detection through enzymatic activity, in *Immunocytochemical Methods and Protocols* (Javois, L. C., ed.), Humana, Totowa, NJ, pp. 155–164.
5. Boenisch, T. (1989) Background, in *Handbook of Immunochemical Staining Methods* (Naish, S. J., et al., eds.), DAKO, CA, Carpenteria, pp. 21–23.
6. Foster, P. S., Hogan, P., Matthaei, K. I., and Young, I. G. (1999) The role of interleukin-5 in allergic airways disease, in *Interleukin-5: From Molecule to Drug Target for Asthma* (Sanderson, C.J., ed.), Marcel Dekker, NY, pp. 127–131.
7. Sehmi, R. and Denburg, J. A. (1999) Bone marrow in allergic disease: the role of interleukin-5 as an eosinophilopoietic factor, in *Interleukin-5: From Molecule to Drug Target for Asthma* (Sanderson, C. J., ed.), Marcel Dekker, NY, pp. 69–64.
8. Shi, H. Z., Xiao, C. Q., Zhong, D., Qin, S. M., Liu, Y., Liang, G. R., et al. (1998) Effect of inhaled interleukin-5 on airway hyperactivity and eosinophilia in asthmatics. *Am. J. Respir. Crit. Care Med.* **157,** 204–209.
9. Walls, C. M., Patel, B., Harte, T. K., Zia-Amirhosseini, P., Mithron, E., Hottenstein, C. S., et al. (1999) SB-240563, An anti IL-5 monoclonal anti-body:Tolerability, activity and pharmacokinetic assessment in patients with asthma. *Eur. Respir. J.* **14,** P1988.
10. Adams, D. H. and Lloyd, A. R. (1997) Chemokines: leucocyte recruitment and activation cytokines. *Lancet* **349,** 490–495.
11. Nocker, R. E. T., Schoonbrood, D. F. M., van der Graaf, E. A., Hack, C. E., Lutter, R., Jansem, H. M., et al. (1996) Interleukin-8 in airway inflammation in patients with asthma and chronic obstructive pulmonary disease. *Int. Arch. Allergy Immunol.* **109,** 183–191.

27

Cytokines in Blister Fluids

Franco Ameglio and Luciano D'Auria

1. Introduction

In the history of clinical pathology, all the body fluids have been employed to examine several types of molecules. Obviously, the serum has always been the principle source of exploration, although other fluids, namely, urine, acqueous humor, cerebrospinal fluid, lymph, and others have also been investigated to obtain information on particular sites linked to the fluid type.

Skin researchers have often carried out numerous tests on cutaneous blister fluids to associate the molecular concentrations analyzed with different pathologic processes, following the idea that the substances causing the lesions or those induced by the lesion triggers might be concentrated in the blisters.

1.1. Pathological Blisters

Blisters may develop from trauma, physical (such as sunburns or other types of radiation) or chemical (insect bites, phytodermatitis, contact with jellyfish) injuries, infectious agents, or autoimmune or allergic processes (1).

Blister fluids may present with transudate or exudate characteristics. The fluid contents vary widely, on the basis of the presence of proteins, cells, and cellular components. The most frequent cells observed are neutrophils, eosinophils, basophils/mast cells, keratinocytes, and T-lymphocytes, depending on the lesion type. In some cases, measuring molecular cell markers rather than the number of the producing cells has been considered a more reliable procedure. This is the case, for instance, for eosinophil cationic protein, myeloperoxidase, and tryptase (2,3).

From: *Methods in Molecular Medicine, vol. 60: Interleukin Protocols*
Edited by: L. A. J. O'Neill and A. Bowie © Humana Press Inc., Totowa, NJ

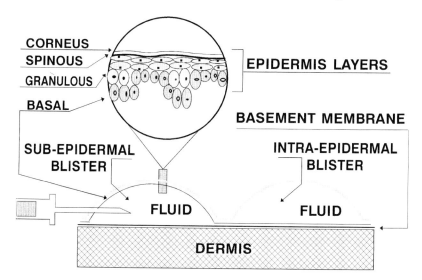

Fig. 1. Pathologic blisters may be of two types, intra- or subepidermal, depending on the histologic site where the blister develops. The mechanisms driving the blister location and development are, at least in part, unknown, and this point therefore represents one of the major targets of the most recent research in this field. Suction blister fluids, a kind of artifactual blister induced by applying a negative pressure to the skin, belong to the subepidermal type. The scheme reported is obviously simplified to the maximum for didactical reasons. More details can be found in any of the good dermatologic textbooks (*1,18*).

1.2. Why Employ Pathologic Blisters?

An analysis of reports exploring blisters (at the time of writing, 218 publications were listed in PubMed, National Library of Medicine, Bethesda, MD) reveals that blister fluid testing is mostly based on local amounts of natural skin compounds. Of particular relevence are the cytokines (*4–8*).

1.3. Classification of Pathological Blisters

To understand blister architecture more easily, a schematic (**Fig. 1**) shows blister types (intraepidermal and subepidermal) on the basis of histologic skin site. All blisters that depend on inflammatory processes are characterized by a more or less altered basement membrane through which both the intercellular fluid proteins and the recruited cells may pass.

1.4. Bullous Dermatoses

Some of the most frequent bullous dermatoses are reported in **Table 1**, which also shows histologic blister sites and the main types of cells recruited within the bulla. Other than pathologic blisters, dermatologic research often uses the suction blisters characterized by subepidermal splitting.

Table 1
Principle Bullous Skin Pathologies

Disease	Blister type	Principle cellular content
Pemphigus vulgaris	Intraepidermal	Acantolytic cells, neutrophils/eosinophils
Bullous (B) pemphigoid	Subepidermal	Eosinophils/neutrophils
Epidermolysis bullosa acquisita	Subepidermal	—
B. eczema	Intraepidermal	Lymphocytes, neutrophils, eosinophils
B. impetigo	Intraepidermal	Neutrophils
B. drug reactions	Intra/subepidermal	Mono/polymorphonuclear cells
B. erythema multiforme	Intra/subepidermal	Mono/polymorphonuclear cells
B. lupus erythematosus	Subepidermal	Mono/polymorphonuclear cells
B. lichen planus	Subepidermal	Mono/polymorphonuclear cells
Burns	Subepidermal	—
Porphyria cutanea tarda	Subepidermal	—

1.5. Suction Blister Fluids

By means of suitable devices capable of inducing a negative pressure on the skin, blisters may be generated on both normal (healthy controls) and lesional or nonlesional skin (patients). The same factors analyzed for pathologic blisters may also be used for suction blister fluids, which may also be generated in normal skin. Fluids of suction blisters may suggest of the soluble substances present in normal or pathologic skin, and also in the absence of bullous diseases *(9–14)*.

1.7. Factors Determining the Passage of Molecules into the Blisters

Previous publications showed that the passage from the external side of the blister to the blister fluid is regulated by the molecular weight of the molecules or their shape, or, by the binding of these molecules to possible carriers. Depending on the integrity of the basement membrane zone, molecules of different molecular weights may spread both from the inside to the outside of the blister or vice versa. Some of the early studies indicated that molecules with a molecular weight of less than 30,000 have a free passage into and from the blisters, whereas their influx is inversely correlated to their molecular weight when this is greater than 30,000 kDa *(15,16)*. The binding of a molecule with other molecules may obviously interfere with this passage.

In a previous study *(17)*, three nonlocally produced molecules, albumin, haptoglobin, and α-1-acid glycoprotein (of hepatic origin), showed lower blister fluid levels than those observed in the sera, confirming that these molecules were partially blocked when they passed through the semipermeable wall. Interestingly, blister fluid/serum ratios were inversely correlated to the theoretical molecular weights of the same molecules. When, molecules synthesized near or in the blisters such as inflammatory cytokines were considered, a direct correlation was found between blister fluid/serum levels and the theoretical molecular weights, suggesting that passage into and out of the blister depended on molecular size.

2. Materials

1. Syringe with large needle.
2. Disinfection tools.
3. Tubes with caps.
4. Graduated pipets and micropipets.
5. Centrifuge.
6. Thermostat.
7. Refrigerator and freezer at –40°C.
8. A microplate reader.
9. Plate washer.
10. ELISA kits for cytokines.

3. Methods
3.1. Blister and Fluid Collection

1. Unless special reasons exist, the blister fluids should be obtained from recently developed lesions, both because the cytokine levels are more elevated and to prevent blister disruption. Some diseases are characterised by stable blisters (bullous pemphigoid [BP]), whereas in others, fluids may rarely be obtained because of the extreme fragility of the blisters (pemphigus vulgaris [PV]) *(1,18)* (*see* **Note 1**).
2. After skin disinfection, the syringe should be inserted near the blister base (where the skin is more resistant) and the fluid aspirated. If more blisters are needed, the needle and syringe must be changed to guarantee aseptic procedure. This operation is painless if the needle does not scratch the blister pavement (*see* **Note 2**). The fluid should be aspirated slowly to avoid blood leakage into the blister.
3. The fluids collected, unless otherwise specified, should be centrifuged (15 min at 800*g* in a routine centrifuge) and filtered (0.22 μm) at 4°C as soon as possible and frozen. Storage temperatures may vary on the basis of the tests to be performed. If a biologic assay is required, samples must be stored at –80°C. Pellets may be used for the cytologic procedures *(19)*. When possible, it is useful to know both the number and the types of fluid cells.
4. The amount of blister fluid may vary greatly from one disease to another *(1)*. In some cases, the blisters are very small, and fluids from more blisters have to be pooled. In these cases, the blisters should have the same duration. Many cytokine concentrations drop over time *(20)*.

3.2. Suction Blistering

1. Suction blistering is a standardized method *(15,21–24)* of obtaining interstitial fluid, migrating inflammatory cells, mediators *(5)*, and pure living epidermal components for transplantation or cell culture *(21)*.

2. Before considering suction blisters, it is important to remember that although they are generally safe and painless, they require a few hours for development during which the subject should remain immobile; they sometimes induce pain in highy sensitive individuals and leave hyperpigmented areas for long periods (even 2 yr). Therefore, an informed consent should be obtained. In the case of blister disruption, as much of the lesion may be infected, a suitable medication is needed. The blister roof should be removed; this portion could be used for other purposes, such as molecular biology *(25)*.

3. As previously reported for pathologic blisters, cytokine concentrations of suction blister fluids must be compared with the serum levels of the same individual *(9)*. When possible (rarely on the lesional skin in inflammatory diseases), the best information is obtained when normal, nonlesional, and lesional skin suction blisters are compared, to rule out possible cytokine induction due to negative pressure. Evident blood contamination is revealed by the hematic aspect of the fluids, although contamination at a minor level may not be detected.

4. If a cytokine determination in a lesional fluid must be compared with serum concentration to establish a local production, the comparison between the lesional and the nonlesional areas may account for a cytokine synthesis linked to clinical disease expression. Finally, comparison with the normal skin guarantees that there is a difference between the diseased and nondiseased skin, as does comparison with suction blister fluids obtained from healthy individuals as controls.

5. A suction blister on nonlesional skin (of patients or healthy subjects) should be generated in an anatomic area where there is a sufficient amount of subcutaneous tissue so that the cup may have an optimal adherence (*see* **Note 3**).

6. In the case of nonbullous diseases or when the spontaneous blisters are very feeble, since they are localized in the more superficial epidermal layers (pemphigus erythematosus, pemphigus foliaceus and pemphigus vegetans), or when the spontaneous bullae are less than 0.5 mm (vesiculobullous diseases, such as linear IgA dermatitis, or Duhring's disease or herpes gestationis) and the aspiration of their content is not possible with any type of needle, suction skin blisters may be generated. A controlled, negative, localized pressure to the skin produces dermoepidermal blisters with a split at the level of the lamina lucida. These are the so-called suction blister fluids. As opposed to pathologic blisters, which are exclusively lesional, suction blister fluids are mainly obtained from the normal or nonlesional skin, even if lesional suction blisters may also be generated, depending on the diseased skin situation. Suction blisters may substitute for a skin biopsy when the presence of soluble molecules is needed with subsequent repetitions over time to monitor patients *(26)*.

3.3. Device for Suction Blistering

1. The first type of device to obtain suction blisters is commercially available, has been improved over the years, and today includes disposable accessories. The blistering device is composed of butenestyrene; it is single packed and γ-sterilized for immediate use. Disposability is dictated by the risks of transmission of human immunodeficiency virus and hepatitis viruses. The device consists of a suction chamber, provided

Table 2
Comparison of Biological vs Immunological Methods
to Detect Cytokine Levels

Biologic methods		Immunologic methods	
Advantages	Limits	Advantages	Limits
Functional measurement	Dosage limited to whole functional molecules	Specific measurement depending on Ab even on molecular components	Nonfunctional measures; molecules with altered epitopes cannot be detected
Complexed cytokines?			Complexed cytokines'
Less expensive if cell cultures are available	Cell culture technology needed	Only ELISA technology	Suitable instrumentation
Frequent interferences due to sample composition	Variations due to cell sensitivity	Reduced interferences due to sample types	Variations due to Ab selection
High sensitivity	Partially nonspecific measures	High sensitivity of new kits	Low sensitivity of old kits
	Variable sample volumes	Low sample volumes	

with an internal adapter with three to five holes of 0.3–0.8 mm size, connected to an electric vacuum pump reaching negative pressures (*see* **Note 4**). At the normal or nonlesional skin level, the fluid is transparent and of a yellowish color. Its composition is similar to that of the lymph/interstitial fluid *(24,27)*. This method has been used to detect several molecules in the skin, some of them of body origin and others representing drugs or drug catabolites administered orally, systemically, or locally *(28–30)*. Obviously, with this approach, no information can be obtained on the cellular source of cytokine production, unless specific cell markers are detected (i.e., eosinophil cationic protein for eosinophils) *(2)*. More recently, another method has been described using syringe suction *(31)*.

3.4. Cytokine Determinations

1. Most of the studies conducted during the last decade to detect cytokine concentrations in pathologic blisters used biologic assays. Since then, enzyme-linked immunosorbent assay (ELISA) tests have in most cases replaced biologic methods. (**Table 2** compares both methods.) Biologic assays generally consist of selection of cells that are sensitive to only one cytokine (when possible) and measuring cell proliferation in the presence of fluids containing the cytokine. Controls must obviously be heavily used. Different reports have highlighted that cytokines may be complexed with other molecules. In this case, both biologic and ELISA methods may or may not detect such cytokine/protein complexes *(32)*. There are several reports in the literature regarding the concentrations of

Table 3
Cytokine Concentrations in Blisters from Different Pathologies

Cytokine	Disease	Blister size[a]	Serum[a]	Reference	Year
IL-1β	PV	7.7–131	<0.3–3.5	*26*	1997
IL-2	BP	9–173	UDL-UDL	*5*	1998
IL-4	PV	<4.1–22.2	<4.1–6.1	*21*	1998
IL-5	BP	76–665	<0.1–112	*2*	1998
IL-6	BP	1725–10,000	0.1–138	*5*	1998
IL-7	BP	<0.035–0.76	0.09–31.6	*22*	1998
IL-8	BP	303–9009	UDL–12	*5*	1998
IL-12	BP	UDL–875	UDL–UDL	*5*	1998
IL-15	BP	36–79	18–40	*23*	1999
IFN-γ	BP	UDL–29	UDL–7	*5*	1998
TNF-α	PV	62–183	0.6–45	*21*	1997
TGF-β1	BP	13–23	0.7–62	*5*	1997

[a]UDL, under detection limit; BP, bullous pemphigoid; PV, pemphigus vulgaris; PCT, porphyria cutanea tarda. Values in pg/mL.

Table 4
Cytokine Concentrations Observed in Psoriatic Sera or Suction Blister Fluids

Cytokine	Ps serum range	NSBF range	Ps SBF range	Reference
IL-1β	UDL–90	UDL	UDL-191	*26*
IL-6	UDL–120	8–15	583–6130	*36*
IL-10	10–99	20–72	3–42	*41*
IFN-γ	UDL–0.08	UDL	UDL–4	*26*
TNF-α	UDL–130	UDL–35	92–491	*25,26*
GM-CSF	UDL–44	UDL	UDL–61	*42*

SBF, suction blister fluid; NSBF, normal SBF; Ps, psoriasis; UDL, under detection limit; values expressed as pg/mL with the exception of IFN-γ, which is expressed in IU/mL.

many cytokines in various types of blisters (*4–14,20,33–42*). **Table 3** reports a list of cytokines recently found in pathologic blisters by employing sensitive commercial kits, along with range of concentrations found.

3.5. Cytokine Concentrations in Normal and Pathologic Suction Blister Fluids

1. Some ranges of cytokine concentrations determined in lesional blister fluids of psoriatic patients are reported in **Table 4**. As expected, authors often report different values obtained with different commercial kits (*see* **Note 5**).

2. The cytokine levels, altered in blister fluids, may be repeatedly measured during the course of therapy. Both interleukin-6 (IL-6) and tumor necrosis factor-α (TNF-α) show a progressive normalization of the values compared with normal suction blister fluids, suggesting that this method may be useful in monitoring treated patients *(26)*.

3.6. Variations from Improvements of Methods

Although only a few years have elapsed since ELISA tests have become commercially available, there has been a dramatic improvement of the kit sensitivities for different cytokines. In some cases, the sensitivity levels changed from 5 µg/mL to 0.1 pg/mL in short periods, permitting the detection of differences between the serum concentrations of patients and healthy controls where previously concentrations in both groups were under the detection limit. There are many of these examples in the literature *(4,12,13)* (*see* **Note 6**). When the blisters are due to inflammatory diseases, the cytokine content is generally very high (**Table 3**). The cytokine concentrations are usually expressed as units per volume, but sometimes it may be important to express the concentrations per mg of total proteins or per amount of cells *(43)*. This is the case of measurements in bioptic homogenates.

3.7. Other Determinations

For each patient and disease type, it is important to record age, sex, disease, stage, blister size, cutaneous localization of the bulla, number of blisters all over the body, mucous membrane involvement, and disease severity score (if available) or other disease markers (if possible). These data may be helpful in examining correlations between the blister content of various components and the disease severity.

Given the relative standardization of the ELISA methods, if the samples must be collected over time, the tests should be performed together to guarantee a correct comparison. The cytokine levels are often very high in inflammatory diseases. **Table 3** may help to select the optimal volumes to use for ELISA determinations. Although ELISAs for cytokines do not differ from those of other determinations, it must be emphasized that the results exceeding the standard curve should not be considered (even if very close to the maximum point). To improve the sensitivity, some commercial kits present a flat curve at the last points; from experience with several repetitions after dilution, it is known that the approximation mistakes may be great. When the results are low, the values under the first point of the curve are not reliable, even if they are closer to the first point than to the zero value. The use of different plot procedures may sometimes create false-positive values.

There are only two ways to resolve the problem: sample concentration or, if available, more sensitive tests. Again, *mixed results obtained with two different kits or different lots should not be considered reliable*, because of the great variability. Only tests performed in the same analytical set with homogeneous reagents should be accepted. In the case of repetition after dilution, some previously determined samples should always be added to be sure of the test reliability. Several commercial kits include at least two types of sample diluents. Obviously, the one most similar to the samples should be used.

Finally, when the basement membrane of the blister is disrupted (this increases with blister aging), molecules larger than those foreseen may cross the barrier. Protein size, shape, and binding with other molecular carriers may also determine cytokine passage from the blood/lymph-interstitial fluid-blister fluid and return *(17)*. In some cases, when the blisters are hematic, the hemoglobin dosage may represent a possible marker of blood contamination.

3.8. Controls for Pathologic Blisters

Although accepted by most researchers in dermatology, it must still be established whether or not a suction blister fluid is a correct control for pathologic blisters (*see* **Note 7**). It is definitely useful to compare the cytokine concentrations with those obtained by measuring the serum levels from blood samples obtained as the same time as the blister fluids. Blister concentrations higher than those of the serum point to local cytokine synthesis; lower concentrations may indicate a block of the mediator production. Sometimes the local presence of inhibitors (carriers that bind cytokines and hide the binding site for the antibody) or catabolic media tors may explain why the blister cytokine amounts are lower than those of the sera.

As previously reported for PV or BP *(20)*, the concentrations of some cytokines observed in recently developed (24-h) blisters were significantly correlated with disease severity/activity. This implies that the skin (lesional biopsy or blister) produces larger cytokine amounts in involved sites, depending on the extension or intensity of the entire disease.

4. Notes

1. When the blister is very small (vesicle), especially if the fluids are coagulated, it is difficult to aspirate the contents. When the blister is larger than 4–5 mm, a 5-mL syringe, with not too subtle a needle, should be employed to avoid needle obstruction by fibrin or cellular debris.
2. Since fluid aspiration eliminates blister tension, the possible local itching and/or pain may disappear.
3. Inducing a suction blister may be a complex procedure in some dermatoses. Perfect adherence of the device cup is mandatory for blister generation. If the skin is xerotic or hyperkeratotic (such as in psoriasis) passage of air, even in minimal amounts, between the edge of the cup and the epidermis can make blister generation impossible. Therefore, selecting areas without desquamation and maintaining the hydrolipidic film, when possible, guarantees successful blistering.

4. It must be emphasized that a slow suction is more reliable since it reduces the possibility of disrupting the basement membrane. In contrast, patients may not tolerate long periods of suction because they are obliged to be immobile, and the negative pressure (which may be painful for sensitive/apprensive subjects) may be uncomfortable.

5. These concentrations may only suggest some indications regarding the range of the expected cytokine levels. Obviously, the numbers may vary widely in other diseases.

6. Measurements in the blister fluids produced contrasting results. Those who employed highly sensitive tests detected cytokine amounts that previous reports defined as negative.

7. We personally believe that a nonlesional suction blister fluid is a correct control for a lesional one but that a normal suction blister cannot be compared with a pathologic one because of different inductive mechanisms.

References

1. Saurat, J. H. (1990) Maladies bulleuses, in *Dermatologie et Venereologie* (Saurat, J. H., Grosshans, E., Laugier, P., and Lachapelle, J. M., eds.), Masson, Paris, pp. 231–276.

2. D'Auria, L., Pietravalle, M., Mastroianni, A., Ferraro, C., Mussi, A., Bonifati, C., et al. (1998) IL-5 levels in the sera and in the blister fluids of patients affected with bullous pemphigoid: correlations with eosinophylic cationic protein, RANTES, IgE and with disease severity. *Arch. Dermatol. Res.* **290,** 25–27.

3. D'Auria, L., Pietravalle, M., Cordiali-Fei, P., and Ameglio, F. (2000) Increased tryptase and myeloperoxidase levels in blister fluids of patients with bullous pemphigoid: correlations with cytokines, adhesion molecules and anti-basement membrane zone antibodies. *Exp. Dermatol.* **9,** 131–137.

4. Ameglio, F., D'Auria, L., Bonifati, C., Ferraro, C., Mastroianni, A., and Giacalone, B. (1998) Cytokine pattern in blister fluids and serum of patients with bullous pemphigoid; relationships with disease intensity. *Br. J. Dermatol.* **138,** 611–614.

5. Grando, S. A., Glukhenky, B. T., Drannik, G. N., Epstein, E. V., Kostromin, A. P., and Korostash, T. A. (1989) Mediators of inflammation in blister fluids from patients with pemphigus vulgaris and bullous pemphigoid. *Arch. Dermatol.* **125,** 925–930.

6. Schaller, J., Giese, T., Ladusch, M., and Haustein, U.-F. (1990) Interleukin-2 receptor expression and interleukin-2 production in bullous pemphigoid. *Arch. Dermatol. Res.* **282,** 223–226.

7. Schmidt, E., Bastian, B., Dummer, R. Tony, H. P., Brocker, E. B., and Zillikens, D. (1996. Detection of elevated levels of IL-4, Il-6, and IL-10 in blister fluid of bullous pemphigoid. *Arch. Dermatol. Res.* **288,** 353–357.

8. Tamaki, K., So, K., Furuya, F., and Furue, M. (1994) Cytokine profile of patients with bullous pemphigoid. *Br. J. Dermatol.* **130,** 128–129.

9. D'Auria, L., Bonifati, C., Mussi, A., D'Agosto, G., De Simone, C., Giacalone, B., et al. (1997) Cytokines in the sera of patients with pemphigus vulgaris: IL-6 and TNF-alpha levels are significantly increased as compared to healthy subiects and correlated with disease activity. *Eur. Cytokine Netw.* **8,** 383–387.

10. Giacalone, B., D'Auria, L., Bonifati, C., Ferraro, C., Riccardi, E., Mussi, A., et al. (1998) Decreased interleukin-7 and transforming growth factor-beta1 levels in blister fluids as compared to the respective serum levels in patients with bullous pemphigoid. Opposite behavior of TNF-alpha, interleukin-4 and interleukin-10. *Exp. Dermatol.* **7,** 157–161.

11. D'Auria, L., Bonifati, C., Cordiali-Fei, P., Leone, G., Picardo, M., Pietravalle, M., et al. (1999) Increased serum interleukin-15 levels in bullous skin diseases: correlation with disease intensity. *Arch. Dermatol. Res.* **291,** 354–356.

12. Takematsu, H., Ohta, H., and Tagami, H. (1991) Determination of tumor necrosis factor in blister fluids of bullous pemphigoid. *Arch. Dermatol. Res.* **283,** 131–132.

13. D'Auria, L., Mussi, A., Bonifati, C., Mastroianni, A., Giacalone, B., and Ameglio, F. (1999) Increased serum IL-6, TNF-alpha and IL-10 levels in patients with bullous pemphigoid: relationships with disease activity. *J. Eur. Acad. Dermatol. Venereol.* **12,** 11–15.

14. Bonifati, C., Ameglio, F., Carducci, M., Sacerdoti, G., Pietravalle, M., and Fazio, M. (1994) Interleukin-1beta, interleukin-6 and interferon-gamma in suction blister fluids of involved and uninvolved skin and in sera of psoriatic patients. *Acta Derm. Venereol. (Stockh.)* **186,** 23–24.

15. Stalder, J. F., Dreno, B., and Litoux, P. (1987) Suction blisters. Technique and applications. *Ann. Dermatol. Venereol.* **114,** 421–423.

16. Fazio, M., Bonifati, C., Alemanno, L., and Ameglio, F. (1994) Differential behaviour of three soluble membrane molercules in sera and suction blister fluids from lesional and non-lesional skin of psoriatic patients: comparison with skin of normal donors. *Eur. J. Dermatol.* **4,** 476–479.

17. D'Auria, L., Pimpinelli, F., Ferraro, C., D'Ambrogio, G., Giacalone, B., Bellocci, M., et al. (1998) Blister fluid/serum ratios of several cytokines evaluated in patients with bullous pemphigoid: relationship with theoretical molecular weights. *J. Biol. Regulat. Homeost. Agents* **12,** 76–80.

18. Lever, W. F. (1990) Non infectious vesicular and bullous diseases, in *Histopathology of the Skin* (Lever, W. F. and Schaumburg-Lever, G., eds.), J.B. Lippincott, Philadelphia, PA, pp. 125–130.

19. Ahokas, T. L., Niemi, K. M., and Halme, H. (1982) Identification of mononuclear cells in suspension from cutaneous infiltrates by a suction blister method. *Acta Derm. Venereol. (Stockh.)* **62,** 377–381.

20. Giacalone, B., D'Auria, L., Ferraro, C., Mussi, A., Bonifati, C., and Ameglio, F. (1998) Bullous pemphigoid blisters of the same duration have similar cytokine concentrations which decrease in older blisters. *Br. J. Dermatol.* **139,** 158–159.

21. Larsen, C. G., Ternowitz, T., Larsen, F. G., and Thestrup-Pedersen, K. (1988) Preparation of human epidermal tissue for functional studies. *Acta Derm. Venereol,* **68,** 474–479.

22. Kiistala, U. and Mustakallio, K. K. (1964) In-vivo separation of epidermis by production of suction blisters. *Lancet* **i,** 1444–1445.

23. Kiistala, U. and Mustakallio, K. K. (1967) Dermo-epidermal separation with suction. Electron microscopy and histochemical study of initial events of blistering on human skin. *J. Invest. Dermatol.* **48,** 466–477.

24. Herfst, M. J. and van Rees H. (1978) Suction blister fluids as a model for intersti-tial fluids in rats. *Arch. Dermatol. Res.* **263**, 325–334.

25. Enk, C. D. and Katz, S. I. (1994) Extraction and quantitation of cytokine mRNA from human epidermal blister roofs. *Arch. Dermatol. Res.* **287**, 72–77.

26. Ameglio, F., Bonifati, C., Pietravalle, M., and Fazio, M. (1994) Interleukin-6 and tumour necrosis factor levels decrease in the suction blister fluids of psoriatic patients during effective therapy. *Dermatology* **189**, 359–363.

27. Groth, S. and Staberg, B. (1984) Suction blisters of the skin: a compartment with physiological, interstitium-like properties. *Scand. J. Clin. Lab. Invest.* **44**, 311–316.

28. Aoyama, H., Sugiyama, H., Ishii, T., Kawauchi, T., Kasauya, T., Nishizaki, A., et al. (1987) Transfer of ofloxacin into suction blister fluid after its oral adminis-tration. *JPN. J. Antibiot.* **40**, 1937–1940.

29. Autio, P., Risteli, J., Haukipuro, K., Risteli, L., and Oikarinen, A. (1994) Effects of an inhaled steroid (budesonide) on skin collagen synthesis of asthma patients in vivo. *Am. J. Respir. Crit. Care Med.* **153**, 1172–1175.

30. Bartholomew, T. C., Summerfield, J. A., Billing, B. H., Lawson, A. M., and Setchell, A. M. (1982) Bile acid profiles of human serum and skin interstitial fluid and their relationship to pruritus studied by gas chromatography mass spectrom-etry. *Clin. Sci.* **63**, 65–73.

31. Mukhtar, M., Singh, S., Shukla, V. K., and Pandey, S. S. (1997) Surgical pearl: suction syrynge for epidermal grafting. *J. Am. Acad. Dermatol.* **37**, 638–639.

32. May, L. T., Viguette, H., and Kenney, G. E. (1992) High levels of complexed interleukin-6 in human blood. *J. Biol. Chem.* **267**, 19,698–19,704.

33. Delaporte, E., Bieber, T., Viac, J., Faure, M., and Nicolas, J. F. (1994) Cytokines epidermique et inflammation cutanée (Review). *Ann. Dermatol. Venereol.* **121**, 836–843.

34. Inaoki, M. and Takehara, K. (1998) Increased serum levels of interleukin-5, IL-6 and IL-8 in bullous pemphigoid. *J. Dermatol. Sci.* **19**, 152–157.

35. Endo, H., Iwamoto, I., Fujita, M., Okamoto, S., and Yoshida, S. (1992) Increased immunoreactive interleukin-5 levels in blister fluids of bullous pemphigoid. *Arch. Dermatol. Res.* **284**, 312–314.

36. Bonifati, C. and Ameglio, F. (1999) Cytokines in psoriasis (Review). *Int. J. Dermatol.* **38**, 241–251.

37. D'Auria, L., Cordiali-Fei, P., and Ameglio, F. (1999) Cytokines and bullous pemphigoid. *Eur. Cytokine Netw.* **10**, 123–133.

38. Schmidt, E., Mittnacht, A., Schomig, H., Dummer, R., Brocker, E. B., and Zillikens, D. (1996) Detection of IL-1alpha, IL-1beta and IL-1 receptor antago-nist in blister fluid of bullous pemphigoid. *J. Dermatol. Sci.* **11**, 142–147.

39. Schmidt, E., Ambach, A., Bastian, B., Brocker, E. B., and Zillikens, D. (1996) Elevated levels of interleukin-8 in blister fluid of bullous pemphigoid compared with suction blisters of healthy control subjects. *J. Am. Acad. Dermatol.* **34**, 310–312.

40. Zillikens, D., Shuessler, M., Dummer, R., Porzsolt, F., Hartmann, A. A., and Burg, G. (1992) Tumour necrosis factor in blister fluids of bullous pemphigoid. *Eur. J. Dermatol.* **2**, 429–431.

41. Mussi, A., Bonifati, C., Carducci, M., Viola, M., Tomaselli, R., Sacerdoti, G., et al. (1994) IL-10 levels are decreased in psoriatic lesional skin as compared to the psoriatic lesion-free and normal skin suction blister fluids. *J. Biol. Regulat. Homeost. Agents* **8,** 117–120.

42. Bonifati, C., Carducci, M., Cordiali-Fei, P., Trento, E., Sacerdoti, G., Fazio, M., et al. (1994) Correlated increases of tumour necrosis factor-alpha, interleukin-6 and granulocyte monocyte-colony stimulating factor levels in suction blister fluids and sera of psoriatic patients. Relationships with disease severity. *Clin. Exp. Dermatol.* **19,** 383–387.

43. Ameglio, F., Bonifati, C., Fazio, M., Mussi, A., Trento, E., Cordiali-Fei, P., et al. (1997) Interleukin-11 production is increased in organ cultures of lesional skin of patients with active plaque-type psoriasis as compared with non-lesional and normal skin. Similarity to interleukin-1beta, interleukin-6 and interleukin-8. *Arch. Dermatol. Res.* **289,** 399–403.

28

Measurement of Cytokines in Synovial Fluid

Fabrizio De Benedetti

1. Introduction

Over the last 20 years, advances in the knowledge of cytokine biology have brought a new dimension to the understanding of pathogenic events in human chronic arthritides, showing promise for future therapeutic approaches. Pathogenetically, it is likely that local and systemic manifestations of rheumatic diseases are consequence of cytokine-mediated cell responses of inappropriate intensity and duration. It is beyond the scope of this chapter to describe in detail the available evidence concerning the role of cytokines in these diseases. This issue has been recently reviewed *(1,2)* and is discussed comprehensively in textbooks of rheumatology *(3,4)*.

Although the actual cytokine concentration in the microenvironment of the inflamed synovium may be higher than cytokine levels detected in the synovial fluid (SF), it is generally accepted that the SF cytokine content reflects cytokine production by the inflamed tissue. In this chapter we focus on the measurement of the so-called proinflammatory cytokines, which are produced essentially by macrophages and synovial fibroblasts, and which are responsible for cell recruitment, fibrosis, and damage to periarticular cartilage and bone (*see* **Table 1**). These cytokines are released in large amounts by the inflamed synovium and can be easily detected in SF. On the other hand, although a vast body of evidence points to a pivotal role of T lymphocytes in the pathogenesis of chronic autoimmune arthritides, and T cells infiltrating the inflamed synovium express several markers of activation, T-cell-derived cytokines are either not detectable or present in very low concentrations in a small percentage of SF samples (**Table 1**). In some instances their production in the inflamed synovium can be demonstrated using sensitive techniques, such as immunocytochemistry or reverse transcriptase polymerase chain reaction (RT-PCR). These techniques are described elsewhere in this book.

From: *Methods in Molecular Medicine, vol. 60: Interleukin Protocols*
Edited by: L. A. J. O'Neill and A. Bowie © Humana Press Inc., Totowa, NJ

Table 1
Synovial Fluid Levels of Cytokines and Their Principal Effects Relevant to the Pathogenesis of Chronic Joint Inflammation and Damage to Joint Tissues[a]

Macrophages and synovial fibroblasts	Levels in synovial fluid	Principal effects relevant to arthritis
IL-1β	++	Induction of chondrocyte production of proteases, PGE_2, NO; inhibition of chondrocyte PG synthesis (cartilage degradation)
		Fibroblast production of proteases and PGE_2
		Induction of chemokine production
IL-6	+++	Osteoclast formation and activation (bone resorption)
		Synovial fibroblast proliferation
		Induction of adhesion molecule expression on endothelium
		Induction of chemokine production T- and B-cell growth factor
TNF-α	++	Activation of macrophages and neutrophils
		Stimulation of proinflammatory cytokine production
		Fibroblast production of proteases and PGE_2
		Induction of adhesion molecule expression on endothelium
		Induction of chemokine production
M-CSF	+	Activation and survival of macrophages
TGF-β	++	Neoangiogenesis
		Proliferation of fibroblasts and fibroblast production
		of extracellular matrix proteins (fibrosis)
IL-8 [b]	++	Recruitment and activation of neutrophils
MCP-1[b]	+++	Recruitment and activation of monocytes/macrophages
T lymphocytes		
IL-2	+/–	Major T-cell growth factor
IL-4	–	Activation of B cells
		Proliferation of T cells
		Inhibition of monocyte production of IL-1, IL-6
IFN-γ	+/–	Activation of macrophages
		Induction of HLA class II expression
		Inhibition of collagen production by chondrocytes

[a]Abbreviations: IFN, interferon; IL, interleukin: M-CSF, monocyte-colony stimulating factor; MCP-1, monocyte chemoattractant protein-1; PG, proteoglycan; PGE_2, prostaglandin E_2; TGF-β, transforming growth factor-β; TNF-α, tumor necrosis factor-α; NO, nitric oxide.
[b]A variety of other chemokines (e.g., RANTES, MIP-1α) can be detected in SF.

Accurate detection and measurement of cytokines in SF is an obvious prerequisite not only for the understanding of their pathogenic role, but also for determining the clinical potential of these molecules. Measurement of cytokines in the SF may provide relevant information on the staging and/or the prognosis of the disease. Moreover, since various therapeutic approaches are now, or will be in the near future, available to readjust a cytokine imbalance by administration of either cytokines or cytokine antagonists, reliable monitoring of cytokine activity in SF may provide an additional measure of the efficacy of these procedures.

Several assays are now available for the measurement of the amount of cytokines present in a wide range of biologic fluids including SF. Biologic assays have been established based on the biologic activities of each cytokine, using either whole animals or cells in vitro. Whole animal-based assays are expensive, often involving a large number of animals; they are also time consuming, imprecise, and require a large volume of the biologic fluid to be tested. These assays played an important role in the early days of cytokine research. Currently, biologic assays are usually performed in vitro using either cultured primary cells or, more often, continuous cell lines. However, none of the biologic assays available fulfill the criteria of specificity, sensitivity, speed, and reliability of an ideal assay. This has stimulated the development of immunoassays or alternative biochemical or immunochemical techniques for the detection and measurement of cytokines. This chapter deals essentially with the measurement of SF cytokines by immunoassays.

A preliminary consideration concerns the definition of cytokine levels in normal SF. Since the amount of SF in a healthy joint is minimal, it is practically (and ethically) impossible, to obtain SF from an healthy individual. To obtain a relevant term of comparison, cytokine levels obtained from patients with chronic inflammatory arthritides are usually compared with those present in noninflammatory conditions, such as osteoarthritis.

1.1. Biologic Assays

As previously mentioned, bioassays are based either on cultured primary cells or on continuous cell lines. Primary cell culture-based assays have two main disadvantages: (1) the separation of the cells from blood or tissues is not, in many instances, straightforward and contamination of the cell preparation can influence the results; and (2) differences due to interdonor variations may represent a problem. Nevertheless, they are useful in research involving newly identified cytokines and in the demonstration of their biologic activities, as well as in experiments aimed at the attribution of a given activity of a biologic fluid (i.e., SF) to a particular cytokine.

One example is provided by the identification of the role of interleukin-6 (IL-6) present in SF in the activation of osteoclasts and in the subsequent bone resorption

(5). In general, cell line-based assays are more economical and produce reliable and accurate estimates of the biologically active cytokine. The main characteristic of bioassays is that they provide an estimation of the net amount of biologically active cytokine present in the biological fluid, i.e., the balance between the cyokine and its natural inhibitors (e.g., soluble cytokine receptors—IL-1 receptor antagonist). However, the major drawback is that bioassays are not specific for a single cytokine. This is the obvious consequence of the redundancy of cytokines. As an example, B9 cells commonly used to measure IL-6 also proliferate in response to other cytokines of the gp130 family (i.e., IL-11 and oncostatin-M). It should also be kept in mind that bioassays may overestimate the amount of a cytokine due to the presence of synergistic interaction between individual cytokines present in the SF. To identify which cytokine(s) is causing the effect on multispecific cells, the common approach is to use antibodies to neutralize a single cytokine specifically.

Biologic assays are usually not as sensitive as immunoassays. One exception is represented by the assay with the murine hybridoma B9 for the measurement of IL-6, which has a sensitivity in the range of 1 pg/mL (6). Nevertheless, for general purposes, IL-6 immunoassays are preferable.

1.2. Immunoassays

Immunoassays are usually quicker and easier to perform than bioassays and therefore represent the method of choice for cytokine measurement, especially given a large number of samples. The amount of SF needed is usually smaller than that needed for bioassays. Conventional competitive radioimmunoassays are usually not sufficiently sensitive to measure physiologic or even pathologic levels of cytokines. The most widely used immunoassays are enzyme-linked immunosorbent assays (ELISAs) based on the two-site principle, by which one antibody is used to capture the cytokine to a solid phase substrate and the other (labeled) is used to reveal the bound cytokine. It is highly preferable that at least one antibody, possibly the one used for capture, be a well-characterized monoclonal antibody. Immunoassays detect the antigenic properties of cytokines. One advantage is that they can be used to distinguish cytokines with the same biologic activity (e.g., IL-1α and IL-1β; and tumor necrosis factor [TNF]-α and TNF-β).

The major drawback of immunoassays is that, in addition to biologically active cytokines, they can detect also partially active or inactive material (i.e., degraded). This often results in a lack of correlation between the amount of cytokines estimated by immunoassays and that estimated by bioassays. A further problem that has to be kept in mind is the possible alteration of the antigenic properties of a cytokine by its binding with other proteins (e.g., soluble receptors), thus masking or modifying the epitopes recognized by the antibodies used in the immunoassays. Moreover, immunoassays may exhibit differential detection of different isoforms of cytokines (variable glycosylation, primary structure variations, etc.).

Therefore, it is not surprising that, with all immunoassays, the specificity and sensitivity of the procedure are essentially determined by the particular couple of antibodies used. Several multicentric studies have demonstrated that use of immunoassays based on different antibodies results in significant variations of cytokine level estimates, even when a single recombinant cytokine preparation is used *(7–10)*. In one study dealing specifically with the measurement of cytokines in SF, it has been demonstrated that ELISAs from different manufacturers showed variations of up to 5–10 times *(11)*. Here, an ELISA–based assay for interleukins in SF is described (*see* **Note 1**).

2. Materials

1. Coating buffer: There are three standard coating buffers; the most appropriate must to be determined experimentally.
   a. Buffer A: Phosphate-buffered saline (PBS), pH 7.4.
   b. Buffer B: 0.03 M sodium carbonate, 0.068 *M* sodium bicarbonate, pH 7.4 (adjust pH with NaOH 1 *M*).
   c. Buffer C: 0.2 *M* sodium phosphate monobasic, 0.2 *M* citric acid, pH 6.0.
2. Blocking buffer: Coating buffer, 1–3% bovine serum albumin (BSA).
3. Assay buffer: PBS, pH 7.4, BSA 1–3% (*see* **Notes 2** and **3**).
4. Wash buffer: PBS, pH 7.4; add Tween-20 to 0.05%.
   With the exception of the coating buffer B (stability less than 1 mo), all these buffers are stable for months if stored at 4°C. Addition of sodium azide (0.02%) or thimerosal (0.02%) does not affect immunoassays.
5. Coating antibody: Dilute in the appropriate coating buffer at 0.5–2.5 µg/mL.
6. Detecting antibody: A biotin-labeled antibody is usually the best option. Dilute in assay buffer at 0.1–0.5 µg/mL.
7. Streptavidin conjugated with horseradish peroxidase (HRP) or alkaline phosphatase (AP). Dilute 1:5000–1:20000 in assay buffer.
8. Substrate: tetramethylbenzidine (TMB) for HRP; p-nitrophenilphosphate (p-NPP) for AP. Prepare according to instructions provided by the manufacturer.
9. Stop solution: Sulphuric acid 0.18 *M* (needed only for the TMB substrate).

3. Methods

1. SF should be collected in sterile nonpyrogenic syringes. Great care should be taken to maintain sterility (in particular for use in bioassays) and to eliminate endotoxin contamination (*see* **Note 4**).
2. For use with immunoassays, EDTA should be added immediately after collection at a final concentration of 5 mg/mL. We use a 100 mg/mL stock solution in distilled water, pH 7.4, adding 50 µL of this stock/mL of SF.
3. Samples should be kept on ice until processed.
4. Separation of SF from cells should be performed as soon as possible (less than 1 h from collection). Since SF is a sticky, viscous liquid similar to egg white, after collection it is highly recommended to perform two sequential centrifugation steps

to clear the SF of cells and other particulate materials. We routinely perform centrifugation at 4°C, the first one at 800*g* for 10 min and the second one in a microfuge at 10,000*g* for 10 min (*see* **Note 5**).

5. The supernatants should be aliquoted and stored at –70°C. Even at this temperature some cytokines (e.g., TNF and IL-1) are unstable, with loss of both biologic and antigenic properties over a prolonged period. Freezing and thawing of samples should be avoided since it results in a significant loss of cytokine activity.

6. Because of its viscosity, it is rather difficult to sterile-filter SF through common 0.45-μm filters. If needed (for bioassays), SF should be diluted at least 1:5 in PBS or culture medium prior to filtration.

7. Because of its consistency, which is like egg white, great care should be taken when pipetting small volumes of SF to prepare dilutions; vortexing is necessary to ensure thorough mixing of these dilutions.

8. Coating the plate: Add 100 μL/well of diluted coating antibody in 96-well polystyrene plates. We routinely use high binding plates (EIA high binding plate from Costar). Cover the plate and incubate overnight at room temperature in a humidified atmosphere. Empty the plate and blot it on paper towels to remove residual coating solution.

9. Blocking the plate: Add 250 μL/well of blocking buffer. Cover the plate and incubate for 1 h at 37°C. Wash the plate three times with wash buffer, possibly using an automated plate-washing apparatus. Empty the plate and blot it on paper towels to remove residual wash buffer.

10. Standard and sample incubation: Prepare dilutions of the standards and samples in assay buffer. Add 100 mL/well in duplicate of the standard curve points and of the samples. Cover the plate and incubate for 4 h at 4°C. This incubation can be performed at room temperature (RT) or at 37°C for shorter times (1–2 h). Wash the plate three times with wash buffer. Empty the plate and blot it on paper towels to remove residual solutions (*see* **Notes 6–8**).

11. Detection: Add 100 μL/well of the detecting antibody solution. Cover the plate and incubate for 2 h at RT. (Some protocols allow for incubation of the samples together with the detecting antibody.) Wash the plate three times with wash buffer. Empty the plate and blot it on paper towels to remove residual detecting antibody. Add 100 μL/well of enzyme-conjugated streptavidin. Cover the plate and incubate for 45 min at RT. Wash the plate five times with wash buffer. Empty the plate and blot it on paper towels to remove residual streptavidin (*see* **Note 9**).

12. Substrate: Add 100 μL/well of substrate solution. The TMB substrate for HRP should be incubated for 20–30 min at RT and the reaction blocked by the addition of 100 μL/well of stop solution. Measure the absorbance at 450 nm in a microplate reader. The p-NPP substrate for AP can be incubated at RT for variable periods from 20 min to overnight. (When performing long incubations, place the plate in a humid chamber protect from light.) Because it is not necessary to stop the reaction, reading of the absorbance (405 nm) can be performed at different times, with the advantage of obtaining acceptable resolutions at different cytokine concentrations.

4. Notes

1. Several companies provide ELISA kits for the measurement of cytokines. As previously mentioned, it is well known that different assays give different cytokine estimates. The present knowledge, as well as our experience, is not sufficient to provide indications on which assay is the best one for a given cytokine. The obvious recommendation is to use the same assay throughout the study. Some companies provide assays in bulk quantity or simply provide the antibodies, as well as the cytokine standard, to be used in the assay. Although it requires some preliminary work to set up the procedure in each individual laboratory, this last option is usually much cheaper. It is preferable to use material from companies providing a cytokine standard that has been calibrated against the international standard. If setting up a home-made ELISA, the home-made standard cytokine preparation should be calibrated against international standards. Information on the available international standard for cytokine measurement, as well the standard themselves, can be obtained from the National Institute for Biological Standards and Controls (NIBSC, P.O. Box 1193, Potters Bar EN6 3QH, UK). Companies selling cytokine kits or antibody pairs to be used in immunoassays provide detailed protocols, and this is usually a good starting point.

2. We and others have found that at least for some TNF-α immunoassays (Endogen, Wolburn, MA; or a home-made assay based on the use of two monoclonal antibodies available from Bohreinger-Mannheim, Mannheim, Germany), the presence of EDTA in the assay buffer increases the recovery of exogenously added recombinant cytokines. Our assay buffer for TNF-α measurement is 20 mM Tris-HCl (pH 7.4), 1% BSA, 10 mM EDTA. However, this needs to be tested with the particular assay in use. Some TNF-α immunoassays are affected by the presence of soluble TNF receptor *(17)* A list of commercially available immunoassays that are not affected by both soluble TNF receptors is provided by Ledur et al. *(9)*.

3. An important issue in immunoassays especially in SF from patients with rheumatic diseases is the possible interference of anti-Ig antibodies (rheumatoid factor) present in SF *(16)*. SF from patients with autoimmune arthritides such as rheumatoid arthritis contain classical IgM rheumatoid factor but may also contain IgG or IgA rheumatoid factor. These Igs can mimick the presence of the antigen by bridging the two antibodies used in the assay, leading to an overestimation of cytokine levels. Classical IgM rheumatoid factor is more efficient than the so-called hidden IgA or IgG rheumatoid factor. Use of polyclonal antibodies, in particular from rabbit, is more prone to these false-positive results. Suppression of the positive interference by rheumatoid factor Igs can be obtained by adding to the assay buffer large amounts of unrelated Igs of the same species of the anti-bodies used in the assays. Usually 100 µg/mL of polyclonal IgG is sufficient. It has been reported that a low percentage of samples, especially those containing high levels of IgM rheumatoid factor, were not completely neutralized by this approach. Grassi et al. *(16)* suggested the use of dithiotreitol, a strong reducing agent, to induce depolymerization of the IgM pentamer.

4. Although there are no extensive studies with SF, it has been shown that significant cytokine (TNF-α, IL-1β, and IL-6) production may occur in peripheral blood in

as little as 2 h at RT, or even at 4°C *(12,13)*. This artifact appears to be due to endotoxin contamination of the collection systems. Different authors have reported significant endotoxin contamination of standard lithium heparin tubes *(14)*. Moreover, heparin has been shown to induce TNF-α production by purified monocytes *(15)*. Therefore, use of heparin should be avoided. It is generally accepted that addition of EDTA reduces or even eliminates cytokine production in vitro after sample collection *(13,14)*.

5. A chloroform extraction procedure has been developed for the processing of biologic fluids prior to IL-1β immunoassays, with the purpose of eliminating interfering factors and therefore increasing the amount of cytokine detected *(18)*. Although this procedure should be used for determination of IL-1β in EDTA/ plasma, we did not find any increase in IL-1β recovery in SF samples.

6. An unresolved issue in SF cytokine measurement by immunoassays is the appropriate diluent for standard curves. The ideal diluent would be SF itself. However, it is almost impossible to obtain normal SF; in physiologic conditions, the amount of SF present in an healthy joint is minimal; some authors have used SF obtained post mortem from healthy subjects, but this is rather complicated. Use of SF from inflamed joints is not advisable due to important variations in individual SF composition. If the sensitivity of the assay allows dilution of the SF sample (*see* below), the standard curve should be diluted in the assay buffer provided by the manufacturer.

7. As may be expected, SF itself interferes with the detection of cytokines due to a possible matrix effect. To minimize the quenching due to this matrix effect, SF samples should be diluted at least 1:5 in the assay buffer provided by the manufacturer. If the sensitivity of the assay is high, a higher dilution should be employed.

8. IL-6 is usually present in very high levels (ng/mL) in SF from inflamed joints. Samples can be diluted up to 1:100, thus practically eliminating the problem of a matrix effect. Interference by the soluble IL-6 receptor and soluble gp130 (the 2 subunits of the IL-6 receptor system that are both present in biologic fluid at ng/mL concentrations) does not appear to be a relevant problem in immunoassays for IL-6. Indeed, a recent study showed that the addition of both soluble receptor molecules did not interfere significantly with nine different immunoassays *(7)*.

9. Particular care should be taken when pipetting streptavidin to avoid contamination of the walls of the well. Moreover, a thorough washing (five times) is necessary to ensure complete removal of unbound streptavidin. These are the most frequent cause of inconsistencies and bad replicates.

References

1. Feldmann, M., Brennan, F. M., and Maini, R. N. (1996) Role of cytokines in rheumatoid arthritis. *Annu. Rev. Immunol.* **14,** 397–440.
2. Feldmann, M., Brennan, F. M., and Maini, R. N. (1998) Cytokines in autoimmune disorders. *Int. Rev. Immunol.* **17,** 217–228.
3. Lotz, M. (1997) Cytokines and their receptors, in *Arthritis and Allied Conditions* (Koopman, W. J., ed.), Williams & Wilkins, Baltimore, MD, pp. 439–478.

4. Dayer, J. M. and Arend, W. P. (1998) Cytokines and growth factors, in *Textbook of Rheumatology* (Kelley, W. N., Harris, E. D., Ruddy, S., and Sledge, C. B., eds.), WB Saunders Company, Philadelphia, PA, pp. 267–286.

5. Kotake, S., Sato, K., and Kim, K. J. (1996) Interleukin-6 and soluble interleukin-6 receptors in the synovial fluids from rheumatoid arthritis patients are responsible for osteoclast-like cell formation. *J. Bone Miner. Res.* **11,** 88–95.

6. Aarden, L. A., De Groof, E. R., Schaap, O. L., and Landsorp, P. M. (1987) Production of hybridoma growth factor by human monocytes. *Eur. J. Immunol.* **17,** 1411–1416.

7. Krakauer, T. (1998) Variability in the sensitivity of nine enzyme-liked immunosorbant assays (ELISAs) in the measurement of human interleukin-6. *J. Immunol. Methods* **219,** 161–167.

8. De Kossodo, S., Houba, V., Grau, G. E., and WHO Collaborative Study Group (1995) Assaying tumor necrosis factor concentrations in human serum. A WHO International Collaborative Study. *J. Immunol. Methods* **182,** 107–114.

9. Ledur, A., Fitting, C., David, B., Hamberger, C., and Cavaillon, J. M. (1995) Variable estimates of cytokine levels produced by commercial ELISA kits: results using international cytokine standards. *J. Immunol. Methods* **186,** 171–179.

10. Mire-Sluis, A. R., Gaines Das, R., and Thorpe, R. (1997) Implications for the assay and biological activity of interleukin-8: results of a WHO International Collaborative Study. *J. Immunol. Methods* **200,** 1–16.

11. Roux-Lombard, P., Steiner, G., and the Cytokine Consensus Study Group of the European Workshop for Rheumatology Research (1992) Preliminary report on cytokine determination in human synovial fluids: a consensus study of the European Workshop for Rheumatology Research. *Clin. Exp. Rheumatol.* **10,** 515–520.

12. Riches, P. and Gooding, R. (1990) In vitro production of cytokines in serum. *Lancet* **336,** 688.

13. Leroux, G., Philippe, J., Offner, F., and Vermeulen, A. (1990) In vitro production of cytokines in blood. *Lancet* **336,** 1197.

14. Riches, P., Gooding, R., Millar, B. C., and Rowbottom, A. W. (1992) Influence of collection and separation of blood samples on plasma IL-1, IL-6 and TNF-alpha concentrations. *J. Immunol. Methods.* **153,** 125–131.

15. Elborn, J. S., Delamere, F. M., and Shale, D. J. (1990) Tumor necrosis factor in normal plasma. *Lancet* **336,** 1015.

16. Grassi, J., Roberge, C. J., Frobert, Y., Pradelles, P., and Poubelle, P. E. (1991) Determination of IL1a, IL-1b and IL2 in biological media using specific enzyme immunometric assays. *Immunol. Rev.* **119,** 125–145.

17. Corti, A., Poiesi, C., Merli, S., and Cassani, G. (1994) Tumor necrosis factor (TNF) alpha quantification by ELISA and bioassay: effects of TNF alpha-soluble receptor (p55) complex dissociation during assay incubation. *J. Immunol. Methods* **177,** 191–198.

18. Cannon, J. G., Van der Meer, J. V. M., Kwiatkoski, D., et al. (1988) Interleukin-1β in human plasma: optimization of blood collection, plasma extraction, and radio-immunoassay methods. *Lymphok. Res.* **7,** 457–466.

29

Measurement of Cytokines in Cerebrospinal Fluid

Toshiyuki Yokoyama

1. Introduction

Cytokines, low-molecular-weight glycoproteins with diverse bioactivities, are produced from local tissues and leukocytes in response to various stimuli and are involved in both physiologic and pathologic events. Cerebrospinal fluid is an informative material used to evaluate cytokine activities associated with a variety of conditions in the central nervous system. Although each cytokine has been well characterized physiochemically, cerebrospinal fluid contains many bioactive substances including cytokines. In addition, it is well known that cytokines show pleiotropy and redundancy. For these reasons, biologic assay of each cytokine in crude fluid is thought to be complex, laborious, time consuming, and inaccurate.

Recently, an immunoassay has been established using specific antibodies against each cytokine. Since radioimmunoassay (RIA) requires the use of radio-labeled compounds and precipitation procedures, enzyme immunoassay (EIA) has been widely used instead. In this chapter, a determination process of human macrophage colony-stimulating factor (M-CSF) concentration in the cerebrospinal fluid is described using the enzyme-linked immunosorbent assay (ELISA) *(1)*. In a previous study *(2)*, this method was used with cerebrospinal fluid samples to evaluate the inflammatory process of aseptic meningitis.

The antibody (horse) specific for human M-CSF is coated onto the microtitrate plate. Standards with known amounts of M-CSF and samples are pipetted into the wells, and any M-CSF is bound by the immobilized antibody. After washing, the second antibody (rabbit) specific for M-CSF is added to the wells and allowed to bind the M-CSF that is bound during the first incubation. After a wash, an enzyme-linked IgG against rabbit IgG (goat) is added to the wells and allowed to bind the second antibody. Following a wash to remove any unbound antibody-reagent, a substrate is added to the wells, and color develops in proportion to the amount of M-CSF bound in the initial step. Intensity of the color is measured. By

From: *Methods in Molecular Medicine, vol. 60: Interleukin Protocols*
Edited by: L. A. J. O'Neill and A. Bowie © Humana Press Inc., Totowa, NJ

comparing the optical density of the samples with the standard curve, the level of M-CSF in the unknown sample is determined.

The preparation and procedure of the ELISA system are described, and then the validity of use of this ELISA for cerebrospinal fluid samples is mentioned as well as general and specific procedural notes.

2. Materials
2.1. Cerebrospinal Fluid

Cerebrospinal fluid should be collected in a plastic tube and immediately centrifuged at 1500g for 20 min in a refrigerated centrifuge to minimize further biologic reaction. The supernatant obtained should be stored at 2–8°C, up to 24 h, or frozen at or below –20°C for longer periods. Repeated freeze-thaw cycles should be avoided.

2.2. Human M-CSF ELISA System

1. A 96-well microtitration plate (Costar 3950) precoated with horse antibody against human M-CSF.
2. Rabbit antibody against human M-CSF: the second antibody.
3. Horseradish peroxidase (HRP)-conjugated goat IgG against rabbit IgG (Bio-Rad): the third antibody.
4. Human M-CSF standard: Available as Leukoprol, four million units (Welfide Corporation, Osaka, Japan), purified from human urine. One unit (U) is defined as the amount of M-CSF necessary to form one colony in the standard murine bone marrow assay *(3)*.

    Calibration: To convert values obtained with the human M-CSF ELISA system to equivalent National Institute for Biological Standards and Control (NIBSC). International Units (IU), use the equation below:

    NIBSC equivalent value (IU) = 0.15 × human M-CSF ELISA system value (U)

5. Sample diluent: 0.25% bovine serum albumin (BSA) in phosphate-buffered saline (PBS).
6. Antibody diluent: 0.25% BSA, 10% immobilized normal horse serum (GIBCO BRL) in PBS.
7. Reaction solution: 0.8 mg/mL *o*-phenylenediaminedihydrochloride (OPD), 0.015% H_2O_2 in 0.1 mol/L citrate buffer.
8. Washing solution: 0.05% Tween-20 in PBS.
9. Acidic stopping solution: H_2SO_4 (2 mol/L).
    Sample diluent, antibody diluent, and washing solution may be stored for up to 1 mo at 2–8°C.

2.3. Preparation of the M-CSF ELISA System (for Reference)

Antibody against human M-CSF (horse and rabbit) is prepared as follows:

1. Immunize a horse and rabbits with a subcutaneous injection of 100 µg (approx 1.5 × 10^7 U) and 10 µg (approx 1.5 × 10^6 U) of human M-CSF emulsified in an equal volume of Freund's complete adjuvant, respectively *(1)*.
2. Administer four further immunizations at 2-wk intervals and collect blood 5 d after the last immunization.

3. Collect crude immunoglobulin fractions against the human M-CSF raised in the sera of the horse or rabbits, using conventional ion-exchange column chromatographic techniques following precipitation by ammonium sulfate at 33% saturation (*4*).
4. Pass the immunoglobulin fractions through a column of human serum-coupled Sepharose 4B to exclude the nonspecific binding materials.
5. Dialyze the immunoglobulin fractions against PBS containing 0.02% sodium azide (NaN_3) to generate the immunoglobulin fractions against human M-CSF, which are frozen at –80°C and stored until use.

2.4. Neutralizing Activity of Antibodies

The neutralizing activity of antibodies is determined using the colony formation assay (*1,5,6*). Serially diluted antibody (0.05 mL) is mixed with the same volume of M-CSF (1000 U) and incubated for 1 h at room temperature in a culture dish. The number of neutralizing units (NU) is calculated from the dilution fold of antibodies, which results in the formation of half the number of colonies obtained in the control experiment, in which normal serum or immunoglobulin solution is added instead of the antibody. In the previous experiment (*1*), the antisera of horse and rabbits contained 5×10^6 NU/mL and 2.7×10^6 NU/mL, respectively, and the immunoglobulin fractions contained 5.8×10^5 NU/A280 (absorbance at 280 nm) and 2.5×10^5 NU/A280, respectively.

2.5. Microtitration Wells

1. Dilute anti-M-CSF immunoglobulin fraction (horse) with PBS containing 0.02% NaN_3 to A280 nm of 0.1 (approx 5.8×10^4 NU/mL in the previous experiment [*1*]) to generate a coating solution for the flat-bottomed, 96-well microtiter plate.
2. Add 0.1 mL of the coating solution per well.
3. Seal the plate and incubate for 24 h at 4°C.
4. Wash each well three times using a fill/empty cycle system; each wash is done with 0.3 mL of washing solution using a microplate washer (Sera Washer MW-96F; Biotec).
5. Put the plate upside down on a piece of tissue paper and rap the bottom of the plate to dry the wells.
6. Fill each well with 0.3 mL of blocking solution (10% immobilized normal horse serum, 0.25% BSA, 0.02% NaN_3 in PBS) to inhibit the nonspecific binding of other proteins.
7. Seal the plate filled with the blocking solution and store at 4°C until use.

3. Methods
3.1. Reagent Preparation

1. Reconstitute human M-CSF, four million units with 500 mL of sample diluent. This reconstitution produces a M-CSF standard of 8000 U/mL. Allow the standard to stand for a minimum of 15 min with gentle agitation before producing a dilution series.
2. Pipet 500 µL of sample diluent into each tube.
3. Pipet 500 µL of the undiluted M-CSF standard (8000 U/mL) into the 4000-U/mL tube and mix thoroughly.

4. Transfer 500 μL from the 4000-U/mL tube to the 2000-U/mL tube and mix thoroughly.
5. Repeat this process successively to complete the twofold dilution series.
6. The undiluted standard serves as the high standard (8000 U/mL).
7. Use the sample diluent as the zero standard (0 U/mL).

3.2. Assay Procedure

See **Note 1** for general points and **Notes 2–6** for important controls.

1. Wash the precoated microtiter plate filled with the blocking solution three times using the fill/empty cycle system to remove the blocking solution.
2. Add 0.1 mL of M-CSF standard or sample per well and incubate overnight at 4°C.
3. After washing and drying, add 0.1 mL of another anti-human M-CSF antibody (rabbit) per well and incubate overnight at 25°C.
4. After washing and drying, add 0.1 mL of HRP-conjugated goat IgG against rabbit IgG (Bio-Rad) per well and allow to stand for 3 h at 25°C.
5. After five washings by the fill/empty cycle system, add 0.1 mL of the substrate solution per well, and shake the plate gently on a microplate mixer for 30 min at room temperature in the dark.
6. Stop the reaction by adding 0.1 mL of 2 N H_2SO_4 per well.
7. The degree of enzymatic turnover of the substrate should be determined within 30 min by reading the color on the automatic microtiter plate reader (Microplate reader 3550; Bio-Rad), using dual-beam wavelenghs of 492 and 690 nm against a blank well in which the sample diluent is added instead of samples.
8. The concentration of human M-CSF in each sample is calculated from the corresponding standard curve.

3.3. Calculation of Results

1. Average the duplicate readings. Subtract the zero standard optical density from the standard or sample optical density.
2. Plot the optical density for the standards vs the concentration of the standards and draw the best curve. A standard curve should be generated and selected for each set of samples to be assayed.

4. Notes

1. General procedure:
   a. Samples and all reagents are allowed to reach room temperature before performing the assay.
   b. Samples and reagents should be thoroughly mixed before use.
   c. Excessive foaming of reagents should be avoided.
   d. Handling the tops of the wells should be avoided both before and after filling.
   e. Standards and samples should be assayed in duplicate.
   f. A separate standard curve should be run for each microtitration plate.
   g. The total dispensing time for each plate should not exceed 30 min.
   h. M-CSF exists in saliva. Precautionary measures to prevent contamination of the reagents should be taken during the assay.
   i. Stopping solution should be added to the plate in the same order as the substrate solution.

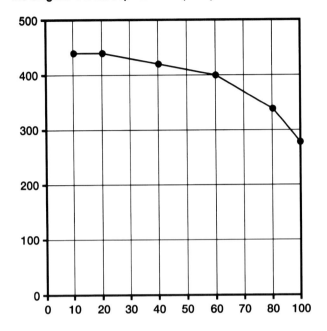

Calculated M-CSF Level in
the Original Cerebrospinal Fluid (U/ml)

Percent of Cerebrospinal Fluid Used in ELISA

Fig. 1. Effect of concentrations of cerebrospinal fluid used in ELISA on calculated M-CSF level in the original cerebrospinal fluid (U/mL). Various concentrations of cerebrospinal fluid were used to determine the original M-CSF level. Values were the means of the duplicated assays. Calculated M-CSF levels were almost constant when the ELISA was carried out using cerebrospinal fluid diluted more than 2.5-fold.

     j. To ensure accurate results, proper adhesion of plate sealers during incubation steps is necessary.
2. Assessing the effect of cerebrospinal fluid on the ELISA:
    a. Because factors in crude biologic fluids nonspecifically interfere with immunoassays, it is necessary to assess the influences of cerebrospinal fluid on the ELISA system. The validity of use of this ELISA for cerebrospinal fluid samples has been mentioned.
    b. Four stored cerebrospinal fluid samples, which were derived from patients suspected of having meningitis (finally diagnosed as gastroenteritis or sinusitis paranasalis) were used. These samples were thus considered to be normal cerebrospinal fluid. M-CSF levels in the four samples (A, B, C, and D) were determined using the ELISA, resulting in 451, 291, 472, and 174 U/mL, respectively. The samples had been arbitrarily diluted 11-fold with the sample diluent in advance (1). Values were means of duplicate assays.
3. Sample C was serially diluted so that rates of the original sample C used in ELISA would be 10, 20, 40, 60, and 80%. The measured concentration was converted into the original sample C value and plotted. As shown in **Fig. 1**, the calculated

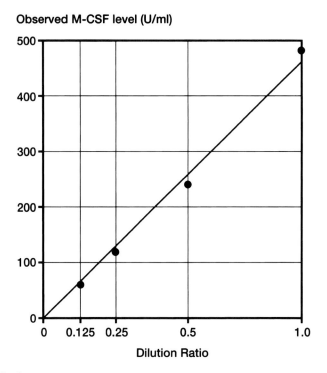

Fig. 2. Dilution test (1). Sample C was serially (×1, ×2, ×4, and ×8) diluted. The measured values made a straight line passing the origin.

M-CSF level in the original sample gradually decreased as the cerebrospinal fluid concentration was increased from 40 to 100%. However, the level was almost constant when the assay was carried out using the samples that had been diluted more than 2.5-fold. This indicates that human cerebrospinal fluid should be diluted more than 2.5-fold for determination of M-CSF level to avoid interference from contaminating proteins.

4. Dilution test (1): Sample C was serially diluted. Before measuring M-CSF levels, each sample was further diluted 11-fold. **Figure 2** shows that the measured values made a straight line passing the origin.

5. Dilution test (2): To make the dilution test for cerebrospinal fluid containing higher levels of M-CSF, each 1 vol of four different M-CSF standards was added to 9 vol of sample A. The final concentrations were 2519, 1546, 887, and 596 U/mL. Each solution was then serially diluted. Before measuring M-CSF levels, each sample was further diluted 11-fold. **Figure 3** shows that the measured values also made a straight line passing the origin for each of the four solutions.

6. Recovery test: The recovery of exogenous human M-CSF in cerebrospinal fluid was studied. One volume of four M-CSF standards with concentrations of 25,077, 12,919, 6113, and 3137 U/mL, was added to 9 vol of each sample (A, B, C, and D). The final

Observed M-CSF level (U/ml)

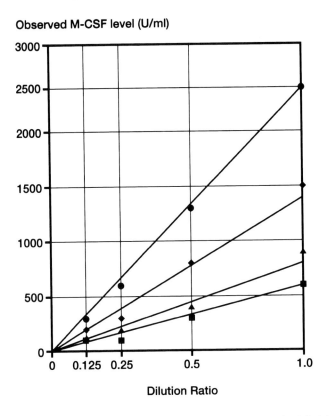

Dilution Ratio

Fig. 3. Dilution test (2). To make the dilution test for cerebrospinal fluid containing higher levels of M-CSF, each 1 vol of four different M-CSF standard solutions was added to 9 vol of sample A. Each solution was then serially (×1, ×2, ×4, and ×8) diluted. Before measuring M-CSF levels, each sample was further diluted 11-fold. This figure shows that the measured values also made a straight line passing the origin for each of the four solutions.

M-CSF concentrations added were theoretically 2508, 1292, 611, and 314 U/mL, respectively. On the other hand, final M-CSF concentrations in the original samples A, B, C, and D were 406, 262, 425, and 157 U/mL, respectively. Before measuring M-CSF levels, each sample was further diluted 11-fold. The M-CSF level was then measured using ELISA. Observed concentrations were converted into original sample values. The recovery rate of the added M-CSF was calculated according to the following formula.

$$\text{recovery rate } (\%) = \frac{\begin{array}{c}\text{observed value} \\ \text{with added M-CSF}\end{array} - \begin{array}{c}\text{calculated value} \\ \text{without added M-CSF}\end{array}}{\text{added M-CSF value}} \times 100$$

The average recovery rates of the added exogenous M-CSF doses (2508, 1292, 611, and 314 U/mL) from the four sample sections were 93.2%, 93.5%, 102.7%, and 89.9%, respectively. Recovery rates were thus good for both lower and higher doses of added exogenous M-CSF.

Acknowledgments

The author is grateful for the excellent technical assistance of Maki Yoshida, Principal researcher, Drug Discovery Laboratories, Welfide Corporation Industries, Ltd. Part of this chapter was taken from **ref. *1*,** with the kind permission of the principal author, Takuji Hanamura, PhD, and the publisher, W. B. Saunders Company.

References

1. Hanamura, T., Motoyoshi, K., Yoshida, K., Saito, M., Miura, Y., Kawashima, T., et al. (1988) Quantification and identification of human monocytic colony-stimulating factor in human serum by enzyme -linked immunosorbent assay. *Blood* **72,** 886–892.
2. Yokoyama, T., Oda, M., Ogura, S., Horiuchi, T., and Seino, Y. (1996) Relationship of interleukin 8 and colony-stimulating factors to neutrophil migration in aseptic meningitis. *Acta Pediatr.* **85,** 303–307.
3. Motoyoshi, K., Suda, T., Kusumoto, K., Takaku, F., and Miura, Y. (1982) Granulocyte-macrophage colony-stimulating and binding activities of purified human urinary colony-stimulating factor to murine and human bone marrow cells. *Blood* **60,** 1378–1386.
4. Onoue, K., Yagi, Y., and Pressman, D. (1964) Multiplicity of antibody proteins in rabbit anti-p-azobenzenearsonate sera. *J. Immunol.* **92,** 173–184.
5. Stanley, E. R. (1985) The macrophage colony-stimulating factor, CSF-1. *Methods Enzymol.* **115,** 565–587.
6. Stanley, E. R., McNeil, T. A., and Chan, S. H. (1970) Antibody production to the factor in human urine stimulating colony formation in vitro by bone marrow cells. *Br. J. Haematol.* **18,** 585–590.

30

Detection of Cytokines in Tears

Archana Thakur and Mark D. P. Willcox

1. Introduction

The tear film provides a refractive optical surface of the eye and nutrients to the underlying epithelial cells; it also contains factors that protect the eye from invasion by foreign particles including microorganisms. The tear film can alter rapidly from a basal state that occurs during the daytime, to the extremes of a rapidly increased lacrimation that occurs during crying (either as the result of physical trauma or emotional trauma) or a cessation of tear flow that occurs during eye closure. During these changes the protein and lipid components of the tear film have been shown to alter dramatically. Antibacterial proteins such as lysozyme and lactoferrin are designated as regulated protein, i.e., their concentration as a function of tear volume does not alter during increased lacrimation (*1*). On the other hand, secretory IgA, the predominant immuno-globulin in tears, is a constitutively secreted protein, i.e., its concentration alters during changes in lacrimation (*1*).

During sleep, lacrimation is switched off, and the tear film changes in a quite dramatic manner so that it can still effectively protect the eye from entrapped microorganisms or other foreign particles. Although concentrations of lysozyme and lactoferrin do not alter during sleep, their amounts relative to the overall total protein in tears actually decreases (*2,3*). On the other hand, the concentration of secretory IgA increases dramatically during sleep, accounting for up to 60% of the total protein in tears (*2*). Along with these changes in protein profiles, the tears are infiltrated with relatively large numbers of polymorphonuclear leukocytes (PMNs) (*3*).

We have recently been studying the contribution of cytokines to the recruitment of PMNs during sleep (*4*). Using tears collected immediately upon eye opening in the morning, we have demonstrated that concentrations of the

From: *Methods in Molecular Medicine, vol. 60: Interleukin Protocols*
Edited by: L. A. J. O'Neill and A. Bowie © Humana Press Inc., Totowa, NJ

cytokines interleukin (IL)-8, IL-6, and granulocyte macrophage colony-stimulating factor (GM-CSF) increase during sleep. These cytokines are also active in tears: our studies have demonstrated that IL-8 is the main protein responsible for recruitment of PMNs and that the GM-CSF in tears can activate PMNs to induce the surface expression of IgA-receptor *(4)*. In addition, we have shown that during asymptomatic wear of contact lenses the concentration of these cytokines, and as a consequence PMN number, can alter *(5)*. Furthermore, during acute inflammatory responses that occur during contact lens wear, the concentrations of IL-8 and GM-CSF increase *(6)*.

Several potential problems are associated with analysis of cytokines levels in tears. One of the limiting factors is the very small quantity of material that can be obtained from the eye. Typically the volume of tears that can be collected on one occasion during the day is approx 5–10 µL; this falls to approx 2 µL immediately on awakening. Tears are in much more abundant supply when subjects are crying; however, as mentioned above, these tears contain altered concentrations of proteins, and crying has the effect of diluting the small amounts of cytokines that may be present in tears. In addition to the amount of tears that can be collected, there are problems with the amounts of cytokines in tears. Therefore, several strategies need to be used.

2. Materials

2.1. Recombinant Cytokines and Antibodies

Purified recombinant cytokines and antibodies against cytokines can be obtained from various commercial sources. Secondary antibodies can be labeled with either biotin or enzymes (peroxidase or phosphatase). Alternatively, hybridomas that secrete appropriate antibodies can be obtained from the American Tissue Culture Collection (ATCC).

2.2. ELISA

1. Phosphate-buffered saline PBS, pH 7.4: 0.14 M NaCl, 2.7 mM KCl, 1.15 mM KH_2PO_4, 8.1 mM Na_2HPO_4; store at 4°C.
2. PBS with 1% (w/v) bovine serum albumin (BSA).
3. Coating buffer: 0.1 M NaHCO$_3$, pH 9.6; store at 4°C.
4. Substrate buffer (*see* **Note 1**): 150 mg 2,2'-azino-*bis* (3-ethylbenzthiazoline-6-sulfonic acid) to 500 mL of 0.1 M citric acid (citrate buffer) in dH$_2$O, pH to 4.35 with NaOH pellets (make fresh as required). For each plate, 10 µL 30% H_2O_2 is added to 11 mL substrate buffer just prior to use. Aliquots of 11 mL substrate buffer can be stored at –20°C.
5. PBS/FCS: PBS with 10% (v/v) fetal calf serum (FCS).
6. PBS/Tween: PBS containing 0.05% (v/v) Tween.
7. 1% (w/v) Sodium dodecyl sulfate (SDS).

2.3. Immunoblotting

1. 15% SDS-polyacrylamide gel (1-mm-thick minigel requires approx 6 mL solution): 3 mL 30% stock acrylamide solution, 1.10 mL 1.5 M Tris-HCl, pH 8.8, 0.03 mL 20% (w/v) SDS, 1.5 mL 60% (w/v) sucrose, 0.318 mL dH$_2$O, 2 µL TEMED, 40 µL 10% (w/v) ammonium persulphate.
2. 3% Stacking gel (requires approx 2 mL solution): 0.3 mL 30% stock acrylamide solution, 0.375 mL 1 M Tris-HCl, pH 6.8, 0.015 mL 20% (w/v) SDS, 0.15 mL 60% (w/v) sucrose, 2.138 mL dH$_2$O, 2 µL TEMED, 20 µL of 10% (w/v) ammonium persulphate.
3. TBS: 20 mM Tris-HCl, pH 7.4, supplemented with 50 mM NaCl.
4. TBS-T: TBS with 0.05% (v/v) Tween-20.
5. TBS-T containing either 1 or 3% BSA. Store at 4°C for up to 6 wk.
6. DAB substrate: Dissolve 10 mg 3,3' diaminobenzidine (DAB) in 15 mL TBS (make fresh as required), and add 12 µL H$_2$O$_2$ just prior to use.
7. Peroxidase-conjugated extra avidin.

2.4. Bioassays

1. HBSS/MOPS/BSA: Hanks' balanced salt solution (HBSS) supplemented with 10 mM 3-[-N-morpholino] propanesulfonic acid (HBSS/MOPS) and 1% (w/v) BSA (make fresh).
2. Methanol 70% (v/v): 700 mL methanol added to 300 mL distilled water. Store at room temperature.
3. Glutaraldehyde 2.5% (v/v): 2.5 mL glutaraldehyde in 97.5 mL PBS (make fresh as required).
4. Trypan blue.
5. Monopoly resolving media (ICN Biomedicals, Aurora, OH).
6. Salines: 0.2% NaCl and 1.6% NaCl.
7. C5a: 100 µg/mL stock (Sigma, St. Louis, MO).
8. Heparinized vacuettes.
9. Hemocytometer.
10. A 96-well Microchemotaxis chamber (Neuro Probe, Cabin John, MD) and 5-µm pore size polycarbonate filters.
11. Diff-Quick stain.
12. Control irrelevant antibody, e.g., rabbit anti-human IgG control antibody.
13. IgM anti-IgA Fc receptor (CD89) monoclonal antibody.
14. Fluorescein isothiocyanate (FITC)-labeled anti-mouse IgM.
15. Anti-IL-8 and anti-GM-CSF antibody (*see* **Subheading 2.1.**).
16. Flow cytomoter and tubes.

3. Methods
3.1. Tear Collection

Conventional methods of tear collection include Schirmer paper strips, cellulose sponges, and glass microcapillaries. Schirmer paper strips and cellulose sponges are limited by unavoidable stimulation of reflex tearing.

Glass microcapillaries are most commonly used, providing efficacious protein recovery, minimal ocular irritation, and little or no reflex tearing. As described in the Introduction, there are basically three tear types; basal open eye, closed eye, and reflex tears. Typically 2–3 µL/min basal tear volume is collected.

1. *Basal open eye tears:* Collect tear samples (without reflex tear stimulation) from the temporal tear meniscus at the lower lid margin (*see* **Note 2**), using calibrated disposable glass microcapillaries of 20 µL capacity.
2. *Closed eye tears:* Collect immediately upon eye opening after overnight sleep, avoiding blinking and reflex tear stimulation during collection. Such samples rich in closed eye *in situ* fluid are referred to as closed eye tears.
3. *Reflex tears:* Collect after stimulating the sneeze reflex with a cotton wool swab.
4. Store tears immediately at –80°C until used.

3.2. Immunoassays for Cytokines

Two main types of immunoassays are used to quantitate cytokines in tears; radioimmunoassay (RIA) and enzyme-linked immunosorbent assay (ELISA). Both immunoassays require availability of specific antibodies. Generally, ELISA is the method of choice for detecting cytokines in tears.

As tears are available in small volumes, multiple antigen detection in a single sample is recommended for ELISA. The multiple antigen detection method was developed by Wakefield and coworkers *(7)*.

3.2.1. Multiple Antigen Detection

1. Dilute tear samples 1:25 in PBS containing 1% (w/v) BSA.
2. Place 110 µL of the diluted tears on an antigen capture ELISA plate, where specific antigen from the sample will be captured while other cytokines/chemokines will remain in the solution.
3. After appropriate incubation, retrieve samples (105 µL) from the ELISA plate wells and place on the next antigen capture ELISA plate.
4. Use a mixture of known amounts of antigens as a control to determine the successive nonspecific loss of antigen during transfer.
5. Approximately 5 µL of sample volume will be lost during transfer.

3.2.2. Tear Cytokine ELISA Protocol

Various pathophysiologic conditions of the eye are associated with increased levels of cytokines/chemokines. One of the noninvasive ways to detect cytokines on the ocular surface is by investigating tears.

1. Dilute purified anticytokine capture antibody (*see* **Notes 3** and **4**) to 2–10 µg/mL in coating buffer. Coat the wells with 50 µL diluted antibody per well.
2. Seal the plate and incubate overnight at 4°C or at least 2 h at 37°C.
3. Wash plate three times with PBS/Tween. For each wash, wells are filled with 400 µL PBS/Tween and allowed to stand for 2 min prior to aspiration. Pound plate on paper towel as a final step.

4. Add 200 µL PBS/FCS per well.
5. Incubate at room temperature for 3 h on plate shaker.
6. Discard blocking buffer and wash three times with PBS/Tween.
7. Add standards and samples diluted (*see* **Note 5**) in PBS/FCS; 100 µL/well in duplicate or triplicate.
8. Incubate at room temperature for 3 h.
9. Wash plate four times with PBS/Tween.
10. Dilute biotinylated anticytokine detecting antibody to 1–5 µg/mL in PBS/FCS. Add 100 µL to each well.
11. Incubate at room temperature for 1 h.
12. Wash six times with PBS/Tween as in **step 3**.
13. Dilute avidin-peroxidase to manufacturer's recommendation in PBS/FCS.
14. Add 100 µL/well. Incubate for 30 min at room temperature.
15. Add 100 µL substrate buffer to each well. Develop for 10–60 min at room temperature. Color development is usually carried out in the dark for most substrates to avoid nonspecific coloration occurring and thus achieve low-background optical densities.
16. Stop reaction by adding 100 µL of 1% SDS. Read plate at OD 405 nm.

3.2.3. Immunoblot Analysis of CE Tears for Cytokines

Immunoblotting can be employed to validate (*see* **Note 6**) the presence of cytokines determined by immunoassay. Validation is based on approximate molecular mass.

1. Prepare 15% SDS-polyacrylamide with 3% stacking gel.
2. Load 10 µL of closed eye tears, open eye tears, or purified human recombinant cytokine (25, 20, 15, 10, or 5 ng/20 µL) onto the gel.
3. Transblot separated proteins in methanol-based buffer onto a nitrocellulose membrane.
4. Block membrane in TBS-T with 3% (w/v) BSA.
5. Incubate for 2 h at ambient temperature.
6. Wash three times with TBS-T for 5 min each time.
7. Incubate with biotinylated anticytokine antibodies at a final concentration of 5 µg/mL in TBS-T containing 1% w/v BSA for 1 h at ambient temperature.
8. Wash three times in TBS-T and incubate with a 1:1000 dilution of peroxidase-conjugated extra avidin for an additional 1 h at ambient temperature.
9. Wash as before and develop by using DAB substrate.

3.3. Bioassays for Tear Cytokines/Chemokines

Cytokine/chemokine bioassays are based on their various biologic effects such as specific cell recruitment, cell proliferation, cytotoxicity, or induction of expression of other cytokine/noncytokine molecules or their receptors. Bioassays can use freshly isolated cells, primary cultures, or continuous, cytokine-dependent cell lines. Bioassays may be as sensitive as an immunoassay, but there are certain limitations (*see* **Note 7**) associated with bioassays. They may be affected by synergistic or antagonistic factors present in samples.

3.3.1. Neutrophil Chemotaxis Bioassay for the Detection of Tear IL-8

Our recent study *(6)* suggests that the presence of high levels of IL-8 in open eye tears of patients experiencing contact lens-related inflammatory responses is associated with stromal infiltration. On the other hand, a study on closed eye tears *(4)* showed that a key role played by this chemokine (IL-8) is as a homeostasis mediator responsible for leukocyte adhesion and emigration into the mucosal surfaces of the eye. The most widely used bioassay for IL-8 activity is assessed by its ability to chemoattract PMNs specifically.

1. Collect peripheral blood into 10-U/mL heparinized vacuettes.
2. Layer blood over monopoly resolving media at a 6:7 ratio of monopoly resolving media and blood by volume.
3. Centrifuge this mixture at 400*g* for 45 min.
4. Collect the upper layer containing peripheral blood mononuclear cells (PBMCs) and the second layer containing the PMNs separately in fresh tubes.
5. Lyse residual red blood cells (RBCs) by adding 0.2% NaCl for 45–60 s, and restore tonicity by adding an equal volume of 1.6 % NaCl.
6. Centrifuge at 350–400*g* for 10 min and resuspend in 2 mL HBSS/MOPS/BSA.
7. Stain with Trypan blue stain to count in a hemocytometer (5 µL of resuspended cells + 45 µL of trypan blue; mix well and take 10 µL of this mixture to count) under ×100 magnification.
8. Assess viability by Trypan blue exclusion.
9. Use only if viability and purity is >95%.
10. Adjust concentration to 2×10^6 cells/mL by adding HBSS/MOPS/BSA.
11. Place 35 µL chemoattractants (tears at 1:35 dilution in HBSS/MOPS/BSA or the positive control C5a at 1 n*M* concentration) and medium (HBSS/MOPS/BSA) alone as a blank in lower wells (*see* **Note 8**) of 96-well microchemotaxis chamber.
12. Cover lower wells with a 5-µm pore size polycarbonate filter.
13. Add 200 µL of cell suspension to the upper wells.
14. Incubate chemotaxis chamber at 37°C for 60 min in a humidified incubator with 5% CO_2.
15. After the incubation period, remove the membrane and wash with PBS.
16. Remove nonadherent cells from the upper side of the membrane by drawing the membrane across a wiper blade three times and rinsing in PBS.
17. Fix membrane in 70% methanol; allow to air-dry.
18. Stain with Diff-Quick.
19. Quantitate neutrophil chemotaxis microscopically by counting the number of cells on the bottom side of the filter in a high power (×400) field.
20. Count at least three fields per duplicate filter and present data as mean number of cells per high power field.

3.3.2. Neutralization of Chemotactic Activity

Tears, closed eye and adverse response (tears collected from inflammatory eye disease or infection eye disease), contain various chemoattractants. Normal healthy closed eye tears only contain neutrophil chemoattractants, i.e., leukotriene B_4 (LTB_4), platelet-activating factor (PAF), IL-8, etc., whereas adverse response tears may also contain mononuclear cell chemoattractants. As mentioned earlier, bioassays are rarely specific (*see* **Note 8**); hence, neutralization with monospecific antibody is crucial for confirming the presence of cytokines in samples.

1. Add anti-IL-8 (final concentration 1 ng/μL) and control irrelevant (rabbit anti-human IgG) antibody to 50 μL of diluted (1:35) tears (closed eye and adverse response).
2. Incubate overnight at 4°C, with an additional 15 min at 37°C after the overnight incubation.
3. Centrifuge samples at 2100g and examine supernatants for their chemotactic activity as described above.

3.3.3. Bioassay for GM-CSFs in Tears Using Flow Cytometry

Classically GM-CSF is assayed by its ability to stimulate the formation of colonies of differentiated cells. In vitro studies have shown that GM-CSF-primed PMNs have a prolonged survival, as well as enhanced synthesis and release of both LTB_4 and PAF *(8,9)*. The presence of GM-CSF during eye closure could be linked with its other physiologic property of regulating host defense functions by activating receptors for IgA on PMNs, thus permitting IgA-mediated phagocytosis. IgA is found in abundance in closed eye tears *(2,3)* and is likely to play an important role in host defense. In vitro examination of the functional role of GM-CSF demonstrated that PMNs treated with closed eye tears showed a 7% increase in IgA receptor expression compared with untreated PMNs. This indicates that GM-CSF present in closed eye tears is functional and may promote IgA-mediated phagocytosis in the closed eye environment. We further tested whether this upregulation in IgA receptors was due to GM-CSF present in tears by adding neutralizing Ab to GM-CSF. These results indicated a significant inhibition of IgA receptor expression on PMNs by anti-GM-CSF antibodies.

1. Separate peripheral blood PMNs from whole blood (*see* **Subheading 3.3.1.**).
2. Suspend in HBSS/ MOPS/BSA to a concentration of 1×10^5 cells/mL.
3. Incubate with tears or GM-CSF (20 and 50 pM as positive control) for 20–40 min at 4 °C.
4. Add monoclonal antibody (IgM) specific for IgA Fc receptor on human PMNs (CD89).
5. Incubated at ambient temperature for 45 min.
6. Wash cells with HBSS/MOPS/BSA, and then incubated with fluorescein isothiocyanate (FITC)-labeled anti-mouse IgM (isotype IgG2a) for 45 min at ambient temperature.
7. After washing once in HBSS/MOPS/BSA, fix PMNs in 2% paraformaldehyde (*see* **Note 9**) in tubes appropriate for the flow cytometer.

8. Acquire sample data on the flow cytometer as soon as possible after staining.
9. Use gating to collect data from positive PMNs (*see* **Note 10**) and to exclude any nonspecific background by using isotypematched FITC-labeled secondary antibody.
10. Collect data from at least 10,000 events from all samples.

3.3.4. Inhibition of IgA Receptor Expression on PMNs

1. Add saturating concentrations of anti-GM-CSF and control irrelevant (rabbit anti-human IgG) antibody with 5 µL closed eye or adverse response tears.
2. Incubate overnight at 4°C with an additional 15 min at 37°C after the overnight incubation.
3. Centrifuge samples at 2100*g*.
4. Examine supernatants for induction of IgA Fc receptors on PMNs.

4. Notes

1. Substrates for ELISA: Various choices of substrates are available for peroxidase- or alkaline phosphatase-labeled antibodies. Substrates for peroxidase enzymes are *o*-dianisidine, 5-aminosalicylic acid, 2,2'-azino-bis (3-ethylbenzthiazoline-6-sulfonic acid), and 3,3',5,5'-tetramethylbenzidine. For alkaline phosphatase-labeled antibodies, *p*-nitrophenyl phosphate can be used.
2. Extreme care should be taken to minimize touching of the lid margins or the corneal surface. Flow rate during tear collection should be monitored by comparing volume of tears collected vs time.
3. The sensitivity of ELISA may be greatly influenced by performance of washing steps and reagent dilutions (immobilized antigen/antibody concentration); therefore checkerboard analysis must be employed to determine the optimal concentration of coating antibody. If antigen concentration is slightly less than the saturating antibody concentration, the standard will provide a sigmoidal curve with a maximum OD plateau at the high antigen concentrations.
4. In general, polyclonal antibodies are better for detecting antibodies than monoclonals.
5. The diluent for immunoassays should be identical for the cytokine standard and for samples. "Recognition" of cytokine is often influenced by overall concentrations of other molecules, e.g., proteins, mucopolysaccharides, etc. A mixture of known amounts of antigens diluted in tears (the reflex type is probably the most appropriate), in which all cytokines are below detectable limits, will determine whether tears interfere with cytokine detection.
6. Tear fluid may contain substances other than cytokines that can "bridge" the first and second anticytokine IgGs and generate false-positives or that may contain cytokine inhibitors, which can lead to false negatives. Therefore, either immunoblotting or bioassay should be performed to verify the immunoassay results.
7. In bioassays, specificity is always uncertain. Specificity for a particular cytokine can be established by using a monospecific neutralizing antibody. Immunoassays can in all cases be used as an alternative to bioassays, although they can additionally detect denatured biologically inactive cytokine molecules and fragments.

8. In chemotaxis assay, the checkerboard analysis should be performed to rule out whether the migratory response of PMNs was largely due to chemotaxis and not to chemokinesis, by confirming that there was significant directed migration when the lower and upper well chemokine concentration was varied.

9. It is important to note that freshly isolated leukocytes may wait for analysis in wash buffer at 4°C, without fixation, for up to 18 h post-staining, without loss of viability. Activated leukocytes may lose viability rapidly, and data should be collected within 5 h post-staining. To preserve cell integrity beyond these time limits, paraformaldehyde fixation may be necessary; however, it is possible that the quality of staining may be diminished by such fixation.

10. Every experiment must include controls. Negative controls are samples of the same cell population treated exactly like the test sample without stimulation.

References

1. Fullard, R. J. and Snyder, C. (1990) Protein levels in non-stimulated and stimulated tears of normal subjects. *Invest. Ophthalmol. Vis. Sci.* **31,** 1119–1126.
2. Sack, R. A., Tan, K. O., and and Tan, A. (1992) Diurnal tear cycle: evidence for a nocturnal inflammatory constitutive tear fluid. *Invest. Ophthalmol. Vis. Sci.* **33,** 626–640.
3. Tan, K. O., Sack, R. A., Holden, B. A., and Swarbrick, H. A. (1993) Temporal sequence of changes in tear film composition during sleep. *Curr. Eye Res.* **12,** 1001–1007.
4. Thakur, A., Willcox, M. D. P., and Stapleton, F. (1998) The proinflammatory cytokines and arachidonic acid metabolites in human overnight tears: homeostatic mechanisms. *J. Clin. Immunol.* **18,** 61–70.
5. Thakur, A. and Willcox, M. (2000) Contact lens wear alters the production of certain inflammatory mediators in tears. *Exp. Eye Res.* **70,** 1–5.
6. Thakur, A. and Willcox, M. (1998) Cytokine and lipid inflammatory mediator profile of human tear during contact lens associated inflammatory diseases. *Exp. Eye Res.* **67,** 9–19.
7. Wakefield, D., McCluskey, P., Roche, N., and Rosio, J. L. (1995) Aqueous humor cytokine profile in patients with chronic uveitis. *Ocular Immunol. Inflamm.* **3,** 203–208.
8. Di Persio, J. F., Billing, P., Williams, R., and Gasson, J. C. (1988) Human granulocyte-macrophage colony stimulating factor and other cytokines prime human neutrophils for enhanced arachidonic acid release and LTB_4 synthesis. *J. Immunol.* **140,** 4315–4322.
9. Wirthmueller, U. A., De Weck, L., and Dahinden, C. A. (1989) PAF production in human neutrophils by sequential stimulation with GM-CSF and the chemotactic factors C5a or fMLP. *J. Immunol.* **142,** 3213–3218.

V

NEWER TECHNIQUES:
INTERLEUKIN SIGNAL TRANSDUCTION, RECOMBINANT INTERLEUKIN PRODUCTION, INTERLEUKIN GENE POLYMORPHISMS, AND THE USE OF cDNA ARRAYS

31

Measurement of Phosphoinositide 3-Kinase Activation by Interleukins

Stephen G. Ward

1. Introduction

Phosphoinositide 3-kinases (PI 3-kinases) are an evolutionarily conserved family of lipid kinases that have attracted much attention over the past 10 years or so (reviewed in ref. *1*). Three PI 3-kinase classes have been defined on the basis of primary structure, regulation, and their in vitro lipid substrate specificity. Class I PI 3-kinases interact with Ras and form heterodimeric complexes with adaptor proteins that link them to different upstream signaling events (*1*). They are able to convert phosphatidylinositol (PtdIns), PtdIns(4)P, and PtdIns(4,5)P_2 into PtdIns(3)P, PtdIns(3,4)P_2, and PtdIns(3,4,5)P_3, respectively, by phosphorylating the D-3 position of the inositol head groups of phosphoinositide lipids (collectively known as D-3 phosphoinositide lipids and shown in **Fig. 1**) (*1,2*).

Class I PI 3-kinases are further classified into the prototypical I_A subclass, which is a heterodimer consisting of the 85 kDa regulatory subunit (responsible for protein-protein interactions mediated via its SH2 domains, SH3 domain, and/or proline rich regions) and a catalytic 110-kDa subunit. The class I_B PI 3-kinases are stimulated by G protein $\beta\gamma$-subunits and do not interact with the SH2-containing adaptors that bind class IA PI 3-kinases. Instead, the only identified member of this family, p110γ, associates with a unique p101 adaptor molecule (*1*). Several lines of evidence suggest that PtdIns(4,5)P_2 is the favored substrate for class 1 PI 3-kinases in intact cells (*1,2*). The class II PI 3-kinases are characterized by the presence of a C-2 domain at the carboxy terminus and predominantly utilize PtdIns and PtdIns(4)P as substrates (e.g., PI3K-C2α), whereas the class III PI 3-kinases utilize only PtdIns as a substrate (e.g., mammalian PtdIns 3-kinase and yeast Vps34p) (*1*). Another D-3 phosphorylated PI lipid is PtdIns(3,5)P_2, which is formed by the consecutive phosphorylation of PtdIns by a PI 3-kinase (presumably a class III enzyme) and of PtdIns(3)P by a PtdIns(3)P 5-kinase (**Fig. 1**) (*3*).

From: *Methods in Molecular Medicine, vol. 60: Interleukin Protocols*
Edited by: L. A. J. O'Neill and A. Bowie © Humana Press Inc., Totowa, NJ

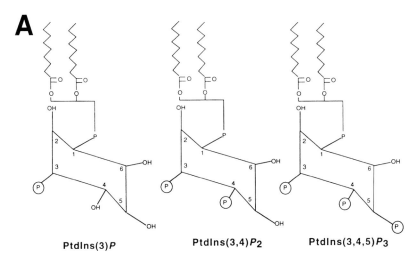

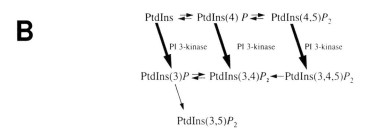

Fig. 1. **(A)** Schematic representation of the structure of D-3 phosphoinositide lipids. **(B)** Routes for synthesis of PtdIns(3)P, PtdIns(3,5)P_2, PtdIns(3,4)P_2, and PtdIns(3,4,5)P_3.

PtdIns is the precursor of all phosphoinositides and constitutes less than 10% of the total lipid in eukaryotic cell membranes **(Fig. 1)**. PtdIns(4)P constitutes approx 5% of cellular phosphoinositide lipids, whereas PtdIns(4,5)P_2 constitutes another 5%. Less than 0.25% of the total inositol-containing lipids are phosphorylated at the D-3 position, consistent with the idea that these lipids exert regulatory functions inside the cell, as opposed to a structural function *(3)*. PtdIns(3)P is constitutively present in eukaryotic cells, and its levels are largely unaltered upon cellular stimulation. In contrast, PtdIns(3,4)P_2 and PtdIns(3,4,5)P_3 are generally absent from resting cells, but their intracellular concentration rises markedly in response to stimulation by a number of interleukins (e.g., IL-2, IL-3, IL-4, IL-10, and IL-13), suggesting a likely function as a second messenger *(1,2)*. Numerous studies using genetics, PI 3-kinase inhibitors, and PI 3-kinase overexpression have implicated PI 3-kinases in the regulation of cell proliferation, survival, metabolism, cytoskeletal reorganization, and membrane trafficking. In addition, the generation and in vitro use of accurate 3-phosphoinositide analogs has led to identification of 3-phosphoinositide binding domains in a diverse range of target molecules *(3,4)*. For instance, the FYVE finger domain binds PtdIns(3)P and is found in proteins involved in different vesicle trafficking events. Moreover, a number of proteins have been identified that directly bind PtdIns(3,4)P_2 and/or PtdIns(3,4,5)P_3 via PH domains. These include protein kinase B (PKB), 3-phosphoinositide-dependent protein kinase (PDK-1), phospholipase Cγ, Bruton's tyrosine kinase (Btk), and exchange factors for the ADP-ribosylation factor (ARF) family of small GTP-binding proteins *(3,4)*.

PI 3-kinase activity can be measured either directly in vitro or *in situ* using techniques that detect the transfer of radiolabeled phosphate from ATP to the D-3 position of the inositol head group of phosphoinositide lipids. Alternatively, PI 3-kinase activity can be measured indirectly by detecting the activity of downstream PI 3-kinase-dependent effector targets (e.g., PKB activity) The latter may involve the use of phospho-specific antibodies that detect the phosphorylated active forms of the effector targets or in vitro assays using appropriate substrates to detect enzyme activity. However, indirect measurements of PI 3-kinase activity are not always appropriate since other upstream signaling pathways may contribute to the regulation of effector activity. Hence, this chapter will deal only with the methods that directly measure lipid kinase activity in vitro or *in situ*. In the first procedure, it is possible to assay specific immunoprecipitated proteins from broken cell lysates (e.g., PI 3-kinase subunits, receptors, receptor component chains, or even cellular proteins) for associated lipid kinase activity under in vitro assay conditions using distinct substrates such as PtdIns *(5–7)*. This assay detects the transfer of the radiolabeled γ-phosphate of ATP to the D-3 position of PtdIns, resulting in the formation of [^{32}P]-labeled PtdIns(3)P. It is also possible to use PtdIns(4)P or PtdIns(4,5)P_2 as in vitro substrates for the prototypical class IA PI 3-kinase (resulting in the formation of [^{32}P]-labeled PtdIns(3,4)P_2 or PtdIns(3,4,5)P_3, respectively), but generally these substrates are much more expensive to buy. The advantages of this procedure are as follows:

1. It can distinguish between various PI 3-kinase subtypes by varying substrate and adding inhibitors to assay buffer that differentially affect lipid kinase activity.
2. It constitutes only a moderate radiochemical hazard since the technique requires use of µCi amounts [^{32}P]-γ-ATP, which are substantially less than those used in the second procedure.
3. It is relatively cheap, quick, and easy to perform.
4. No specialized apparatus is required.

The disadvantages are as follows:

1. Regulatory properties and precise substrate specificities of the PI 3-kinase(s) may be critically distorted by the assay conditions and the nature of lipid presentation used.

2. It may detect other lipid kinases such as PI 4-kinases that coassociate with immunoprecipitated proteins or other lipid kinases that nonspecifically associate with protein A-Sepharose beads.
3. Requires separation of extracted lipids by thin-layer chromatography (TLC), which poorly resolves specific D-3 phosphoinositides such as PtdIns(3)*P* from the other single phosphate-containing inositol lipid PtdIns(4)*P*.
4. Accurate quantitation requires a phosphoimager, which may not be readily available. Alternatively, the relevant regions of the silica gel may be scraped from the TLC plate into scintillation liquid followed by β-scintillation counting, but this is tedious and potentially hazardous and can lead to loss of material; thus, it can be inaccurate.

In situ measurement of PI 3-kinase activity relies on metabolic labeling of intact cellular pools of ATP with [^{32}P]Pi followed by lipid extraction *(8,9)* and separation of the [^{32}P]-labeled glycerophosphoryl derivatives of D-3 phosphoinositide lipids by high-performance liquid chromatography (HPLC) analysis *(10)*. The advantages of this procedure are as follows:

1. It allows highly quantitative detection of all phosphoinositide lipids with good resolution. Thus, one sample can provide a large amount of information concerning the effects of receptor-induced effects on all the inositol-containing phospholipids.
2. It allows sensitive detection of picomole amounts of D-3 phosphoinositides.

However, there are also several disadvantages, as follows:

1. It requires the use of mCi amounts of [^{32}P]Pi, which means extra precautions must be taken with handling and storage of samples because of the radiochemical hazard.
2. Analysis of the deacylated lipid extracts requires the use of an elaborate and specialized HPLC apparatus to resolve the glycerol derivatives (GroPIns(3)*P*, GroPIns(3,5)*P*$_2$, GroPIns(3,4)*P*$_2$, and GroPIns(3,4,5)*P*$_3$ from [^{32}P]-labeled contaminants.
3. It does not necessarily distinguish between the lipid kinase activity of various different isoforms and subtypes of the PI 3-kinase family.
4. It is time consuming and expensive, and generates a great deal of liquid radioactive waste.

2. Materials
2.1. In Vitro Measurement Of PI 3-Kinase Activity

Solutions 1–5 can be prepared from analytical grade reagents dissolved in autoclaved deionized water. The solutions are stored at 4°C and are stable for up to 3 mo.

1. Lysis buffer: 1% (v/v) Nonidet P-40, 100 m*M* NaCl, 10 m*M* iodoacetamide, 10 m*M* NaF, 20 m*M* Tris-HCl, pH 7.4. Prior to use, the buffer is supplemented with the protease inhibitors phenyl methyl sulfonyl fluoride (PMSF) (1 m*M*), leupeptin (1 µg/mL), pepstatin (1 µg/mL), and antipain (1 µg/mL).

2. Phosphate-buffered saline (PBS), pH 7.4: Dissolve 80 g NaCl, 2.0 g KCl, 11.5 g Na_2HPO_4, and 2.0 g KH_2PO_4 in 900 mL distilled water. Adjust pH to 7.4 with 1 M NaOH if necessary. Make volume up to 1 L with distilled water. Dilute 1 in 10 with distilled water for use.

3. Washing buffer: 0.5 M LiCl, 100 mM Tris-HCl, pH 7.4.

4. Lipid kinase assay buffer: 5 mM $MgCl$, 0.25 EDTA, 20 mM HEPES (pH 7.4).

5. 1 mCi (37 MBq) $[\gamma\text{-}^{32}P]$-ATP (3000 Ci/mmol).

6. 1 N HCl.

7. Chloroform/methanol (1:1 v/v) and methanol/1 N HCl (1:1 v/v).

8. Protein A- and protein G-Sepharose.

9. PtdIns and phosphatidylinositol (PtdSer) in solid form, which will be used for preparation of lipid kinase substrate mixture; PtdIns(4)P and PtdIns(4,5)P_2 (1 mg/mL in chloroform stored for up to 6 mo at –20°C) can be used as standards for TLC separation of phospholipids.

10. 1.5-mL Screw-top Sarstedt tubes.

11. Probe sonicator.

12. Perspex radiation shields and waste containers.

13. Silica gel 60 TLC plates (19 × 19 cm) sprayed with 1% (w/v) potassium oxalate and air-dried.

14. TLC tank containing 1-propanol: 2 N acetic acid (65:35 v/v).

15. Whatman 3MM paper cut to size of TLC tank.

16. Iodine.

17. XAR 5 film (Kodak), exposure cassettes, X-ray film developer.

18. 100 µM ATP: make up fresh just before use.

2.2. In Situ *Measurement of D-3 Phosphoinositide Lipids*

Solutions and organic solvent mixtures 1–7 should be prepared from analytical grade reagents.

1. Sterile phosphate-free balanced salt solution supplemented with sodium bicarbonate and 20 mM HEPES, adjusted to pH 7.4 with 10 N sodium hydroxide. Store at 4°C for up to 1 mo.

2. Fetal calf serum (FCS) that has been dialyzed overnight against saline to remove any phosphate from the FCS. Should be sterile filtered and stored in aliquots at –20°C. Working aliquots can be stored at 4°C for 1 mo.

3. 100 mL Chloroform/methanol/H_2O (32.6:65.3:2.1 v/v/v). Make up fresh before use.

4. Chloroform containing 10 µg/mL Folch lipids. Make up fresh just before use.

5. 2.4 M HCl, 5 mM tetrabutylammonium sulphate. Make up fresh just before use.

6. 25% Methylamine in H_2O/methanol/N-butanol (4:4:1 v/v).

7. N-butanol/petroleum ether (bp 40–60°C)/ethyl formate (20:4:1 v/v).

8. 1.25 M $(NH_4)_2HPO_4$ adjusted to pH 3.8 with H_3PO_4. This buffer should be filtered through Whatman 2 µm cellulose nitrate filters before use. The solution is stored at room temperature and is stable for up to a month. It should, however, be degassed by refiltering and bubbling through with either He or N_2 for 30 min before use.

9. 10 mCi (370 MBq) [^{32}P]-Pi (8500–9120 Ci/mmol), 10 µCi (370 kBq) [^{3}H]-PtdIns (10–20 Ci/mmol), 5 µCi (370 kBq) [^{3}H]-PtdIns(4)P (1–5 Ci/mmol), and 5 µCi (370 kBq) [^{3}H]-PtdIns(4,5)P_2 (1–5 Ci/mmol).
10. Buffer B: 1.25 M (NH$_4$)$_2$HPO$_4$, adjusted to pH 3.8 with H$_3$PO$_4$ at 25°C.
11. 1.5-mL Screw-top Sarstedt tubes.
12. HPLC system equipped with Partisphere strong anion exchange (SAX) columns (Whatman) and connected to either an on-line β-radiodetector or a fraction collector. If a fraction collector is used, it will be necessary to quantitate fractions using a β-scintillation counter.

3. Methods
3.1. In Vitro Measurement of PI 3-Kinase Activity

1. Immunoprecipitates should be prepared using either protein A or G-Sepharose depending on IgG subclass of antibody employed (*see* **Note 1**).
2. Wash immunoprecipitates three times in lysis buffer (*see* **Note 2**), twice in PBS, twice in washing buffer, once in water, and once in lipid kinase assay buffer. Resuspend immunoprecipitates in 40 µL of lipid kinase buffer and place at room temperature (*see* **Note 2**).
3. Weigh out 1 mg of solid form PtdIns and 1 mg of solid form PtdSer and make a 1-mL mixture in 1 mM EDTA, 25 mM HEPES, pH 7.4. The mixture of lipids will form small aggregates, which should be dispersed by sonication (*see* **Note 3**).
4. Add 50 µL of the sonicated PtdIns/PtdSer mixture to the immunoprecipitates. Initiate reaction by adding a mixture of 10 µCi [γ-^{32}P]-ATP and 100 µM ATP in a volume of 10 µL.
5. Incubate at room temperature, agitating every minute or so. It is advisable to perform time-course experiments to investigate linearity of the reaction, but 15–20-min incubation periods are usually sufficient.
6. Stop the reaction by adding 100 µL 1 N HCl. To extract the lipids, add 200 µL of chloroform/methanol (1:1), vortex for 20 s, and centrifuge for 5 min to separate phases.
7. Recover and wash the lower chloroform phase by placing in a new tube containing 400 µL methanol/1 N HCl (1:1 v/v). Vortex and centrifuge to separate phases (1000g, 5 min).
8. Transfer the lower chloroform phase to a new tube and dry *in vacuo* (*see* **Note 4**).
9. Resuspend dried lipids in 50 µL chloroform and spot onto a dry TLC plate previously impregnated with 1% (w/v) potassium oxalate (*see* **Note 5**). Spot 5–10-µL drops at a time, and dry each drop using a low-power hair dryer. It is also advisable to spot on 10 µL of standard PtdIns(4)P and PtdIns(4,5)P_2 solutions as standards (*see* **Note 6**).
10. Place TLC plate into TLC tank containing 1-propanol: 2 N acetic acid (65:35 v/v) and Whatman 3MM paper that has been saturated with the running solvent (*see* **Notes 7** and **8**).
11. Once the solvent front has reached the top, remove the TLC plate, air-dry, and place in TLC tank containing iodine to stain the substrate PtdIns and standard PtdIns(4)P and PtdInd(4,5)P_2. Remove from iodine tank and expose to X-ray

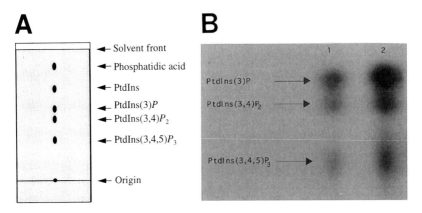

Fig. 2. **(A)** Schematic representation of a TLC separation of D-3 phosphoinositide lipids using 1-propanol/2 *N* acetic acid (65:35 v/v) as a running solvent. **(B)** A representative section of an autoradiograph of a TLC separation of D-3 phosphoinositide lipids derived from in vitro lipid kinase assay of p85 immunoprecipitates using PtdIns as a substrate. Immunoprecipitates are derived from either resting (*lane 1*) or IL-13-stimulated (*lane 2*) HT-29 cells.

film at $-70°C$ to identify phosphoinositide lipids (*see* **Note 9**). An example of a typical TLC separation of the D-3 phosphoinositide lipid products of an in vitro PI 3 kinase assay is shown in **Fig. 2**.

3.2. In Situ *Measurement of D-3 Phosphoinositide Lipids*

1. Cells must be depleted of phosphate prior to labeling with $[^{32}P]Pi$ by washing three times in 50 mL phosphate-free balanced salt solution. Between washes, cells are incubated at $37°C$ for 10 min. (*see* **Note 10**).
2. After phosphate depletion, cells are resuspended in balanced salt solution supplemented with 5% dialyzed FCS and 20 m*M* HEPES. After addition of $[^{32}P]Pi$, cells are incubated at $37°C$ for appropriate times (*see* **Note 11**).
3. After incubation at $37°C$, the cells are washed three times in 50 mL phosphate-free balanced salt solution to remove unincorporated $[^{32}P]Pi$. Cells are then resuspended at required cell concentration in balanced salt solution at approx 2×10^7 cell/mL.
4. Stimulate 120-µL aliquots at $37°C$ in 1.5-mL screw-top Sarstedt tubes.
5. Terminate incubations by addition of 500 µL chloroform/methanol/H_2O (32.6/65.3/ 2.1. v/v) to produce a homogenous primary extraction phase (*see* **Note 12**).
6. Separate phases by addition of (a) 200 µL chloroform containing 10 µg/mL Folsch lipids; and (b) 200 µL 2.4 *M* HCl, 5 m*M* tetrabutylammonium sulphate. Vortex and centrifuge (1000*g*, 5 min) to separate phases.
7. Remove lower phase (approx 800 µL) carefully into fresh 1.5-mL Sarstedt tube (*see* **Note 4**) already containing 400 µL 0.1 *M* HCl, 5 m*M* EDTA. Vortex and centrifuge (1000*g* 5 min) to separate phases.

8. Remove lower phase into clean Sarstedt tubes and dry *in vacuo* (*see* **Note 13**).
9. Once dried, the extracted lipids must be deacylated by the addition of 1 mL 25% (w/v) methylamine/methanol/*N*-butanol (4:4:1) followed by incubation in a 53°C water bath for 40 min. This procedure yields glycerophosphoryl derivatives of the inositol-containing lipids. Samples are then cooled rapidly on ice for 5 min and dried *in vacuo* (*see* **Note 13**).
10. Add 0.5 mL H_2O followed by 0.6 mL *N*-butanol/petroleum ether (bp 40–60°C)/ethyl formate (20:4:1 v/v) to the dried deacylated lipids. Vortex and centrifuge (1000*g*, 5 min). Carefully remove the upper organic phase and discard. Wash the lower water-soluble phase with a further 0.6 mL of *N*-butanol/petroleum ether (bp 40–60°C)/ethyl formate mix. Vortex, centrifuge, and discard upper phase as above. Dry lower phase *in vacuo*.
11. Redissolve pellet in 100 µL H_2O (*see* **Note 14**), and analyze deacylated [^{32}P]-labeled lipids by HPLC using a 12.5-cm Whatman Partisphere SAX column. Samples are eluted from the column using a gradient based on buffer A (water) and buffer B at a flow rate of 1 mL/min: 0 min, 0% B; 5 min, 0% B; 45 min, 12% B; 60 min, 30% B; 61 min, 100% B; 65 min, 100% B; 66 min, 0% B; 90 min, 0% A and B.
12. Eluates can be analyzed with an on-line radiodetector or collected in fractions (0.5 mL) and quantitated by β-scintillation counting (*see* **Note 15**). Eluted peaks are compared with retention times for standards prepared from commercial [^{3}H] phosphoinositides and [^{32}P]-labeled D-3-phosphoinositides prepared as described in **Subheading 3.1.** An example of a typical HPLC separation of the glycerophosphoryl inositol lipid products from a [^{32}P]Pi-labeled leukemic cell line is shown in **Fig. 3**.

4. Notes

1. Antibody can be directed against a specific PI 3-kinase subunit (e.g., p85 α/β, p110 α/β/δ, etc.), or subunits of the respective interleukin receptors under analysis and cellular proteins (e.g., *Src*-like tyrosine kinases), which may coassociate with PI 3-kinase(s). Alternatively, the assays may be performed on any peptide fragments (suitably immobilized on beads) that have been used to precipitate receptor chains or cellular proteins.
2. Many lipid kinases are sensitive to detergents *(11,12)*. Do not use sodium dodecyl sulfate (SDS) in lysis buffers since SDS kills lipid kinase activity. Moreover, Nonidet P-40 inhibits PI 3-kinase activity but potentiates PI 4-kinase activity. It is therefore crucial to remove all detergent from the immunoprecipitates by thoroughly washing them in 1-mL vol of the indicated solutions prior to assaying them for associated lipid kinase activity. Immunoprecipitates are generally washed by pelleting protein A/G beads by centrifugation (1000*g*, 3 min), aspirating 90% of the supernatant, and adding 1 mL of the next washing solution. During the last washing step, after aspirating 90% of the supernatant, the remaining 10% of the supernatant should be removed using a flat-ended Hamiltion syringe, with minimal disruption of the protein Sepharose A/G beads. It is critical to keep all washing buffers on ice and to perform all centrifugation steps at 4°C to minimize risk of protease and phosphatase activity, which may interfere with PI 3-kinase activity.

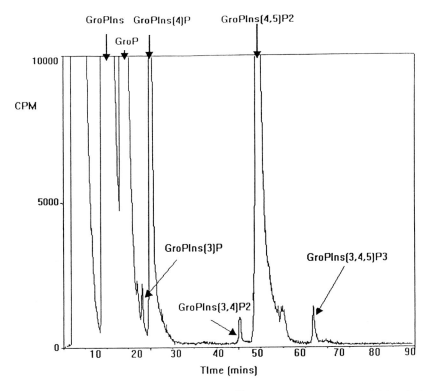

Fig. 3. HPLC elution profile of deacylated (^{32}P)-labeled phosphoinositides derived from IL-13-activated HT-29 cells.

3. Sonication should be performed on ice with a probe sonicator (usually during the immunoprecipitation step). Typically, three 10-s bursts interspersed by periods of 30 s is sufficient. However, the precise sonication time will depend on the power of the particular sonicator and whether it is in tune. The PtdIns appears cloudy at first and should eventually clear. Sonicating too long results in oxidized, precipitated lipid. Do not store the substrate mixture, but rather make up sufficient amounts of PtdIns/PtdSer mixture for the assay and discard any excess. The sonicated mixture of PtdIns and PtdSer may be further diluted as required, to obtain optimal substrate concentration.
4. Generally, the lower phase can be removed using a 200-μL gel loading tip immersed through both the upper and lower phases so that the tip rests on the bottom of the tube. The lower phase can then be carefully removed from the bottom upward, exerting care to avoid taking any upper phase. It is important to take care during the removal of the lower phase, as any loss of material or removal of different volumes between samples will lead to inaccuracies between samples.
5. TLC plates can be impregnated with 1% potassium oxalate by simple immersion or by spraying. Plates should be air-dried and can be stored for at least 2 mo until use.

6. The lipid samples should be loaded 3 cm from the bottom of the plate. Upon placing the TLC plate in the tank, the solvent front should be allowed to be at least 1–2 cm from the top of the TLC plate. This takes 5–6 h depending on the solvent mixture used, although plates can be left to run overnight without any detrimental effect.

7. Five to six hours prior to placing a loaded TLC plate into the tank, the running solvent mixture should be prepared and added to the TLC tank containing Whatman 3MM paper cut to the size of the tank. The volume of solvent depends on the size of the TLC tank, but usually the solvent volume should be sufficient to immerse the bottom 1–2 cm of the TLC tank once the 3MM is saturated. For best results, TLC running solvent should be made fresh for each assay, although if absolutely necessary, the solvent mixture can be left for 2–3 d in a TLC tank as long as a tight-fitting cover is placed on the top of the tank to prevent evaporation of solvent. Other solvent mixtures may be used such as chloroform/methanol/acetone/acetic acid/H_2O (40:13:15:12:8 v/v/v/v) or chloroform/methanol/10 M ammonium hydroxide (45:35:10 v/v/v). These different solvent mixtures allow good separation of PtdIns(3)P, PtdIns(3,4)P_2, and PtdIns(3,4,5)P_3. The R_f values for each lipid vary depending on the solvent mix used, so migration of lipids should always be compared with that of standard PtdIns, PtdIns(4)P, and PtdIns(4,5)P_2.

8. The 1-propanol/2 N acetic acid running solvent for TLC allows good separation of PtdIns(3)P, PtdIns(3,4)P_2, and PtdIns(3,4,5)P_3, although PtdIns(3)P and PtdIns(3,4)P_2 are not resolved too well from PtdIns(4)P or PtdIns(4,5)P_2, respectively. This may be a problem when immunoprecipitated proteins coassociate with other lipid kinases such as PtdIns 4-kinase. In such circumstances, it may be appropriate to use the following TLC separation system to separate PtdIns(3)P from PtdIns(4)P *(13)*. Silica gel 60 plates are immersed face up for 10 s with gentle stirring in CDTA solution. This solution is prepared by stirring a mixture of 0.9 g CDTA in 30 mL 0.33 M NaOH followed by the addition of 60 mL ethanol. After immersion in CDTA solution, the plates are air-dried and then activated for 10 min at 110°C. The TLC developing solution is prepared by stirring together methanol (35 mL), chloroform (32 mL), and pyridine (24 mL) in a bottle in a fume hood (to avoid exposure to harmful pyridine). Add 6.3 g boric acid and shake until dissolved. Add 4 mL water and 1.6 mL concentrated formic acid and tranfer solution to the TLC tank. Saturate tank using Whatman 3MM paper attached to the tank walls. Plate should be air-dried 2–3 h prior to autoradiography. It is important to note that iodine detection of the separated lipids is impossible due mainly to pyridine on the TLC plate. In this borate system, PtdIns migrates with an R_f of 0.82, whereas the R_f of PtdIns(3)P is 0.51 and the R_f of PtdIns(4)P is of 0.46 *(13)*.

9. The identity of phosphoinositide lipids can be verified in four ways: (a) comparison with known "cold" standards that are identified by iodine staining; (b) comparison with radiolabeled standards that are identified by autoradiography; (c) HPLC analysis of the radiolabeled phosphoinositide lipids after the lipids have been recovered from the plate by scraping and subsequently deacylated (*see* **Subheading 3.2.9.**); and (d) sensitivity of in vitro lipid kinase activity to PI 3-kinase inhibitors such as

wortmannin *(14)* and LY294002 *(15)* or reagents such as adenosine (inhibits PtdIns 4-kinase but does not affect PI 3-kinase) *(11)* and Nonidet P-40 (inhibits PI 3-kinase, but potentiates PtdIns 4-kinase activity) *(11,12)*. These inhibitors and reagents can be added to the lipid kinase assay mixture at approprate concentrations (*see* **Subheading 3.1.4.**). The entire procedure from performing cell stimulations to obtaining the first exposed autoradiograph should take 2 d.

10. Balanced salt solution is cell dependent, but for leukemic T-cell lines such as Jurkat cells, phosphate-free DMEM (Gibco) is appropriate.
11. Concentrations of cells and [^{32}P]Pi are cell dependent, but 2×10^8 and 1 mCi/mL is suitable for labeling of Jurkat cells. Incubation times for metabolic labeling are also cell dependent and may vary from 60 min to several hours.
12. Samples may be stored at –20°C at this stage.
13. Once the [^{32}P]-labeled lipids have been separated into chloroform, they should not be stored but rather dried *in vacuo* immediately followed by deacylation. Similarly, after deacylation, the cooled lipid extracts should be dried immediately *in vacuo*. This drying step can be performed overnight, and the deacylated samples can then be stored at –20°C if necessary prior to washing with *N*-butanol/petroleum ether (bp 40–60°C)/ethyl formate (20:4:1 v/v). Time for drying of samples after deacylation can vary from 4 to 10 h depending on type of SpeedVac employed.
14. Redissolved [^{32}P]-labeled phosphoinositide lipid solutions should be centrifuged (1000*g*, 2 min) and/or filtered (0.45-µ*M* filter) to remove any debris prior to HPLC separation on a Partisphere SAX column. The time-scale from radiolabeling of cells to a point at which the lipid extracts are ready for HPLC analysis should be 1.5–2 d.
15. One sample takes a minimum of 90 min to elute from the HPLC column. Time to obtain quantitation of radiolabeled lipids depends on whether an on-line β-radiodetector is used (in which case, analysis can be almost instantaneous) or whether 1-mL eluate fractions are collected. In respect to the latter, scintillation liquid must be added to all the fractions in scintillation vials followed by β-scintillation counting, which requires each sample to be counted for 5–10 min. The entire procedure from performing cell stimulations to obtaining the complete HPLC and radiodetection analysis of the [^{32}P]-labeled lipids can take 3–5 d depending on the number of samples and the method of radiodetection.

References

1. Vanhaesebroeck, B., Leevers, S., Panayatou, G., and Waterfield, M. D. (1997) Phosphoinositide 3-kinases: a conserved family of signal transducers. *Trends Biochem. Sci.* **22,** 267–271.
2. Fruman, D. A., Meyers, R. E., and Cantley, L. C. (1998) Phosphoinositide 3-kinases. *Annu. Rev. Biochem.* **67,** 481–507.
3. Rameh L. E. and Cantley L. C. (1999) The role of phosphoinositide 3-kinase lipid products in cell function. *J. Biol. Chem.* **274,** 8347–8350.
4. Leevers, S. Vanhaesebroeck, B., and Waterfield, M. D. (1999) Signalling through phosphoinositide 3-kinases: the lipids take centre stage. *Curr. Opin. Cell Biol.* **11,** 219–225.

5. Whitman, M., Downes, C. P., Keeler, M., Keller, T., and Cantley, L. (1988) Type 1 phosphatidylinositol kinase makes a novel inositol phospholipid, phosphatidylinositol 3-phosphate. *Nature* **33,** 644–646

6. Varticovski, L., Druker, B., Morrison, D., Cantley L., and Roberts, T. (1989) The colony stimulating factor-1 receptor associates with and activates phosphatidylinositol 3-kinase. *Nature* **342,** 699–701.

7. Morgan, S. J., Smith, A. D., and Parker, P. J. (1990) Purification and characterisation of bovine brain type I phosphatidylinositol kinase. *Eur. J. Biochem.* **191,** 761–767.

8. Jackson, T., Stephens L., and Hawkins P. T. (1992) Receptor specificity of growth factor-stimulated synthesis of 3-phosphorylated inositol lipids in Swiss 3T3 cells. *J. Biol. Chem.* **267,** 16,627–16,636.

9. Stephens, L., Jackson, T., and Hawkins P. T. (1993) Synthesis of phosphatidylinositol 3,4,5-trisphosphate in permeabilised neutrophils regulated by receptors and G proteins. *J. Biol. Chem.* **268,** 17,162–17,172.

10. Stephens, L., Hawkins P. T., and Downes C. P. (1989) Metabolic and structural evidence for the existence of a third species of polyphosphoinositide in cells: D-phosphatidyl-*myo*-inositol 3-phosphate. *Biochem. J.* **259,** 267–276.

11. Carpenter, C. L. and Cantley, L. C. (1990) Phosphoinositide 3-kinases. *Biochemistry* **29,** 11,147–11,156.

12. Ward, S. G., Reif, K., Ley, S., Fry, M. J., Waterfield, M. D., and Cantrell, D. A. (1992) Regulation of phosphoinositide kinases in T cells: evidence that phosphatidylinositol 3-kinase is not a substrate for T cell antigen receptor-regulated tyrosine kinases. *J. Biol. Chem.* **267,** 23,862–23,869.

13. Walsh, J. P., Caldwell, K. K., and Majerus, P. W. (1991) Formation of phosphatidylinositol 3-phosphate by isomerisation from phosphatidylinositol 4-phosphate. *Proc. Natl. Acad. Sci. USA* **88,** 9184–9187.

14. Ui, M., Okada, T., Hazeki, K., and Hazeki, D. (1995) Wortmannin is a unique probe for an intracellular signalling protein phosphoinostide 3-kinase. *Trends Biochem. Sci.* **20,** 303–307.

15. Vlahos, C. J., Matter, W. F., Hui, K. Y., and Brown R. F. (1995) A specific inhibitor of phosphatidylinositol 3-kinase 2-(4-morpholinyl)-8-phenyl-4H-1-benzopyran-4-one (LY294002). *J. Biol. Chem.* **269,** 5241–5248.

32

Analysis of Interleukin-2 Signaling Using Affinity Precipitations and Polyacrylamide Gel Electrophoresis

Paul Brennan and Verónica Athié-Morales

1. Introduction

Interleukin-2 (IL-2) was first discovered and characterized as T-cell growth factor *(1)*. It is responsible for the growth of T cells and thus plays an important role in the proper functioning of the immune system. IL-2 has a high affinity receptor consisting of an α-, β-, and γ-chain. The γ- chain is shared with a number of other cytokines such as IL-3 and IL-7, which also play a role in cell growth *(2)*. The IL-2 receptor β- chain also comprises part of the receptor for IL-15.

The initial IL-2 intracellular signaling event that can be measured is a change in protein tyrosine phosphorylation. One of the easiest ways to investigate this is by resolution of proteins by polyacrylamide gel electrophoresis (PAGE) and detection with anti-phosphotyrosine antibodies. In the case of IL-2 these phosphotyrosine events are caused by oligomerization of the IL-2 receptor, which brings together the Jak1 and Jak3 tyrosine kinases, associated with the β- and γ- chains respectively *(3–7)*. This is shown schematically in **Fig. 1**. The standard method for phosphotyrosine Western blotting is described here.

IL-2 signaling pathways following tyrosine phosphorylation include activation of the Ras-mitogen activated protein (MAP) kinase pathway *(8–10)*, activation of STAT transcription factors, particularly STAT3 and STAT5 *(11–14)*, and activation of the phosphatidylinositol 3-kinase (PI 3-kinase) pathway *(15,16)*; as shown in **Fig. 1**. The small G-protein Ras activates the serine-threonine kinase Raf, leading to the classical mitogen-activated kinase cascade. A method for assaying active Ras is described. STAT transcription factors are activated by tyrosine phosphorylation, which can be measured using the phosphotyrosine antibody in Western blotting. They are also phosphorylated on serine residues. An affinity precipitation method allowing analysis of STAT DNA binding is described.

From: *Methods in Molecular Medicine, vol. 60: Interleukin Protocols*
Edited by: L. A. J. O'Neill and A. Bowie © Humana Press Inc., Totowa, NJ

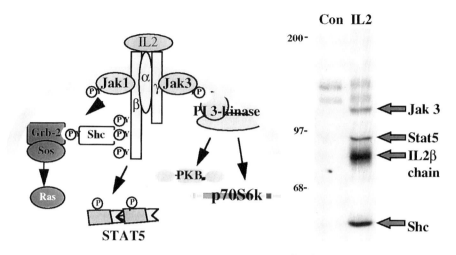

Fig. 1. Interleukin-2 signaling schematic and example phosphotyrosine Western blot performed as described in **Subheading 3.1.** Kit225 cells were stimulated for 1 h with 20 ng/mL IL-2. Con, control.

Finally, the activation of PI 3-kinase can be studied by analysis of the serine phosphorylation of some of its downstream pathways such as the serine-threonine kinase protein kinase B (PKB), also called Akt *(17,18)*. Another commonly measured PI 3-kinase effector is the serine kinase p70S6kinase *(19,20)*.

The techniques discussed and described have been used by the authors to study IL-2 signaling. Peripheral blood lymphocytes or T-cell lines were used. However, the techniques can be easily applied to other cell types and used to investigate kinetics of activation and protein localization. They can also be applied to other stimuli. Various examples of these and similar applications of the techniques can be found in the literature *(3,14,21–23)*.

As in the case of phosphotyrosine, various changes in phosphoserine can also be measured using specific antibodies in Western blotting. This approach has been utilized to analyze the activity of all three of the pathways discussed. One of the best characterized phosphospecific antibodies currently available is the phospho-MAP kinase antibody, which is useful for monitoring the MAP kinase signaling pathway. Another is the phosphospecific antibody for PKB/Akt, which can be used for monitoring activity of the PI 3-kinase pathway *(24)*. Various antisera are also available for measuring phosphorylation of STAT proteins *(23,25,26)*. **Table 1** shows the antibodies that have been used successfully by the authors. More antibodies are becoming commercially available every month, providing an excellent source of new reagents.

Affinity precipitation of active molecules from cell lysates and the subsequent analysis of these molecules by PAGE and Western blotting is a useful extension of the techniques described above. This method concentrates the active molecules and provides a sensitive way of determining the activity of the signaling pathway in question. One example is the affinity precipitation of active Ras *(27)*. When the G-protein Ras is activated by the exchange of GDP to GTP, it can interact with the serine/threonine kinase Raf *(28)*. Thus, the activation of Ras can be measured by affinity precipitation of active Ras from cell lysates with the Ras binding domain from the kinase Raf-1 fused to glutathione *S*-transferase *(27)*. Following precipitation with glutathione agarose beads, the proteins are eluted into reducing sample buffer and resolved by PAGE. Ras is detected using a specific antibody. Because this interaction with Raf-1 only occurs when Ras is active, only active Ras is found in the affinity precipitation. This method is described. It is important to remember that phosphorylation does not always correlate with activity so often it is necessary to measure activity by various methods.

STAT complexes capable of binding DNA and their phosphorylation status can be investigated by a method involving DNA affinity precipitation. The affinity matrix in this case is a double-stranded oligonucleotide corresponding to a high-affinity binding site for STATs. When this is incubated with cell lysates, STATs capable of binding DNA will be precipitated. These complexes are released from the beads, resolved by PAGE, and transferred onto membranes; the proteins are then detected by specific antibodies.

To summarize, methods are described to generate total cell lysates. These lysates can be resolved by PAGE and Western blotting using phosphospecific antibodies. Furthermore, they can be used in affinity precipitations to investigate the activity of various molecules in commonly activated signaling pathways. Data using interleukin-2 (IL-2) as an example are shown to illustrate the techniques.

2. Materials
2.1. Generation of Total Cell Lysates

1. 2X Total lysis buffer (store at 4°C): 100 mM HEPES, pH 7.4, 10 mM NaF, 10 mM iodoacetamide, 150 mM NaCl (*see* **Note 1**).
2. 10% Nonidet P-40 (store at room temperature for up to 6 mo).
3. 1000X Small peptide inhibitors (SPI): 1 mg/mL each of pepstatin, chymostatin, leupeptin, and antipain in DMSO; store at –20°C in aliquots.
4. 100X Phenyl methyl sulfonyl fluoride (PMSF): 100 mM in ethanol (store at 4°C).
5. 100X Na$_3$VO$_4$ (sodium orthovanadate): 100 mM in H$_2$O (store at –20°C) (*see* **Note 2**).
6. Acetone.
7. 3X Reducing sample buffer (RSB): 9% sodium dodecyl sulfate (SDS), 187.5 mM Tris-HCl, pH 6.8, 30% glycerol, 10% 2-mercaptoethanol.

2.2. PAGE

1. 30% (w/v) Acrylamide 0.8% bisacrylamide stock solution (available from National Diagnostics). **Warning:** *Acrylamide is a neurotoxin—always wear gloves.*
2. 1 M Tris-HCl, pH 8.8, and 1 M Tris-HCl, pH 6.8.
3. 20% (w/v) SDS.
4. H_2O.
5. Ammonium persulfate: Make fresh as 10% w/v solution.
6. N, N, N', N'-Tetra-methylethylenediamine (TEMED).
7. Gel apparatus (*see* **Note 3**).
8. Gel running buffer: 190 mM glycine, 25 mM Tris-HCl, 0.1% (w/v) SDS.
9. Molecular weight markers: Prestained molecular weight markers, available from GibcoBRL or Amersham, are recommended.

2.3. Western Blotting: A, Transfer

1. Transfer apparatus: We recommend wet transfer (*see* **Note 4**).
2. Polyvinylidene diflouride (PVDF) membranes (Immobilon P, Millipore).
3. Methanol.
4. Transfer buffer: 10 mM 3-(cyclohexylamino)-1-propanesulfonic acid (CAPS), pH 11.0.
5. Filter paper.

2.4. Western Blotting: B, Detection

1. Apparatus for agitation (for example, rocking platform).
2. Containers for incubation of blocking reagent, antibody, and washing.
3. 10X phosphate-buffered saline (PBS): 80 g NaCl, 2 g KCl, 11.5 g $Na_2HPO_4.7H_2O$, 2 g KH_2PO_4.
4. Blocking reagent: 3% (w/v) Bovine serum albumin in PBS.
5. Anti-phosphotyrosine antibodies: Recommended antibodies are 4G10 (Upstate Biotechnology) and PY20 (ICN Laboratories) (*see* **Note 5**).
6. PBS with 0.05% (v/v) Tween-20 (PBS-T).
7. Secondary antibody: Mouse Ig, horseradish peroxidase-linked whole antibody (from sheep) on Rabbit IG, horseradish peroxidase-linked whole antibody.
8. Parafilm.
9. Enhanced chemiluminiscent reagent (Amersham).
10. Film (X-Omat S from Kodak).
11. Cassettes with intensification screens for exposure of film.

2.5. Affinity Precipitation of Active Ras

1. Reagents for PAGE and Western blotting as mentioned above are also required for this technique.
2. 1X Lysis buffer: 50 mM HEPES, pH 7.4, 10 mM NaF, 10 mM iodoacetamide, 75 mM NaCl. Store at 4°C.
3. GST-RBD (Ras binding domain): Amino acids 1–149 of human c-Raf in pGex-KG; generates a 42-kDa fusion protein *(27)*. Fusion protein should be prepared from standard protocols and stored at –80°C.

4. Glutathione agarose beads (GAB) (*see* **Note 6**). Store at 4°C.
5. Anti-Ras (pan) mouse monoclonal antibody (Oncogene).
6. 10% Nonidet P-40 (*see* **Subheading 2.1.**).
7. PMSF, Na₃VO₄, and SPI (*see* **Subheading 2.1.**).
8. 1 *M* MgCl₂ (*see* **Note 7**).
9. Secondary antibody: Mouse Ig, horseradish peroxidase-linked whole antibody (from sheep).

2.6. DNA Affinity Precipitation of STATs

1. Reagents for PAGE and Western blotting as mentioned above are also required for this technique.
2. 2X oligonucleotide binding lysis buffer: 100 m*M* Tris-HCl, pH 7.9, 0.2 m*M* EDTA, 20 m*M* NaF, 20% glycerol. Store at 4°C.
3. Biotinylated double-stranded oligonucleotide: 0.1 mg/mL in TE (10 m*M* Tris-HCl, 1 m*M* EDTA, pH 8.0) with 75 m*M* NaCl. Store at 4°C (*see* **Note 8**).
4. Streptavidin-conjugated agarose beads: 50% slurry in PBS/0.05% sodium azide. Wash three times in PBS with 0.05% sodium azide and store at +4°C.
5. Anti-STAT antibodies (**Table 1**).
6. 2.5 *M* NaCl (*see* **Note 9**).
7. 10% Nonidet-P40 (described in **Subheading 2.1.**).
8. PMSF, Na₃VO₄, and SPI (described in **Subheading 2.1.**).
9. 100 m*M* Dithiothreitol (100X). Store at –20°C.

3. Methods
3.1. Analysis of Phosphotyrosine Changes

This method describes the steps involved in generating total lysates, SDS-PAGE, and Western blot analysis with phosphotyrosine antibodies. The SDS-PAGE and Western blotting is also used for all the other techniques.

1. Make buffer up fresh immediately before use. Use 1/2 vol 2X total lysis buffer and add NP-40 (to 1%, 1/10 dilution), SPI, PMSF, and Na₃VO₄. Make up extra volume with H₂O. Note that PMSF is only stable for about 30 min in aqueous solution (*see* **Note 1**).
2. Stimulate cells as desired (*see* **Note 10**).
3. Terminate stimulation by addition of cells to ice-cold PBS.
4. Spin at 190*g* for 5 min in refrigerated centrifuge.
5. Decant supernatant and resuspend cells in ice-cold total lysis buffer (500 µL for 5×10^6 cells).
6. Place sample on ice for 30 min.
7. Spin samples at 12,000*g* for 5 min and remove supernatant (lysate) into 0.7 vol of acetone for protein precipitation. Place samples at –20°C for 1 h (*see* **Note 11**).
8. Centrifuge sample at 12,000*g* for 5 min, remove supernatant, and resuspend protein pellet in 100 µL reducing sample buffer.
9. Run sample on relevant polyacrylamide gel (7.5% gel is recommended, but this depends on the size of the proteins to be analyzed): 7.5% gel recipe: 7.5 mL 30%

Table 1
Antibodies Used Successfully[a]

Antigen	Conc.	MW (kDa)	% Gel	Positive control	Time	Secondary antibody	Source
PhosphoERK 1/2 (pThr 183/pTyr 135)	100 ng/mL	42, 44	15	PdBu (50 ng/mL)	O/N, 4°C	anti-rabbit	Promega
Pan ERK2	125 ng/mL	42, 44	15		O/N, 4°C	anti-mouse	Transduction Laboratories
PhosphoPKB (pS 473)	1:1000	65	7.5	Vanadate	O/N, 4°C	anti-rabbit	New England Biolabs
Pan PKB	1 μg/mL	65	7.5		2 h, RT	anti-rabbit	Upstate Biotechnology
PhosphoSTAT5 (pY 694)	1:1000	92	7.5	IL-2	O/N, 4°C	anti-rabbit	New England Biolabs
Pan STAT5	1 μg/mL	92	7.5	IL-2	1 h, RT	anti-mouse	Transduction Laboratories
PhosphoSTAT3 (pS 721)	1 μg/mL	89	7.5	IFN-α	1 h, RT	anti-rabbit	Upstate Biotechnology
PhosphoSTAT3	1:1000	89	7.5	IFN-α	O/N, 4°C	anti-rabbit	New England Biolabs
Pan STAT3 (pY 705)	250 ng/mL	89	7.5	IFN-α	O/N, 4°C	anti-mouse	New England Biolabs
Pan STAT1	100 ng/mL	91	7.5	IFN-α	1 h, RT	anti-mouse	Transduction Laboratories

[a]Conc., concentration; O/N, overnight.

(v/v) acrylamide/bisacrylamide mix, 11.2 mL 1 *M* Tris-HCl, pH 8.8, 11.2 mL of H$_2$O, 150 μL 20% (w/v) SDS, 100 μL fresh 10% (w/v) ammonium persulfate, and 20 μL TEMED. For stacking gel: 3.3 mL 30% (v/v) acrylamide/bisacrylamide mix, 2.5 mL 1 *M* Tris-HCl, pH 6.8, 14 mL H$_2$O, 100 μL 20% SDS, 100 μL fresh 10% ammonium persulfate, and 20 μL TEMED. Pour gel immediately—10-cm gels are recommended.

10. Transfer gel onto PVDF membrane (for 4 h at 70 V using a wet transfer method).
11. Block membrane with 3% BSA for 1 h at room temperature.
12. Incubate membrane with 1 μg/mL of 4G10 and PY20 antibody for 1 h at room temperature.
13. Wash three times in PBS-T.
14. Incubate with 1:1000 dilution of mouse Ig, horseradish peroxidase-linked whole antibody (from sheep) for 1 h at room temperature.
15. Wash three times with PBS-T.
16. Develop using enhanced chemiluminesence (ECL) as recommended by Amersham.

3.2. Use of Phosphospecific Antibodies

This section uses the techniques of generating total lysates, PAGE, and Western blotting described in the previous section. It is best to test the phosphospecific antibodies on freshly prepared PVDF membranes. These can then be stripped of antibody and reanalyzed with different antibodies. A typical result is shown in **Fig. 2**.

1. Membranes as described in **Subheading 3.1.** can be used with a variety of phosphospecific antibodies to molecules involved in IL-2 signaling pathways. **Table 1** shows the relevant percentage gels and the antibody conditions.
2. Membranes should be sequentially checked with the phosphoantibody and with the "pan" antibody that reacts with phosphorylated and nonphosphorylated protein to ensure equal loading (*see* **Note 12** for stripping protocol).
3. Recommended conditions require the loading of approximately 1×10^7 T-cell equivalents per lane (*see* **Note 10**).
4. Run the relevant percentage gel (**Table 1**).
5. Transfer as recommended (*see* **Subheading 3.1.** and **Note 4**).
6. Block membrane with 3% BSA for 1 h at room temperature.
7. Incubate membrane with the antibodies recommended (*see* **Table 1**) either for 1 h at room temperature or overnight at 4°C.
8. Wash three times with PBS-T.
9. Add appropriate secondary antibody coupled with horseradish peroxidase (recommended concentrations 1:1000 mouse Ig, horseradish peroxidase-linked whole antibody [from sheep] or 1:5000 rabbit Ig, horseradish peroxidase-linked whole antibody [from donkey]), for 1 h at room temperature.
10. Wash three times with PBS-T.
11. Develop using ECL reagent from Amersham.

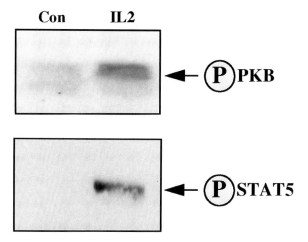

Fig. 2. PhosphoPKB and phosphoSTAT5 Western blot. Human peripheral blood lymphocytes were stimulated with 20 ng/mL IL-2, and total lysates were generated and resolved on a 7.5% gel. Western blotting and antibody detection were performed as described in **Subheading 3.2.** Con, control.

3.3. Affinity Precipitation of Active Ras

This elegant method describes the affinity precipitation steps involved in measuring active Ras, first described by Taylor and Shalloway *(27)*, in response to cytokines such as IL-2. Once the affinity step is completed and the samples have been resuspended in reducing sample buffer, PAGE and Western blot are essentially identical to that described in **Subheading 3.1.** and are not discussed further. A typical result is shown in **Fig. 3**.

1. Make up fresh lysis buffer (LB) at 4.0 mL per sample. Add Nonidet P-40 to 1%, MgCl to 10 mM (final concentration), and inhibitors as recommended above.
2. Wash quiescent cells once.
3. Count the cells and resuspend to desired cell concentration in 1 mL RPMI-1640. We commonly use $1.5–2 \times 10^7$ cells/sample.
4. Place 1-mL samples at 37°C for 10 min.
5. Activate at 37°C according to each assay. A good positive control for the activation of Ras is phorbol 12,13 di-butyrate (PdBu) (50 mg/mL).
6. Stop activation by placing samples on ice. Keep samples on ice or work in cold room from this step.
7. Spin for 1 min at 12,000g, 4°C.
8. Remove supernatant and lyse by adding 1 mL freshly made ice-cold 1 × LB (1 mL per maximum up to 2×10^7 cells).
9. Vortex to resuspend the pellet. *Do not allow the tube to warm up.*
10. Lyse for 20 min (*see* **Note 13**), at 4°C, mix rotating.

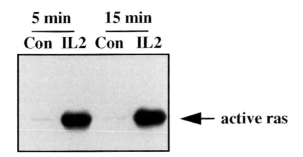

Fig. 3. Precipitation of active Ras from IL-2-stimulated peripheral blood lymphocytes as described in **Subheading 3.3.** Con, control.

11. Spin for 5 min at 12,000*g*, 4°C, to eliminate cell debris.
12. Transfer all the supernatant that corresponds to total lysate, approx 1 mL, to a fresh tube containing glutathione-agarose beads (GAB).
13. Preclear with 10 µL GAB (50% in PBS, 2 m*M* EDTA).
14. Incubate for 15 min, at 4°C, mix rotating.
15. Spin for 5 min at 6000*g*, 4°C. Transfer supernatant to a fresh tube and add 10 µL GST-RBD previously coupled to GAB (*see* **Note 13**).
16. Perform binding for 2 h, 4°C, mix rotating.
17. Spin for 5 min at 6000*g*, 4°C.
18. Allow the beads to settle.
19. To wash the beads:
    a. Eliminate the supernatant *very carefully* with a Gilson pipet; beads are *very delicate* and float easily. A remainder of up to approx. 0.1 mL can be left.
    b. Add 1 mL LB.
    c. Invert and flick the tubes to resuspend the beads.
    d. Spin at 6000*g*, 5 min, 4°C.
    e. Wash the beads by this method three times.
20. Eliminate the supernatant as thoroughly as possible. It is recommended to use a Hamilton syringe to remove the buffer as completely as possible. Hamilton syringes will allow removal of all the buffer without affecting the beads.
21. Add 50 µL 2.5X RSB. (Samples can be frozen at –20°C at this step.) Boil for 10 min in a hot block (remember to make a hole in the lid of the sample). Also boil the molecular weight markers.
22. Spin for 5 min at 6000*g*, 4°C.
23. Load the whole sample on a 15% SDS-PAGE gel.
24. Transfer the gel.
25. Western blotting is performed as described previously for phosphotyrosine using the pan Ras antibody (1:500, overnight at 4°C; secondary: mouse Ig, horseradish peroxidase-linked whole antibody [from sheep], 1:5000 for 1 h at room temperature). Ras is detected as a band of 21 kDa. This antibody recognizes all known isoforms of Ras.

3.4. Affinity Precipitation of Active STAT Complexes

Although in many aspects this method is very similar to that used for the affinity precipitation of active Ras, it has been reproduced in full here to avoid any confusion. Once the affinity step is completed and the samples have been resuspended in reducing sample buffer, PAGE and Western blot are essentially identical to that described in **Subheading 3.1.** and are not discussed further. A typical result is shown in **Fig. 4**.

1. Make up fresh LB: 4.0 mL per point. Add Nonidet P-40 to 1%, NaCl to 150 mM (final concentration; *see* **Note 9**), DTT to 1 mM, and inhibitors as recommended above.
2. Cells should be stimulated as desired; 2×10^7 peripheral blood lymphocytes per sample is normally used. A good positive control for STAT5 is 20 ng/mL IL-2.
3. Stop activation by placing samples on ice. Keep samples on ice or work in cold room from this step.
4. Spin for 1 min at 12,000g, 4°C.
5. Remove supernatant and lyse cells by adding 1 mL freshly made ice-cold 1X oligonucleotide binding lysis buffer (1 mL per maximum of 2×10^7 cells).
6. Vortex to dissolve pellet. *Do not allow the tube to warm up.*
7. Lyse for 20 min (*see* **Note 14**), 4°C, mix rotating.
8. Spin for 5 min at 12,000g, 4°C, to eliminate cell debris.
9. Incubate for 15 min, 4°C, mix rotating.
10. Spin at 6000g, 5 min, 4°C. Take supernatant (lysate) into a fresh tube and add 30 µL of prewashed streptavidin-agarose beads + 1 µg of required 5' biotinylated oligonucleotide, normally 10 µL from a 0.1-µg/µL stock.
11. Perform binding for 2 h, 4°C, mix rotating.
12. Spin for 5 min at 6000g, 4°C.
13. Allow the beads to settle. If the proteins remaining in the supernatant after the oligonucleotide binding are to be compared with the bound proteins, the supernatant can be acetone precipitated at this stage (refer to **Subheading 3.1., step 7**).
14. To wash the beads:
    a. Eliminate the supernatant *very carefully* with a Gilson pipet; the beads are *very delicate* and float easily. A remainder of up to approx 0.1 mL can be left.
    b. Add 1 mL oligonucleotide binding lysis buffer.
    c. Invert and flick the tubes to resuspend the beads.
    d. Spin at 6000g, 5 min, 4°C.
    e. Wash the beads by this method three times.
15. Eliminate the supernatant as thoroughly as possible. It is recommended to use a Hamilton syringe to remove the buffer as completely as possible. Hamilton syringes will allow removal of all the buffer without affecting the beads.
16. Add 50 µL 2.5X RSB. (Samples can be frozen at –20°C at this step.) Boil for 10 min in a hot block (remember to make a hole in the lid of the sample). Also boil the molecular weights markers.
17. Spin at 6000g, 5 min, 4°C.

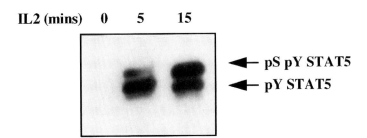

Fig. 4. Precipitation of active STAT5 from IL-2-stimulated peripheral blood lymphocytes as described in **Subheading 3.4.** The lower band represents STAT5 that has been tyrosine phosphorylated (pY), and the upper band represents STAT5 that has been serine and tyrosine phosphorylated (pS pY).

18. Load the whole sample on to a 7.5% gel to perform SDS-PAGE. Care needs to be taken when loading the gels as beads can block the tip and loading becomes very difficult. Some researchers load the samples with Hamilton syringes.
19. Perform Western blotting. The STAT complexes can be detected using specific antibodies (antibodies for STAT3 and STAT5 are described in **Table 1**).

4. Notes

1. Many different types of lysis buffers are used, particularly for generating total cell lysates. It is important to understand the purpose of the various components. Usually either Tris or HEPES is used, as both of these buffers have good buffering capacity at physiologic pH. Nonidet P-40 (NP-40) is a standard detergent used to permeabilize the membranes. It does not form the large micelles that can occur in other detergents, so usually large-membrane linked protein complexes do not cause abnormal coprecipitations. Both SPIs and PMSF are inhibitors of proteolysis. However, SPIs are reversible but stable in aqueous solution whereas PMSF is irreversible and very unstable. Sodium orthovanadate (Na_3VO_4) is a tyrosine phosphatase inhibitor. It is particularly important for assays that depend on phosphotyrosine interactions.
2. Preparation of Na_3VO_4: Weigh 1.84 g per 100 mL of solution to be made up. Dissolve in approx 80 mL of H_2O. Alter pH to 10 with 1 M HCl (solution should turn bright yellow). Boil until clear. Allow to cool to room temperature. Check pH and adjust again if necessary with NaOH. Boil again. Allow to cool to room temperature until solution is clear. Make up to full volume. Filter, aliquot, and store at –20°C.
3. Gel apparatus varies from laboratory to laboratory, but protocols are fairly standard. In case of doubts, researchers are recommended to read the advice from manufacturers and to take extreme care as electricity is very dangerous.
4. Two methods for the transfer of proteins from a polyacrylamide gel to a membrane are commonly used—wet transfer and semidry transfer. The wet transfer is thought to be the best to transfer proteins of a wide range of size evenly. However, it generally takes longer, approx 4 h and requires substantially more transfer buffer. Semidry transfer is thought to be optimal only for small to medium

sized proteins (less than 100 kDa) but is quicker (1 h) and generally requires substantially less transfer buffer. The transfer buffer recommended here is for wet transfer only. A typical semidry transfer buffer is 48 mM Tris-HCl, 39 mM glycine, 20% methanol, 0.037% SDS.

5. Many different suppliers are available for antiphosphotyrosine antibodies. 4G10 and PY20 are thought to bind to phosphotyrosine in different amino acid sequences. Thus, certain proteins will react better with one antibody compared with to the other. Often they are used separately.

6. The glutathione-agarose beads are supplied as a lyophilized powder and must be rehydrated in PBS. Incubate for 1 h at room temperature. Wash four times in PBS + 0.05% sodium azide. Resuspend to 50% v/v slurry. Store at 4°C.

7. Ras GTP binding is Mg^{2+} dependent, and thus this reagent is essential.

8. Oligonucleotides are normally supplied single stranded. Complementary strands can be used to make double-stranded oligonucleotides by the following method: Make up 1 mg/mL of each of the 5' and the 3' complementary strand oligonucleotides in 10 mM Tris-HCl, pH 8, 1 mM EDTA (TE). Mix equal volumes. Incubate for 10 min at 95°C in a water bath. Turn off the water bath and leave it cooling down to reach room temperature. This gives a 1 mg/mL stock. To use, dilute to 0.1 mg/mL with TE + 75 mM NaCl. The oligonucleotide sequence derived from the FcγR-GAS (GRR), GTATTTCCCAGAAAAGGAAC (29) has been used to affinity purify STAT5 (14,23) very successfully, but other oligonucleotide sequences may be optimal for different proteins.

9. STAT DNA binding is sensitive to high concentrations of NaCl. The optimum salt concentration varies for each STAT but is particularly a problem for STAT4. A high concentration of NaCl is required to "salt" transcription factors from DNA in the nucleus. Thus, it is best to lyse the cells with a high NaCl concentration but to dilute the lysate prior to performing the oligonucleotide affinity precipitation. Lysis in 150 mM NaCl is recommended. DNA binding is best in 15 mM NaCl.

10. The amount of cell lysate that should be loaded on the gel, and therefore the number of cells required for lysis, varies according to cell type, available material, and sensitivity of the antibodies used. Some laboratories perform protein assays and load a known amount of protein extract, whereas others prefer to load equal cell numbers. The experiments shown here have used 5×10^6 to 1×10^7 cells, which is equivalent to 250–500 μg of protein.

11. The acetone precipitation step has two functions: The first is to remove the detergent to prevent competition with SDS, which is required for SDS-PAGE. The second is as a method for concentrating the samples. It is also possible to precipitate proteins in trichloroacetic acid. Some researchers prefer to lyse directly into 1% SDS lysis buffer. However, with lymphocytes, this causes the DNA to come out of solution and separation by ultracentrifugation must be performed before loading on a gel. In the case of easily degraded proteins this method can prevent degradation better than 1% NP-40 lysis buffers even when high concentrations of protease inhibitors are present.

12. For stripping and detection of membranes, incubate the membrane in 50 mL stripping buffer (100 mM 2-mercaptoethanol, 2% SDS, 62.5 mM Tris-HCl, pH 6.8) for 30 min at 55°C with agitation, and then wash membranes twice for 5 min in PBS-T.

13. To couple the fusion protein to GAB: Couple 1 mg of protein per 100 mL of a 50% suspension GAB. Final concentration of protein on beads is 10 mg/mL. Incubate dialyzed fusion protein with corresponding volume of GAB in a 15-mL Falcon tube rotating for 2 h at 4°C. Wash three times in PBS-EDTA, using 15-s spins at 470g and let beads settle for 2 min before removing the supernatant. Keep first supernatant in case binding was not completed. Wash once in storage buffer (50 mM HEPES, pH 7.4, 50 mM NaCl, 50% glycerol). To remove the storage buffer, spin at 850g for 1 min and wait at least 10 min for the beads to settle down (the buffer contains 50% glycerol). Resuspend in a small volume of storage buffer and transfer into minifuge tubes. Wash once more with storage buffer. Resuspend at 50% slurry with storage buffer and keep at –20°C. At this stage, beads are ready to use for affinity precipitation experiments. To test coupling efficiency: Take 5 mL of coupled beads and add 20 mL of RSB. Boil for 10 min and run in an SDS-PAGE minigel. A clear band the size of the fusion protein should be visible. Coupling is stable for one to two months at –20°C. It is recommended to couple small amounts of protein/beads and repeat the procedure when required.

14. Times shown for precipitations are the minimum incubation times required to get good results. Reasonably longer times do not affect the reactions.

References

1. Smith, K. A. (1988) Interleukin-2: inception, impact and implications. *Science* **240,** 1169–1176.
2. Nelson, B. H. and Willerford, D. M. (1998) Biology of the interleukin-2 receptor. *Adv. Immunol.* **70,** 1–81.
3. Beadling, C., Guschin, D., Witthuhn, B. A., Ziemiecki, A., Ihle, J. N., Kerr, I. M., and Cantrell, D. A. (1994) Activation of JAK kinases and STAT proteins by interleukin-2 and interferon-α, but not the T cell antigen receptor, in human T lymphocytes. *EMBO J.* **13,** 5605–5615.
4. Johnston, J., Kawamura, M., Kirken, R., Chen, Y., Blake, T., Shibuya, K., et al. (1994) Phosphorylation and activation of the Jak-3 Janus kinase in response to interleukin-2. *Nature* **370,** 151–153.
5. Miyazaki, T., Kawahara, A., Fujii, H., Nakagawa, Y., Minami, Y., Liu, Z.-J., et al. (1994) Functional activation of Jak1 and Jak3 by selective association with IL-2 receptor subunits. *Science* **266,** 1045–1047.
6. Russell, S., Johnston, J., Noguchi, M., Kawamura, M., Bacon, C., Friedman, M., et al. (1994) Interaction of IL-2R β and γ chains with Jak1 and Jak3: implications for XSCID and XCID. *Science* **266,** 1042–1045.
7. Witthuhn, B., Silvennoinen, O., Miura, O., Lai, K., Cwik, C., Liu, E., and Ihle, J. (1994) Involvement of the Jak-3 Janus kinase in signalling by interleukins 2 and 4 in lymphoid and myeloid cells. *Nature* **370,** 153–157.
8. Fairhurst, R. M., Daeipour, M., Amaral, M. C., and Nel, A. E. (1993) Activation of mitogen-activated protein kinase/ERK-2 in phytohaemagglutin in blasts by recombinant interleukin-2: contrasting features with CD3 activation. *Immunology* **79,** 112–118.

9. Izquierdo, M., Leevers, S. J., Williams, D. H., Marshall, C. J., Weiss, A., and Cantrell, D. A. (1994) The role of protein kinase C in the regulation of extra cellular signal regulated kinase by the T cell antigen receptor. *Eur. J. Immunol.* **24,** 2462–2468.

10. Turner, B., Rapp, U., App, H., Greene, M., Dobashi, K., and Reid, J. (1991) Interleukin-2 induces tyrosine phosphorylation and activation of p72-74 Raf-1 kinase in a T cell line. *Proc. Natl. Acad. Sci. USA* **88,** 1227–1232.

11. Lin, J.-X., Migone, T.-S., Tsang, M., Friedmann, M., Weatherbee, J. A., Zhou, L., et al. (1995) The role of shared receptor motifs and common Stat proteins in the generation of cytokine pleiotropy and redundancy by IL-2, IL-4, IL-7, IL-13, and IL-15. *Immunity* **2,** 331–339.

12. Hou, J., Schindler, U., Henzel, W. J., Wong, S. C., and McKnight, S. L. (1995) Identification and purification of human Stat proteins activated in response to interleukin-2. *Immunity* **2,** 321–329.

13. Johnston, J. A., Bacon, C. M., Finbloom, D. S., Rees, R. C., Kaplan, D., Shibuya, K., et al. (1995) Tyrosine phosphorylation and activation of Stat5, Stat3, and Janus kinases by interleukin-2 and interleukin-15. *Proc. Natl. Acad. Sci. USA* **92,** 8705–8709.

14. Beadling, C., Ng, J., Babbage, J. W., and Cantrell, D. A. (1996) Interleukin-2 activation of STAT5 requires the convergent action of tyrosine kinases and a serine/threonine kinase distinct from the Raf-1/Erk2 MAP kinase pathway. *EMBO J.* **15,** 1902–1913.

15. Remillard, B., Petrillo, R., Maslinski, W., Tsudo, M., Strom, T. B., Cantley, L., and Varticovski, L. (1991) Interleukin-2 receptor regulates activation of phosphatidylinositol 3-kinase. *J. Biol. Chem.* **266,** 14,167–14,170.

16. Reif, K., Burgering, B. M. T., and Cantrell, D. A. (1997) Phosphatidylinositol 3-kinase links the interleukin-2 receptor to protein kinase B and p70 S6 kinase. *J. Biol. Chem.* **272,** 14,426–14,438.

17. Franke, T. F., Kaplan, D. R., Cantley, L. C., and Toker, A. (1997) Direct regulation of the *Akt* proto-oncogene product by phosphatidylinositol-3,4-bisphosphate. *Science* **275,** 665–668.

18. Datta, K., Bellacosa, A., Chan, T. O., and Tsichlis, P. N. (1996) Akt is a direct target of the phosphatidylinositol 3-kinase. *J. Biol. Chem.* **271,** 30,835–30,839.

19. Kozma, S. C. and Thomas, G. (1994) p70s6k/p85s6k: mechanism of activation and role in mitogenesis. *Semin. Cancer. Biol.* **5,** 255–260.

20. Han, J. W., Pearson, R. B., Dennis, P. B., and Thomas, G. (1995) Rapamycin, wortmannin, and the methylxanthine SQ20006 inactivate p70s6k by inducing dephosphorylation of the same subset of sites. *J. Biol. Chem.* **270,** 21,396–21,403.

21. Turner, H., Reif, K., Rivera, J., and Cantrell, D. A. (1995) Regulation of the adapter molecule Grb2 by the FceR1 in the mast cell line RBL2H3. *J. Biol. Chem.* **270,** 9500–9506.

22. Brennan, P., Babbage, J. W., Burgering, B. M. T., Groner, B., Reif, K., and Cantrell, D. A. (1997) Phosphatidylinositol 3-kinase controls E2F transcriptional activity in response to interleukin-2. *Immunity* **7,** 679–689.

23. Ng, J. and Cantrell, D. A. (1997) STAT3 is a target for multiple serine kinases in T cells; integrating interleukin2 and T cell antigen receptor signals. *J. Biol. Chem.* **272,** 24,542–24,549.

24. Watton, S. J. (1999) Akt/PKB localisation and 3'phosphoinositide generation at sites of epithelial cell-matrix and cell-cell interaction. *Curr. Biol.* **9,** 433–436.
25. David, M., Petricoin, E. III, Benjamin, C., Pine, R., Weber, M. J., and Larner, A. C. (1995) Requirement for MAP kinase (ERK2) activity in interferon α- and interferon β-stimulated gene expression through STAT proteins. *Science* **269,** 1721–1723.
26. Wen, Z. and Darnell, J. E., Jr. (1997) Mapping of Stat3 serine phosphorylation to a single residue (727) and evidence that serine phosphorylation has no influence on DNA binding of Stat1 and Stat3. *Nucleic Acids Res.* **25,** 2062–2067.
27. Taylor, S. J. and Shalloway, D. (1996) Cell cycle-dependent activation of Ras. *Curr. Biol.* **6,** 1621–1627.
28. Rommel, C. and Hafen, E. (1998) Ras—a versatile cellular switch. *Curr. Opin. Gen. Dev.* **8,** 412–418.
29. Larner, A. C., David, M., Feldman, G. M., Igarashi, K., Hackett, R. H., Webb, D. S. A., et al. (1993) Tyrosine phosphorylation of DNA binding proteins by multiple cytokines. *Science* **261,** 1730–1733.

33

Applications for Green Fluorescent Protein in Cell Signaling

Paul Brennan and Emmanuelle Astoul

1. Introduction

The discovery of green fluorescent protein (GFP) as a naturally fluorescing protein and its subsequent modification to allow easy detection with standard fluorescent equipment such as the fluorescence-activated cell sorter (FACS) has revolutionized our ability to detect the presence of transfected proteins and to determine their location in whole cells and in organisms. GFP was found in the bioluminescent jellyfish *Aequorea (1,2)*. It has since been modified to change its excitation and emision *(3–5)*. Expression vectors are now supplied commercially that allow proteins to be tagged easily *(6,7)*. Furthermore, it is a small protein, only 29 kDa, and the DNA encoding it can be easily modified using polymerase chain reaction to introduce any restriction sites for any subcloning work required.

This chapter discusses some of the applications of GFP used by researchers in studying signal transduction in cell lines. The first and second sections deal with GFP as a transfection marker and one of the applications. The third section discusses protein translocation upon receptor stimulation. The methodology is described, and some examples are discussed. Recently transcription factors have been tagged with GFP, and their translocation from cytosol to the nucleus has been analyzed *(8)*. A similar approach has been used to analyze the translocation of kinases from cytoplasm to plasma membrane *(9–13)*. This type of analysis has also been used to investigate domains of proteins *(13)*.

Other applications that have not been described include using GFP in polycystronic viruses to check effective infection *(14)*. GFP has also been used in a large number of organism such as fruit flies *(15)*, *Dictyostelium (15)*, and mice *(16)*, generating exciting pictures *(17)*. Many of the newest applications are discussed in the newsgroup: bionet.molbio.proteins.fluorescent.

From: *Methods in Molecular Medicine, vol. 60: Interleukin Protocols*
Edited by: L. A. J. O'Neill and A. Bowie © Humana Press Inc., Totowa, NJ

2. Materials

2.1. Cell Electroporation and Analysis by FACS

1. Cells (*see* **Note 1**).
2. Purified GFP expression vector (*see* **Note 2**): We use pEFGP-C1 vector from Clontech (Palo Alto, CA; store at –20°C in 10 m*M* Tris-HCl, containing 1 m*M* EDTA).
3. Electroporation cuvets (*see* **Note 3**).
4. Electroporator: We use a Bio-Rad Gene Pulser.
5. Suitable cell culture media and fetal calf serum (FCS); store at 4°C.
6. Tubes for use in FACS machine.
7. Phosphate-buffered saline (PBS).
8. FACS machine.

2.2. Analysis of Transfected Cells for Expression of Cell Surface Molecules

1. All the reagents described in previous section.
2. Ficoll (*see* **Note 4**) from Nycomed Pharma (Oslo, Norway).
3. Antibodies for detection of cell surface markers (for example, intercellular adhesion molecule [ICAM]-phycoerythrin); store at 4°C.

2.3. Analysis of Protein Translocation by Confocal Fluorescence Microscopy

1. Electroporation equipment (described above).
2. 35-mm Glass-bottomed dishes (MatTek).
3. Inverted confocal microscope (Zeiss Laser Scanning Microscope 5.10) equipped with a warm chamber and CO_2 apparatus.
4. Zeiss LSM software.
5. Hanks' medium, or Dulbecco's modified eagle's medium (DMEM), *without* phenol red; store at 4°C.

3. Methods

3.1. Transfection of Kit225 Cells

The method described has been successfully used for transfection of the interleukin-2 (IL-2)-dependent cell line Kit225 (*see* **Fig. 1**, for example). It can be applied to any cell line. It is necessary to experiment with the conditions to optimize them for a particular cell line (*see* **Note 5**). Examples of this transfection technique applied to Jurkat T cells *(18,19)*, A20 B cells (described below and in **ref.** *12*) and the rat basophilic leukemia cell line RBL2H3 can be found in the literature *(8,20)*.

1. Spin down cells and count. Use $1.0-1.5 \times 10^7$ cells/sample.
2. Mix DNA (*see* **Note 6**) and cells in a final volume of 0.6 mL RPMI-1640 medium containing 10% FCS in an Eppendorf tube and transfer to electroporation cuvet.
3. Check voltage and capacity and electroporate at 320 V, 960 µFD. This should

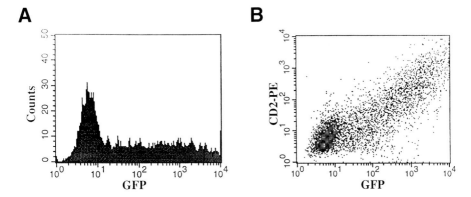

Fig. 1. **(A)** Kit225 cells transfected with 10 μg of an expression vector for GFP analyzed as described in **Subheading 3.1.** This figure shows variable levels of expression of GFP from a population of cells. **(B)** Kit225 cells cotransfected with a expression vector for GFP (10 μg) and an expression vector for rat CD2 (10 μg). CD2 was detected with a phycoerythrin-conjugated antibody to rat CD2. This figure demonstrates the principle of cotransfection.

give a time constant of about 15–16 ms. If this is lower than 12 or higher than 27, something is very wrong (such as volume too low).

4. After transfection, transfer, using a pastet, to a 6-well plate. Add 8–10 mL and divide in two for ± IL-2 treatment.
5. Allow time for expression (*see* **Note 5**), and analyze by FACS. Cells should be placed in a FACS tube and analyzed in the relevant fluorescence channel (FL1 in a Becton Dickinson FACS Caliber). Nontransfected cells should be used as a negative control and gates should be set so that the nontransfected cells appear between 10^0 and 10^1 of the FACS. Transfected cells expressing GFP will appear, demonstrating a clear green fluorescence as shown in **Fig. 1**.

3.2. GFP and Analysis of Transfected Cells for Cell Surface Molecule Expression

Many uses can be made of GFP as a cotransfection marker. These include cell cycle analysis of transfected cells (*see* **Note 7**). Another use is to follow the induction (regulation) of a cell surface molecule by a transfected signaling molecule, such as oncogenic ras. Cytoplasmic GFP will only be found in living and transfected cells, allowing the exclusion by FACS of cells nonrelevant for the study. The modulation of the surface molecule expressed, possibly regulated by the transfected protein, can then be detected with fluorescence-labeled antibodies.

1. Transfect cells as suggested in **Subheading 3.1.**
2. Dead cells can be separated by Ficoll if this is necessary (*see* **Note 4**). Layer cells

in media above half a volume of Ficoll. Centrifuge at 800g for 15 min without the brake. Wash twice with PBS.

3. Add antibody for required cell surface marker (PE or tricolor conjugated) (*see* **Note 8**).
4. Wash samples three times with PBS.
5. Analyze by FACS (compensation will be necessary; *see* **Note 9**).

3.3. Observation of Protein Translocation by Real-Time Confocal Microscopy

The main advantage of the use of a GFP-fused protein vs fluorescence-coupled antibodies is the possibility of analyzing living cells. That property allows the study of protein localization under dynamic conditions (*see* **Fig. 2** for an example). The following protocol is optimized for A20 cells:

1. Transfect the cells (*see* **Note 10**) using standard procedure. We use electroporation of 1×10^7 cells in 500 µL of RPMI containing 10–40 µg of DNA (*see* **Note 5**), at 310 V and 960 µF using the Bio-Rad gene pulser apparatus.
2. After transfection, cells are resuspended at 1×10^6/mL in complete RPMI and cultured in glass-bottomed dishes (*see* **Note 11**) for 8–18 h to allow cells to adhere and express sufficient level of the chimeric protein.
3. Gently rinse the dishes twice with warm medium (containing no phenol red) before analysis. Cover the cells with 2 mL of this medium and mount it in the prewarm chamber of the confocal microscopy. If you plan a long experiment time, the chamber should be filled with an appropriate concentration of CO_2 (5–10%).
4. Samples are detected with a 63×1.4 NA oil immersion objective and excited with an argon laser emitting at 488 nm. Set the focus, fluorescence intensity, and contrast parameters before adding any stimulus.
5. Be prepared to add the stimulus directly in the dish *very gently* at the surface of the medium, avoiding making waves.
6. Use the "time series" option in the Zeiss LSM software to set the interval you want between images and the number of image. Record the first image just before stimulation. When this initial image is scanned, quickly but very steadily move the camera to access the sample, add the stimulus, and replace the camera. Then let the scanning work automatically.
7. Images can be saved as "galleries" showing on the same page every scan, as individual files for each scan, or even as animated films.

4. Notes

1. Cells: The efficiency and optimum conditions vary according to cell type and should be determined by varying the voltage and amount of DNA used. The authors have used many different T-cell lines and the B-cell line A20. Other transfection methods are commonly used for other cell types such as calcium phosphate (*21*), DEAE-dextran (*22*), and various lipsome-based techniques (*23*).
2. DNA: Many laboratories recommend cesium chloride-purified DNA, as large quantities of highly pure DNA can be generated. However, it is also common to

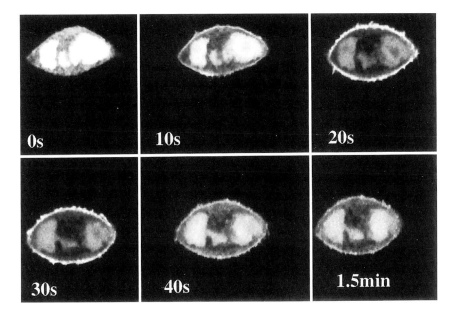

Fig. 2. The mouse B-lymphoma cell line A20 transfected by GFP fused to the lipid-binding PH domain of Akt/PKB, at different time points after stimulation through its antigen receptor. Real-time confocal analysis allows kinetic analysis of the very rapid PKB translocations.

    use some of the commercially available DNA purification methods such as those available from Quiagen and Promega. The amount of DNA required for each transfection varies according to cell type.

3. Cuvets: 0.4-mm cuvets for cell electroporation are expensive. Manufacturers recommend single use, but many laboratories wash and reuse them. Cuvets can be soaked in washing-up liquid and then washed using a bottle scrubber. They should then be sterilized in ethanol for about 20 min and washed twice in sterile media.

4. Electroporation of T-cell lines can cause a lot of cell death. The dead cells can nonspecifically bind antibody, making analysis difficult. It is possible to separate dead cells from live ones using Ficoll. When cells in media are layered over Ficoll and centrifuged at 800g, without using the brake, the dead cells are found below the Ficoll and the live cells are found at the Ficoll media interface. This manipulation may result in substantial loss of cells. Thus, a balance between the problems of cell loss and cell number required for the experiment requires some optimization on the part of the researcher.

5. The limiting factor of these experiments is the expression of the GFP-tagged protein. The level of expression depends on the expression vector used, the amount of DNA (*see* **Note 6**), and the time allowed for expression. Severe overexpression can result in problems, such as the formation of inclusion bodies.

It may then be useful to reduce the concentration of transfecting DNA and the time of expression after transfection to limit accumulation of the protein. This is less of a problem when using GFP as a cotransfection marker.

6. The amount of DNA depends on the level of expression required. Most T-cell lines transfect well with between 10 and 40 µg of DNA. Transfected GFP from a CMV-driven expression vector requires only a small amount of DNA to be detectable. If multiple cuvets are prepared using the same DNA, pool contents, and then divide into aliquots for stimulation. For multiple plasmid transfection, transfect all DNA at the same time.

7. For analysis of cell cycle with GFP, it is possible to label cells with bromodeoxyuridine (BrdU) as normal before staining, then fix the cells in 1% paraformaldehyde, and treat with 2 M HCl/0.5% Triton in H_2O for 15 min. This results in significant loss of green fluorescence from the GFP (reduction to 10%), although it can still be detected. It may be possible to use other BrdU staining protocols more efficiently in combination with GFP.

8. For analysis of cell surface molecule expression, optimal concentration of antibody depends on the number of cells stained and the quality of the antibody. Directly conjugated commercial antibodies are usually used at concentrations between 0.2 and 2 µg/mL. Use 200 µL for approx 1×10^6 to 5×10^6 cells.

9. For FACS analysis, the GFP-expressing cells can be very bright. Researchers should be careful to compensate carefully, especially when using phycoerythrin-conjugated antibodies.

10. For real-time confocal microscopy, choose a cell that seems to adhere strongly as the stimulation and the movement of the camera after stimulation might make it move. If possible, favor cells that are less round.

11. After transfection for real-time confocal microscopy, seed a lot of plates for each stimulus you want to use, as the risk of the cell moving and ending out of focus is quite high, especially on long-term time series.

References

1. Morin, J. G. and Hastings, J. W. (1971) Energy transfer in a bioluminescent system. *J. Cell. Physiol.* **77,** 313–318.
2. Shimomura, O., Johnson, F. H., and Saiga, Y. (1962) Extraction, purification and properties of aequorin, a bioluminescent protein from the luminous hydromedusan, *Aequorea. J. Cell. Comp. Physiol.* **59,** 223–227.
3. Cormack, B. P., Valdivia, R., and Falkow, S. (1996) FACS-optimized mutants of the green fluorescent protein (GFP). *Gene* **173,** 33–38.
4. Heim, R., Cubitt, A. B., and Tsien, R. Y. (1995) Improved green fluorescence. *Nature* **373,** 663–664.
5. Heim, R. and Tsien, R. Y. (1996) Engineering green fluorescent protein for improved brightness, longer wavelengths and fluorescence resonance energy transfer. *Curr. Biol.* **6,** 178–182.
6. Clontech (1999) *Living Colors User Manual*, vol. PT2040-1, Clontech, Palo Alto, CA, pp. 16–17.

7. Clontech (1996) *New Living Colors Vectors.* CLONTECHniques XI, Clontech, Palo Alto, CA, pp. 20–23.

8. Turner, H., Gomez, M., McKenzie, E., Kirchem, A., Lennard, A., and Cantrel, L. D. A. (1998) Rac-1 regulates nuclear factor of activated T cells (NFAT) C1 nuclear translocation in response to Fcepsilon receptor type 1 stimulation of mast cells. *J. Exp. Med.* **188,** 527–537.

9. Sakai, N., Sasaki, K., Ikegaki, N., Shirai, Y., Ono, Y., and Saito, N. (1997) Direct visualization of the translocation of the gamma-subspecies of protein kinase C in living cells using fusion proteins with green fluorescent protein. *J. Cell Biol.* **139,** 1465–1476.

10. Feng, X., Zhang, J., Barak, L. S., Meyer, T., Caron, M. G., and Hannun, Y. A. (1998) Visualization of dynamic trafficking of a protein kinase C betaII/green fluorescent protein conjugate reveals differences in G protein-coupled receptor activation and desensitization. *J. Biol. Chem.* **273,** 10,755–10,762.

11. Meller, N., Liu, Y.-C., Collins, T. L., Bonnefoy-Berard, N., Baier, G., Isakov, N., et al. (1996) Direct interaction between protein kinase C theta (PKC theta) and 14-3-3 tau in T cells: 14-3-3 overexpression results in inhibition of PKC theta translocation and function. *Mol. Cell. Biol.* **16,** 5782–5791.

12. Astoul, E., Watton, S., and Cantrell, D. (1999) The dynamics of protein kinase B regulation during B cell antigen receptor engagement. *J. Cell Biol.* **145,** 1511–1520.

13. Watton, S. J. (1999) Akt/PKB localisation and 3' phosphoinositide generation at sites of epithelial cell-matrix and cell-cell interaction. *Curr. Biol.* **9,** 433–436.

14. Cheng, L., Fu, J., Tsukamoto, A., and Hawley, R. G. (1996) Use of green fluorescent protein variants to monitor gene transfer and expression in mammalian cells. *Nature Biotechnol.* **14,** 606–609.

15. Brand. (1995) GFP in *Drosophila. Trends Genet.* **11,** 324–325.

16. Ikawa, M., Kominami, K., Yoshimura, Y., Tanaka, K., Nishimune, Y., and Okabe, M. (1995) Green fluorescent protein as a marker in transgenic mice. *Dev. Growth Differ.* **37,** 455–459.

17. Matus, A. (1999) Introduction: GFP illuminates everything. *Trends Cell Biol.* **9,** 43.

18. Genot, E., Cleverley, S., Henning, S., and Cantrell, D. (1996) Multiple p21ras effector pathways regulate nuclear factor of activated T cells. *EMBO J.* **15,** 3923–3933.

19. Reif, K., Lucas, S., and Cantrell, D. (1997) A negative role for phosphatidylinositol 3-kinase in T cell antigen receptor function. *Curr. Biol.* **7,** 285–293.

20. Turner, H. and Cantrell, D. A. (1997) Distinct Ras effector pathways are involved in FcεR1 regulation of the transcriptional activity of Elk-1 and NFAT in mast cells. *J. Exp. Med.* **185,** 43–57.

21. Chen, C. A. and Okayama, H. (1988) Calcium phosphate-mediated gene transfer: a highly efficient transfection system for stably transforming cells with plasmid DNA. *Biotechniques* **6,** 632–638.

22. Rosenthal, N. (1987) Identification of regulatory elements of cloned genes with functional assays. *Methods Enzymol.* **152,** 704–709.

23. Sambrook, J., Fritsch, E. F., and Maniatis, T. (1989) *Molecular Cloning: A Laboratory Manual*, Cold Spring Harbor Laboratory, Cold Spring Harbor, NY.

34

Use of *Pichia pastoris* for Production of Recombinant Cytokines

Kevin P. Murphy, Csaba Pazmany, and Mark D. Moody

1. Introduction

An understanding of the structure and function of cytokines requires the availability of milligram to gram amounts of highly purified and biologically active cytokines. A variety of expression systems have been used to produce recombinant proteins, including *Escherichia coli*, *Pichia pastoris*, baculovirus, and poxvirus systems. The *P. pastoris* expression system is particularly well suited for the production of recombinant cytokines. The relative merits of the *P. pastoris* expression system compared with others have been reviewed elsewhere (*1–3*). In summary, *P. pastoris* offers the potential for high yields of biologically active recombinant cytokines at relatively low production costs. In contrast to *E. coli*, with which folding problems often lead to inclusion body formation, the expressed proteins are properly folded and can be secreted into the media. In addition, unlike bacterial systems, *P. pastoris* is capable of high-mannose type N-linked glycosylation (without the hyperglycosylation problems of *Saccharomyces cerevisiae*) (*4,5*). Another reason for choosing *P. pastoris* over bacterial expression systems is that the yeast cells are not a source of endogenous endotoxin, as is the case with *E. coli*. This is particularly important for recombinant cytokines: contaminating endotoxin could stimulate cells to produce inflammatory cytokines.

1.1. Characteristics of Cytokines Produced Using P. pastoris

Our laboratory has produced over a dozen different cytokines (**Table 1**). Bioassays have shown that all the recombinant cytokines are biologically active (with the exception of rat interleukin-6 [IL-6], which suffered from aggregation problems), and gel filtration analysis has shown that all are in the correct quarternary structure, for example, human (h) IL-17 forms a dimer, porcine tumor necrosis factor-α (TNF-α) forms a trimer, and porcine (p) IL-1β exists as a monomer. We have

From: *Methods in Molecular Medicine, vol. 60: Interleukin Protocols*
Edited by: L. A. J. O'Neill and A. Bowie © Humana Press Inc., Totowa, NJ

Table 1
Characteristics of Recombinant Cytokines Produced by *Pichia pastoris*

Cytokine	Yield[a] mg/L	Amino acid sequence (predicted MW)	SDS PAGE (apparent MW; kDa)	Gel filtration (apparent MW; kDa)	Quanternary structure	Glycosylation
Porcine IFN-γ	7	16,700	16 and 22.1	65.6	Dimer	Yes
Porcine TNF-α	5	17,678	17.7	49.2	Trimer	No
Porcine IL-1-β	3	17,575	18.8	21	Monomer	No
Porcine IL-4	0.1	12,520	10.4[a]	25	Monomer	Yes
Porcine IL-6	2	20,927	22.5	25	Monomer	No
Rat IL-6	100	20,702	21.7	n.d.	Monomer	No
Porcine IL-8	32	9097	9.9	25	Dimer	No
Human IL-17	1	15,500	16 and 20	39	Dimer	Yes
Murine IL-17	8	15,300	16 and 20	40	Dimer	Yes

[a]Apparent MW of nonglycosylated form.

found that several of these cytokines are glycosylated (**Fig. 1**); in the case of hIL-17, the glycosylation is very similar to that observed in hIL-17 produced by mammalian cells (*6*). The proteins are greater than 95% pure (**Fig. 2**), and the yield of the purified recombinant cytokines is typically in the range of 1–30 mg/L of shake flask culture (**Table 1**), although the yield of pIL-4 is considerably less, only 100 µg/L.

2. Materials
2.1. Yeast Strains

We have chosen to use mut^s strains of *P. pastoris* for all our work. Mut^s strains are deficient in the major alcohol oxidase gene, and thus utilize methanol more slowly than the mut$^+$ strains. Mut^s strains do not require careful control of methanol addition during culture, making them more suitable for shake-flask cultures, in which continous feeding of methanol is not practical. For most of our work we have used the mut^s strain KM71H (*6*). We developed this *Pichia* strain with a repaired *his*4 gene so that we can use the pPICZα and pPICZ9 plasmids (which do not encode the *his*4 gene) and still grow the transformants in media formulations without the addition of histidine. This was necessary because the mut^s strain KM71 (available from Invitrogen [Carlsbad, CA]) is deficient in histidine synthesis. This histidine deficiency of KM71 allows for the selection of recombinant yeast when transformed by plasmids (such as pPIC9) that encode the *his*4 gene.

2.2. Plasmids and cDNA

The pPICZα and pPIC9 plasmids (available from Invitrogen) are commonly used as vectors for the transformation of *P. pastoris*. The pPIC9 plasmid encodes ampicillin resistance for the selection of *E. coli* transformants, and a gene for histidine synthesis for the selection of recombinant *P. pastoris* clones. The pPICZα plasmids encode resistance to zeocin for selection of both *E. coli* and *P. pastoris* recombinants. Because the plasmids do not share the same multiple cloning site, it is not possible to use the same cloning strategy for the both plasmids. We constructed a new plasmid for transferring genes into *P. pastoris*, pPICZ9, so that we may use the same cloning strategy for both plasmids (*6*). The pPICZ9 plasmid was made by the replacement of the 1.25-kb *Bgl*II-*Not*I fragment of pPICZαA with the 1.24-kb *Bgl*II-*Not*I fragment of pPIC9, which contains the 5'AOX1 gene sequence, the α-factor secretion signal, and a multiple cloning site. We routinely grow all recombinant plasmids in the *E. coli* strain JM109 (supplied by Promega, Madison, WI) using Luria-Bertani medium (LB), LB plus ampicillin (for pPIC9 based plasmids), or low-salt LB plus zeocin (for pPICZ9-based plasmids) (*see* **Subheading 2.3.**).

The cDNA molecules used for the cloning of porcine interferon-γ (pIFN-γ), pTNF-α, pIL-1β, pIL-6, and pIL-8 were the kind gift of Dr. Michael Murtaugh (University of Minnesota, St. Paul, MN). The cDNA used for the cloning of rat IL-6 was the kind gift of Dr. Jack Gauldie (McMaster University, Hamilton, Ontario).

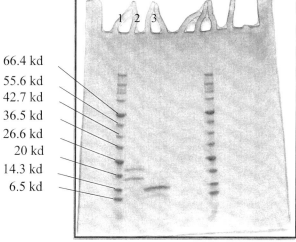

Fig. 1. *N*-linked glycosylation of porcine IFN-γ was demonstrated by the ability of PNGaseF to reduce the apparent molecular weight of the 16- and 21-kDa bands to a single band of approx 14 kDa. *Lane 1*, molecular weight markers; *lane 2*, pIFN-γ control; *lane 3*, pIFN-γ treated with PNGase F.

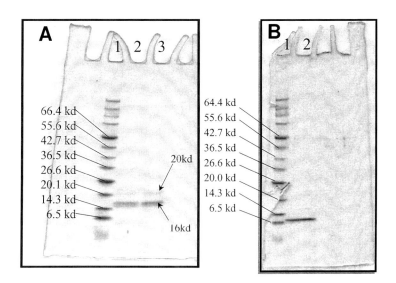

Fig. 2. **(A)** Coomassie stained SDS-PAGE analysis of purified mIL-17. *Lane 1*, molecular weight markers; *lanes 2* and *3*, gel filtration fractions of mIL-17. The arrows indicate the positions of the 20-kDa glycosylated mIL-17 (approx 15% of total protein) and the 16-kDa nonglycosylated mIL-17. **(B)** Coomassie stained SDS-PAGE analysis of purified pIL-8. *Lane 1*, molecular weight markers; *lane 2*, purified pIL-8.

2.3. Media

For routine growth and shake-flask scale production of *P. pastoris* we have used the media formulations of buffered minimum gylcerol medium (BMGY), buffered minimum methanol medium (BMMY), minimum dextrose medium (MD), yeast extract peptone dextrose medium (YPD), and YPD plus zeocin, which are described in the *Pichia* Expression Kit manual (version D) and the pPICZα A,B,C manual (version A) (published by Invitrogen).

1. BMGY medium: 1% yeast extract, 2% peptone, 100 mM potassium phosphate, pH 6, 4×10^{-5}% biotin, 1.34% yeast nitrogen base (with ammonium sulfate and without amino acids), and 1% glycerol.
2. BMMY medium: 1% yeast extract, 2% peptone, 100 mM potassium phosphate, pH 6, 4×10^{-5}% biotin, 1.34% yeast nitrogen base (with ammonium sulfate and without amino acids), and 0.5% methanol.
3. MD medium: 4×10^{-5}% biotin, 1.34% yeast nitrogen base (with ammonium sulfate and without amino acids), and 2% glucose.
4. YPD medium: 1% yeast extract, 2% peptone, 2% glucose. Zeocin was added to YPD for a final concentration of 100 µg/mL.
5. LB medium: 1% tryptone, 0.5% yeast extract, and 1% NaCl.
6. Low-salt LB plus zeocin medium: 1% tryptone, 0.5% yeast extract, 0.5% NaCl, and 25 µg/mL zeocin.
7. The base-salt medium for use in fermentation vessels is that described in the *Pichia* fermentation guidelines (Invitrogen and by Siegel and Bricrly *(7)*, except that the trace salt solution is formulated as follows; 0.09 mM cupric sulfate, 0.53 mM sodium iodide, 8 mM zinc chloride, 2.1 mM cobalt chloride, 2 mM manganese sulfate, 20 mM ferrous sulfate, 0.04 mM sodium molybdate, 1.9 mM biotin, and 0.33 mM boric acid.

2.4. Buffers

100 mM Sodium citrate buffer, pH 4.5, was used for all chromatography procedures except where noted.

2.5. Other Materials

Polymerase chain reactions (PCR) were performed using the *Pfu* polymerase (Stratagene, La Jolla, CA). The antibiotic zeocin was from Invitrogen.

3. Methods
3.1. Molecular Cloning of Cytokines into Transfer Plasmids

We have used two approaches in the molecular cloning of recombinant cytokines. When available, we have used cDNA as the source of DNA to be engineered into the *P. pastoris* transfer plasmid. When cDNA was unavailable, we constructed synthetic cDNA as described below *(8)*.

A

N-terminal primer

Invertase signal sequence   pTNFα sequence

           M L L Q A F L F L L A G F A A K I S A L R S S S.........

GCG GAT CC **ACC ATG** CTT TTG CAA GCT TTC CTT TTC CTT TTG GCT GGT TTT GCA GCC AAA ATA TCT GCA CTC AGA TCA TCG TCT CA

BamHI   Kozak

C-terminal primer

CG GAA TTC <u>TCA</u> CAG GGC AAT GAT CCC AA

   Eco RI   Stop

B

N-terminal Primer   Kex2   <u>Ste13</u>   <u>Ste13</u> mIL-17 Sequence

                                                               T V K A A A

5' ACA **CTC gAg** *AAA AgA gCT gAA gCT* <u>**ACT gTC AAg CT gCT gCT AT** 3'</u>

         Xho I

C-Terminal Primer

5' Cg **gAA TTC TCA** ggC AgC TTg TCT gAC AAT AgA 3'

     Eco R1   <u>**STOP**</u>

3.1.1. Secretion Signals and Recombinant Cytokine Processing

We used both the invertase and the α-factor sequences to direct the secretion of our recombinant cytokines. For cloning pTNFα cDNA into the pPIC9 plasmid, we employed an N-terminal primer that encoded the *Saccharomyces cerevisiae* invertase signal sequence *(9)* with a Kozak sequence at the N-terminal methionine *(10)* (**Fig. 3A**). The yeast alpha-factor signal sequence (included in the pPIC9 and pPICZ9 transfer vectors) was used for the other cytokines (**Fig. 3B**). When using these secretion signals, we engineered the first amino acid of the mature secreted cytokine to be directly downstream and in-frame with the last amino acid of the secretion signal. By designing the N-terminal primer in this manner, we are able to engineer the cytokine so that in many cases (pTNF-α, pIL-8, murine [m]IL-17, and hIL-17) the cytokine is secreted with the natural N-terminal amino acid (**Fig. 4**). For pIFN-γ and pIL-1β, there is incomplete processing of the glutamic-alanine residues of the α-factor signal sequence by the Ste13 protease (**Fig. 4**). The pIL-6 secreted protein is processed at a site that results in the removal of the first two amino acids of the predicted mature protein (**Fig. 4**). This "incorrect" processing of pIFN-γ, pIL-1β, and pIL-6 appears to be of little consequence, as these recombinant cytokines are biologically active.

3.1.2. Construction of the Expression Plasmids

Cytokine cDNAs for pIL-1β, pIL-6, and pIL-8 were amplified by PCR using primers with the appropriate restriction sites (*Xho*I and *Eco*RI) for the directional cloning into pPIZ9, in-frame with the α-factor signal sequence (pIL-6 was cloned into pPIC9) (**Fig. 3B**). The C-terminal primers encoded a stop codon to terminate translation after the last amino acid. The PCR product was purified using the Geneclean kit (Bio 101, Vista, CA), digested with *Xho*I and *Eco*RI, purified

---

Fig. 3. (**A**) PCR primers used for amplification of the pTNF-α cDNA to be cloned into pPIC9. The nucleotides of the Kozak sequence and the initiating methionine are shown in bold. The nucleotides of the translation stop codon are underlined. The amino acids of the invertase signal sequence are indicated by italics. Amino acids corresponding to mature pTNF-α are underlined. (**B**) PCR primers for amplification of the synthetic mIL-17 cDNA to be cloned into pPICZ9. The nucleotides of *Xho*I and *Eco*RI restriction sites (bold) were included in the primers so that the PCR-amplified hIL-17 sequence could be inserted into the pPICZ9 vector. Amino acids of the α-factor secretion signal that are downstream of the pPICZ9 *Xho*I site (italics) were encoded in-frame with the first six amino acids of mature mIL-17 (underlined) in the N-terminal primer. The Kex2 and Ste13 signal cleavage sites are indicated by arrows. The C-terminal primer encodes a stop codon after the codon for the last mIL-17 amino acid.

Porcine TNFα N-terminal Analysis
- Processing site of the Invertase signal/pTNFα protein
  AGFAAKISA LRSSSQTDK...
- Sequence analysis result

  LRSSSQTDK...

Porcine IL-8 N-terminal Analysis
- Processing sites of the α–factor/pIL-8 protein

  Kex2 Ste13 Ste13 Porcine IL-8
  VSLEKR EA EA ARVSAELRCQ...
- Sequence analysis result

  ARVSAELRCQ...

Murine IL-17 N-terminal Analysis
- Processing sites of the α-factor/mIL-17 protein

  Kex2 Ste13 Ste13 murine IL-17
  VSLEKR EA EA TVKAAAIIPQS...
- Sequence analysis result

  TVKAAAIIPQS...

Porcine IFNγ N-terminal Analysis
- Processing sites of the α–factor/pIFNγ protein

  Kex2 Ste13 Ste13 Porcine INFγ
  VSLEKR EA EA QAPFFKEITI
- Sequence analysis result

  n+4   EAEAQAPFFKEITI...
  n+2   EAQAPFFKEITI...

Porcine IL-6 N-terminal Analysis
- Processing sites of the α-Factor/pIL-6 protein

  Kex2 Ste13 Ste13 Porcine IL-6
  VSLEKR EA EA TPGRLEEDAKGD...
- Sequence analysis result

  n-2   GRLEEDAKGD...

Fig. 4. N-terminal sequence analysis of purified recombinant cytokines. The underlined amino acids are the predicted N-terminal amino acids for the mature cytokines.

again using the Geneclean kit, and ligated into the pPICZ9 plasmid vector, which had been digested with *Xho*I and *Eco*RI and treated with calf intestinal alkaline phosphatase. For cloning human and mouse IL-17, for which no cDNA was readily available, we constructed synthetic cDNAs by following the method of Dillon and Rosen *(6,8)*. Briefly, the hIL-17 and mIL-17 amino acid sequences were used to generate a set of six overlapping oligonucleotides (*see* **Note 1**), and a mixture of the oligonucleotides (60 ng each) was amplified in an eight-cycle PCR using *Pfu* polymerase to generate the complete coding sequence. The cDNA products of these reactions were amplified in a second round of PCR using primers (**Fig. 1**) with the appropriate restriction sites (*Xho*I and *Eco*RI) for the directional cloning into pPICZ9.

After ligation of the PCR products into the pPICZ9 plasmid, the ligation mixture was transformed into *E.coli* JM109, and colonies were selected on LB zeocin media. A clone containing the correct cytokine coding sequence in the transfer vector plasmid was identified by restriction digest analysis of the plasmid DNA and confirmed by sequencing the plasmid DNA using the 5' alcohol oxidase (AOX), 3'AOX, and α-factor primers available from Invitrogen. (*see* **Note 2** for potential problems).

3.2. Introduction of the Expression Plasmid into P. pastoris

3.2.1. Linearization of the Expression Plasmid

Once the correct DNA sequence of the expression plasmid is confirmed, the plasmid is then linearized and electroporated into the *P. pastoris* strain KM71H as described in the Invitrogen *Pichia* Expression Kit instruction manual (version D). Expression plasmids for cytokines cloned into pPIC9 (pIL-6 and pTNF-α) are linearized with *Sal*I, and cytokines cloned into pPICZ9 are linearized with *Sac*I or *Bst*XI.

3.2.2. Preparation of Competent Cells for Electroporation

1. Inoculate 5 mL BMGY medium with a single colony of *P. pastoris* and culture overnight at 30°C in a 50-mL tube with shaking at 250 rpm.
2. Transfer the 5-mL overnight culture into 200 mL of BMGY medium in a 2L-baffled flask, and incubate at 30°C with shaking at 250 rpm until the OD600 of the culture reaches 1–2.
3. Pellet the cells in 500-mL sterile centrifuge bottles at 500g at 10°C for 10 min.
4. Suspend the cell pellet with 500 mL of ice-cold, double-distilled sterile water.
5. Pellet the cells in 500-mL sterile centrifuge bottles at 500g at 10°C for 10 min.
6. Suspend the cell pellet with 50 mL of ice-cold, double-distilled sterile water.
7. Pellet the cells in a 50-mL sterile tube at 500g at 10°C for 10 min.
8. Suspend the cell pellet with 20 mL of ice-cold sterile 1 M sorbitol.
9. Pellet the cells in a 50-mL sterile tube at 500g at 10°C for 10 min.
10. Suspend the cell pellet with 1 mL of ice-cold sterile 1 M sorbitol, and store the cells on ice.

3.2.3. Transformation of P. pastoris by Electroporation

1. Add 5–20 µg of the linearized expression plasmid in a volume of 10 µL of water to a chilled 0.2-cm electroporation cuvet.
2. Add 80 µL of *P. pastoris* suspended in 1 *M* sorbitol to the cuvet, mixing carefully to avoid bubbles in suspension.
3. Store on ice for 5 min.
4. Pulse the cells as recommended by the manufacturer of the electroporation equipment. We use an Electroporator II (Invitrogen) with the capacitance set at 50 µF and the resistance set at 100 Ω.
5. Immediately after electroporation, place the cuvet on ice and add 0.5–1 mL ice-cold 1 *M* sorbitol.
6. Spread aliquots of the transformation mixture on selective plates containing 1 *M* sorbitol (YPD zeocin plates are used for pPICZ9-based plasmids, and MD plates are used for pPIC9-based plasmids). We suggest plating aliquots of 10, 50, and 100 µL of the electoporation cell suspension.
7. Incubate plates for 3 d at 30°C until colonies form.

3.3. Expression Clone Screening

The following method is used for screening clones for expression of the protein of interest.

1. Pick colonies and grow overnight in 50 mL of BMGY medium in 500-mL baffled flasks at 30°C with shaking at 225 rpm.
2. Pellet the cells (10 min at 4000*g*) and suspend in induction media containing methanol (BMMY).
3. Incubate the BMMY culture (30°C and 225 rpm) for 24–48 h. Feed the cultures with 0.1% (vol/vol) methanol at intervals of approx 12 h.
4. Pellet the cells and concentrate fivefold samples of culture media with a Centricon-10 ultrafiltration device (Millipore, Bedford, MA).
5. Examine the concentrated culture media samples by Coomassie stained sodium dodecyl sulfate-polyacrylamide gel electrophoresis (SDS-PAGE) gel, and identify clones producing the protein of interest by observation of a band of the appropriate size.
6. Confirm the identity of the protein by amino acid sequencing (*see* **Subheading 3.7.**).
7. Prepare a master clone stock by storing a fresh culture of the positive clone at –70°C in BMGY media containing 15% glycerol.

3.4. Shake-Flask Production of Recombinant Cytokines

1. Grow 500 mL BMGY medium shake-flask cultures of the *P. pastoris* expression clone overnight at 30°C in 2-L baffled flasks (225 rpm) to an OD600 of 15–20.
2. Pellet the cells by centrifugation (10 min at 4000*g*),and suspend in 100 mL of BMMY medium (containing 0.01% Antifoam 204 [Sigma, St. Louis, MO]) to induce cytokine production.
3. Because the methanol is metabolized by the cells, feed the cells by adding methanol to the BMMY (0.1% [vol/vol]) at 12–16-h intervals.

4. After 24–48 h of induction, remove the cells by centrifugation (10 min at 4200*g*) and clarify the cell-free medium containing the secreted cytokine by 0.2-μm filtration.

3.5. Purification of Recombinant Cytokines

The recombinant cytokines are typically purified to greater than 95% purity by using a combination of ion-exchange chromatography followed by gel-filtration (**Fig. 2**).

1. Dilute 2L of the 0.2-μm filtered media with an equal volume of 100 m*M* sodium citrate, pH 4.5.
2. Load the material onto 1 mL HiTrap SP or Q columns (Amersham Pharmacia, Piscataway, NJ) at a flow rate of 5 mL/min. Wash the column with 10 mL of citrate buffer. Elute the protein with 10 mL citrate buffer containing NaCl and collect in 1-mL fractions. The appropriate NaCl concentrations for the wash and elution buffers must be determined empirically, but they typically range from 50 to 1000 m*M*.
3. Examine the fractions by Coomassie stained SDS-PAGE, and pool those fractions containing the cytokine.
4. Further purify the pooled fractions by gel-filtration using a Sephacryl 100 26/60 column (Amersham Pharmacia) at a flow rate of 5 mL/min. Examine the fractions by Coomassie stained SDS-PAGE, and pool those fractions containing the cytokine.
5. *See* **Note 4** for particular problems with pIL-6.

3.6. Fermentation Production of Recombinant Cytokines

We perform 10-L fermentation as follows.

1. Grow a 500-mL starter culture of the expression clone overnight in BMGY at 30°C in a 2-L baffled flask (225 rpm) to an OD_{600} of 10–20.
2. Pellet the cells (10 min at 4200*g*) and suspend in 500 ml of base salt medium. Use these cells to inoculate 6.5 L of base salt fermentation medium in a 10-L fermentation vessel (BioFlo 3000; New Brunswick, Edison, NJ).
3. Add antifoam 204 (Sigma) to a final volume of 0.01%.
4. Maintain the following parameters during the fermentation; temperature at 30°C, dissolved oxygen at 30%, pH at 5.0, and agitation from 500 to 800 rpm.
5. Grow the *P. pastoris* culture as a batch culture for 20 h to an OD_{600} of 75–100. After this initial growth, add 50% glycerol to the vessel at a rate of 84 mL/h for a 20-h period. The resulting culture typically reaches an OD_{600} of over 150.
6. Induce the production of recombinant cytokine in these cells by the addition of 35 mL of methanol at a rate of 3.5 mL/min. Feed additional methanol at 7 mL/h for 24 h until the fermentation is stopped and the culture is pumped from the vessel.
7. Remove the cells from the culture by centrifugation (10 min at 4200*g*) and clarify the cell-free media containing the secreted cytokine by 0.2-μm filtration.
8. The clarified media is stored frozen at –20°C or processed immediately for purification using methods similar to those used for the shake-flask cultures except that larger chromatography columns are used.

3.7. Analysis of Processing of the Secretion Signal of the Recombinant Cytokines

N-terminal amino acid sequencing of the cytokines was performed by Edman chemistry. Protein samples for analysis are subjected to SDS-PAGE and electroblotted onto a PDVF membrane. The membrane is stained with Coomassie blue and the bands of interest are excised for analysis.

3.8. Glycosylation Analysis

Because *P. pastoris* is capable of both N-linked and O-linked glycosylation *(5)*, it is important to examine recombinant cytokines for glycosylation. N-linked glycosylation of the purified cytokines was examined by digestion of the sample with peptide-*N*-glycosidase F (PNGase F; Glyco,Novato, CA) (**Fig. 1**). O-linked glycosylation of the purified cytokines was examined by digestion of the sample with *N*-acetyl neuraminidase (NANase) and *O*-glycosidase (Glyco). (We did not observe O-linked glycosylation of any of the recombinant cytokines.) The digestions were performed overnight at 30°C in the buffer conditions suggested by Glyco.

3.9. Protein Concentration Determination

Accurate determination of cytokine protein concentration is essential, particularly when these proteins are used to calibrate enzyme-linked immunosorbent assays (ELISAs). The BCA method, Bradford method, or Lowry method may be used to estimate protein concentration. However, such methods rely on the calibration of a standard curve of bovine serum albumin or a similar protein. Because the protein of interest may behave differently than the standards in these assays, the results provide only an estimate of true protein concentration.

We have obtained reliable results of protein concentration by measuring the absorbance at 280 nm in 6 *M* guanidine HCl. The extinction coefficient for the protein can be calculated using a program available at the Swiss Prot website (http://expasy.hcuge.ch/sprot/protparam.html), which uses the method of Gill and von Hippel *(11)*. For this method to be reliable, it is necessary that the protein preparation be free of other proteins or substances that have absorbance at 280 nm (such as the "brown stuff" contaminant; *see* **Note 3**). When we compared the concentrations calculated using absorbance at 280 nm with the concentrations determined by the BCA method (Pierce) or Bradford method (Pierce, Rockford, IL) (using bovine serum albumin as a standard), we found that all methods gave similar results (values typically differ by 20%).

3.10. Molecular Weight Determination

The apparent molecular weight of recombinant cytokines was determined using precast 4–20% acrylamide gels (Novex, San Diego, CA). Proteins for use as molecular weight markers were purchased from New England Biolabs (Beverly, MA).

The apparent molecular weight of the cytokines in solution was determined by gel-filtration chromatography. The elution volume of a 100-μL sample of purified purified cytokine was measured on a Superdex 75 column (10×30 cm) (Pharmacia) run at a flow rate 0.5 mL/min. This column was calibrated with blue dextran, ribonuclease A, chymotrypsinogen, ovalbumin, and albumin (Pharmacia).

3.11. Lyophilization of Cytokines

Lyophilization is a commonly employed method to preserve recombinant proteins. Samples of purified cytokines were lyophilized after the addition of trehalose to a final concentration of 15%. Because lyophilization can affect the structure and activity of proteins, it is important to confirm that the recombinant cytokine has similar biologic activity before and after lyophilization. It is also important to check that lyophilization does not lead to aggregation of the recombinant cytokines. Therefore we used gel-filtration chromatography as an analytical method to determine the molecular weight of the preparation.

4. Notes

1. One strategy to increase protein expression levels is to alter the DNA sequence of the gene to utilize yeast codon preferences. We have not found evidence to support this approach. When constructing synthetic genes we have chosen for the preferred codons for *S. cerevisiae (12)*. Although we have not performed direct study of the effect of mammalian and yeast codons on expression levels, we have consistently observed comparable expression levels whether proteins were encoded using mammalian or yeast codons preferences (**Table 1**).

2. When screening *E. coli* clones that were transformed with plasmids generated from the ligation of pIL-6 and pTNF-α into the pPIC9 expression vector, we observed altered plasmids that lacked approx 5 kb of sequence. Although these plasmids often contained the cytokine insert, they lacked vector sequences that are needed for successful introduction into *P. pastoris*. These rearrangements of pPIC9-based plasmids were seen in approx 50% of transformants. We never observed this problem when using the pPICZ9 plasmid vector.

3. We, and other users of the *Pichia* system, have observed the copurification of a contaminant that we call "brown stuff." During the initial purifications of pTNF-α, we observed a faint brown color associated with the TNF-α protein. Analysis by Coomassie stained SDS-PAGE of this preparation showed only the TNF-α protein.

However, careful examination of these gels showed a brown band that migrated at the dye front. Although SDS-PAGE showed that the brown contaminant was smaller than the TNF-α, it was not removed during gel-filtration—indicating that it was "sticking" to the TNF-α. Further evidence that the brown contaminant was binding to the TNF-α was found when the TNF-α band was blotted onto nitrocellulose and analyzed by N-terminal amino acid sequencing. This N-terminal sequencing showed that, in addition to the expected TNF-α sequence, a contaminating sequence was detected. The sequence of the contaminant matched that of collagen. We also performed N-terminal sequencing on a blot of the brown material migrating near the dye front of the gel. This material had the same "collagen-like" sequence. We hypothesized that the most probable source of the "collagen-like" material was the peptone that is a component of the BMGY and BMMY media is peptone; peptone contains large amounts of collagen fragments. When we prepare pTNF-α in fermentation media (which contains no peptone, and thus no collagen), we find that the TNF-α preparation does not have a brown color, nor do we detect collagen fragments by N-terminal sequencing.

Because we wished to develop purification methods for cytokines using BMGY and BMMY media in shake-flasks, it was important to develop purification methods that would eliminate the copurification of the collagen fragments. The simple elimination of peptone from the BMMY media was not an option, as we found that this greatly reduced the yield of protein. We did find that purification methods that exposed the protein and BMMY medium to high salt concentrations drove the association of the protein and the collagen fragments together. By avoiding high concentrations of ammonium sulfate and NaCl, we found that the collagen fragments did not bind to the TNF-α. By following the purification methods described in **Subheading 3.5.**, we produced recombinant cytokines without any collagen contamination. However, we caution *P. pastoris* users to be alert for such contamination.

4. The aggregation of secreted protein posed a challenge during the production of rat IL-6. This cytokine was secreted into media at levels equal to 100 mg per liter. Cation exchange chromatography produced protein that was greater than 95% pure by SDS-PAGE. Unfortunately, gel-filtration revealed that this protein had formed aggregates found in the void volume. Despite changes in media, buffer ionic strength, and purification protocols, we were unable to avoid this aggregation problem. pIL 6 also exhibited a tendency to form high-molecular-weight aggregates. However, for this protein, avoidance of high-ionic-strength buffers and protein concentrations above 500 µg/mL prevented the formation of aggregates.

These two examples of cytokine aggregation demonstrate the benefit of including gel-filtration as both an analytical tool and a purification method. It is also important to examine cytokine solutions that have been prepared from lyophilized preparations for aggregation.

Acknowledgments

This work was supported in part by USDA award 97-33610-4031.

References

1. Ratner, M. (1989) Protein expression in yeasts. *Biotechnology* **7,** 1129–1133.
2. Cregg, J. M., Verdick, T. S., and Raschke, W. C. (1993) Recent advances in the expression of foreign genes in *Pichia pastoris*. *Biotechnology* **11,** 905–910.
3. Buckholz, R. G. and Gleeson, M. A. G. (1991) Yeast systems for the commercial production of heterlogous proteins. *Biotechnology* **9,** 1067–1072.
4. Grinna, L. S. and Tschopp, J. F. (1989) Size distrubution and general structural features of N-linked oligosaccharides from the methyltrophic yeast, *Pichia pastoris. Yeast* **5,** 107–115.
5. Kukuruzinska, M. A., Bergh, M. L. E., and Jackson, B. J. (1987) Protein gylcosylation in yeast. *Annu. Rev. Biochem.* **56,** 915–944.
6. Murphy, K. P., Gagne, P., Pazmany, P., and Moody, M. D. (1998). Expression of human interleukin-17 in Pichia pastoris: purification and characterization. *Protein Exp. Purif.* **12,** 208–214.
7. Siegel, R. S. and Brierley, R. A. (1989) Methylotophic yeast *Pichia pastoris* produced in high-density fermentations with high cell yields as a vehicle for recombinant protein production. *Biotechnol. Bioeng.* **34,** 403–404.
8. Dillon, P. J. and Rosen, C. A. (1990) A rapid method for the construction of synthetic genes using the polymerase chain reaction. *Biotechniques* **9,** 299–300.
9. Tsschopp, J. F., Sverlow, G., Kosson, R., Craig, W., and Grinna, L. (1987) High level secretion of glycosylated inveratse in the methylotrophic yeast *Pichia pastoris. Biotechnology* **5,** 1305–1308.
10. Kozak, M. (1984) Compilation and analysis of sequences upstream from the translational start site in eukaryotic mRNAs. *Nucleic Acids Res.* **12,** 857–872.
11. Gill, S. C. and von Hippel, P. H. (1989) Calculation of protein extinction coefficients from amino acid sequence data. *Anal. Biochem.* **182,** 319–326.
12. Bennetzen, J. L. and Hall, B. D. (1982). Codon selection in yeast. *J. Biol. Chem.* **257,** 3026–3031.

35

Analysis of Single Nucleotide Polymorphisms in the Interleukin-1B Gene Using 5' Nuclease Assays

Emad M. El-Omar

1. Introduction

Interleukins are soluble peptide molecules that mediate the interaction between immunocompetent and haematopoietic cells and between the immune and neuroendocrine systems *(1)*. They are produced by a variety of activated cells and exert their biological activities by binding to specific receptors on target cells. Interleukin-1β is the archetypal pleiotropic cytokine being produced by many cells and exerting its biological effects on almost all cell types *(2)*. Interleukin-1β is a very potent proinflammatory cytokine and is involved in the host's response to many antigenic challenges.

Recently, it has become apparent that genetic polymorphisms in many genes could account for inter-individual variations in the expression of the genes' products. Most genomic variation is attributable to single nucleotide polymorphisms (SNPs) which are stable biallelic sequence variants distributed at a frequency of approx 1 in every 1000 base pairs throughout the genome. Using association and linkage studies, SNPs have been utilized in mapping disease genes, tracking population history and exploring human identity. A range of high-throughput methods for typing SNPs is now widely available *(3)*. These include PCR followed by restriction fragment length polymorphism analysis (PCR-RFLP), single-strand conformation polymorphism (SSCP), heteroduplex analysis, DNA chips, and primer extension. The major disadvantage of these methods is their dependence on post-PCR molecular biology steps and most require some form of gel or capillary electrophoresis. Two recent methods, 5' nuclease assays and molecular beacons, obviate the need for post-PCR molecular biology steps and the need for electrophoresis as allelic

From: *Methods in Molecular Medicine, vol. 60: Interleukin Protocols*
Edited by: L. A. J. O'Neill and A. Bowie © Humana Press Inc., Totowa, NJ

discrimination occurs during the PCR. In this chapter, we discuss the 5'
fluorogenic nuclease assay (TaqMan), which in our experience offers the best
and most economical high throughput SNP genotyping method. As an example
of the use of this technology, we will describe the genotyping of three SNPs
within the interleukin-1B *(IL-1B)* gene *(4)*. These biallelic polymorphisms
represent C-T base transitions at positions -511, -31 and +3954 base pairs from
the transcriptional start site.

1.2. Principle Behind Allelic Discrimination Using 5' Nuclease Assays

For biallelic systems, each 5' nuclease assay requires the design of two
fluorogenic allele-specific probes *(5–7)*. The probes are selected so that one
matches the wild-type sequence (traditionally designated allele 1), and the other
matches the mutant sequence (designated allele 2). The 5' end of each probe is
labeled with a fluorescent reporter dye and at the 3' end with the quencher dye
6-carboxytetramethylrhodamine (TAMRA). In our experience, best results
were obtained by using 6-carboxyfluorescein (FAM) as the reporter dye for the
wild-type sequence and VIC for the mutant sequence *(8)*. In the PE Biosystems
TaqMan platform, the reporter dye VIC has recently replaced the reporter dyes
JOE (2,7-dimethoxy-4,5-dichloro-6-carboxyfluorescein) and HEX (hexachloro-
6-carboxyfluorescein) because VIC has a more equivalent intensity to that of
FAM and because its narrower spectrum has less overlap with FAM. Both quali-
ties improve signal processing and thus allelic discrimination *(9)*. In solution,
the proximity of the dyes on each intact probe allows the quencher (TAMRA) to
absorb energy from the reporter dye through fluorescent resonance energy
transfer. During PCR amplification, the fluorogenic probe is cleaved by the 5'
nuclease activity of the *Taq* polymerase thus liberating the reporter dye and causing an increase in its fluorescence intensity *(5)*. An increase in reporter fluorescence indicates that the probe-specific target has been amplified. Mismatches
between a probe and its target sequence reduce probe hybridization efficiency
and subsequent cleavage. An allele is detected as significantly increased intensity of its reporter dye over background. The fluorescence dye 6-carboxy-X-
rhodamine (ROX) is included in each assay to normalise 2 variation in signal
strength among wells *(8)*. Using the example above, a significant increase
in FAM or VIC fluorescent signal indicates homozygosity for the FAM- or
VIC-specific allele. If both signals are increased, this indicates heterozygosity.

The fluorescence is measured post-PCR using the ABI PRISM® 7700
Sequence Detection System. In addition to having a built-in thermal cycler, the
7700 system has a 488 nm laser directed via fiber optic cables to each of the 96
sample wells. The laser excites the dyes and the fluorescence emission travels
back through the cables to a CCD camera detector. For each sample, the CCD

camera collects the emission data between 520 nm and 660 nm once every few seconds. This range encompasses the peak emission wavelengths of FAM (535 nm), VIC (550 nm) and TAMRA (580 nm), and ROX (605 nm). The system measures fluorescence directly in the PCR reaction tubes (96-well plates with optical caps specifically designed for high optical transmission). The Sequence Detection System (SDS) software analyses the data by first calculating the contribution of each component dye to the experimental spectrum. The reporter signal is then normalised to the fluorescence of an internal reference dye. These internal controls are based on reactions run on the same plate that contain no DNA template (NTC), and known allele 1 and allele 2 templates. Scores for alleles 1 and 2 are then calculated on a scale of 0–1, and these scores are finally normalized for extent of reaction. The final output plot identifies four distinct clusters of samples: homozygotes for allele 1 (1,1), homozygotes for allele 2 (2,2), heterozygotes (1,2), and no amplification samples (No Amp) *(5)*. These clusters are visually defined by genotype-specific colors.

2. Materials

2.1. Reagents

1. TaqMan® universal PCR master mix: This reagent is suitable for all TaqMan DNA applications including allelic discrimination. It is supplied in a 2X concentration and contains AmpliTaq Gold" DNA polymerase, AmpErase" UNG, Passive Reference 1, and optimized proprietary buffer components. Recommended storage conditions are 2–8°C, enabling use direct from the refrigerator. In the 25 µL PCR reaction volume, the final concentration of the TaqMan master mix is 1X.
2. Primers (Operon Technologies) and probes (PE Biosystems) were designed using the Primer Express software supplied by PE Biosystems. The method for designing primers and probes is provided in **Subheading 3**. The primer and probe sequences used for the three *IL-1B* biallelic polymorphisms are given in **Fig. 1**. For all three *IL-1B* assays, the optimal final probe and primer concentrations were 200 nmol/L and 900 nmol/L, respectively.
3. DNA samples used in our studies were genomic in origin and were collected from ongoing epidemiological studies on the pathogenesis of gastric cancer *(4)*.
4. MicroAmp® optical 96-well reaction plates and optical caps.

2.2. Hardware

The ABI PRISM 7700 Sequence Detector provides the instrumentation for detecting the fluorescent signal during thermal cycling. If the reaction is run real-time, the 7700-s built-in thermal cycler must be used. However, for most established and robust assays, the thermocycling could be performed on any PCR machine with the 7700 being used for endpoint analysis only. This has the advantage of increasing throughput to a great extent. We used the real-time function during the initial stages of optimizing and validating the assays.

IL-1B-31

Probes

IL-1B-31 (C)   5'-TCG CTG TTT TTA TGG CTT TCA AAA GCA G-3'

IL-1B-31 (T)   5'-CCT CGC TGT TTT TAT AGC TTT CAA AAG CAG A-3'

Primers

IL-1B-31-F   5'-CCC TTT CCT TTA ACT TGA TTG TGA-3'

IL-1B-31-R   5'-GGT TTG GTA TCT GCC AGT TTC TC-3'

IL-1B-511

Probes

IL-1B-511 (C)   5'-TGT TCT CTG CCT CGG GAG CTC TCT G-3'

IL-1B-511 (T)   5'-CTG TTC TCT GCC TCA GGA GCT CTC TGT C-3'

Primers

IL-1B-511-F   5'-TCC TCA GAG GCT CCT GCA AT-3'

IL-1B-511-R   5'-TGT GGG TCT CTA CCT TGG GTG-3'

IL-1B+3954

Probes

IL-1B+3954(C)   5'-CAG AAC CTA TCT TCT TCG ACA CAT GGG ATA AC-3'

IL-1B+3954(T)   5'-CAG AAC CTA TCT TCT TTG ACA CAT GGG ATA ACG-3'

Primers

IL-1B+3954-F   5'-CCT AAA CAA CAT GTG CTC CAC ATT-3'

IL-1B+3954-R   5'-TGC ATC GTG CAC ATA AGC CT-3'

Fig. 1. *IL-1B* TaqMan probe and primer sequences.

The real-time function is also essential during the phase of defining allelic control samples as described later. Once the assay was optimized and allelic controls were available, we used the GeneAmp PCR System 9700 (PE Biosystems) for thermocycling and the 7700 for endpoint analysis only (*see* **Note 1**).

3. Methods
3.1. Designing TaqMan® Probes and Primers

The Primer Express software (PE Biosystems) guides the user through the various steps of probe and primer design. The user imports the working DNA sequence (in any format) into the software and most of the subsequent steps are self-explanatory. There are a number of important criteria that have to be satisfied in order to maximize success of the assay. Most of these are selected automatically by the software, but the user must manually satisfy a few others (italicized), as described below. These criteria are derived from the PE Biosystems literature that accompanies the SDS software *(9)*.

3.1.1. Criteria for Selecting Allelic Discrimination Probe Sequences

1. Ensure that the polymorphic site *lies in the middle one-third of the probe* and preferably equidistant from the 5' and 3' ends.
2. No G on the 5' end. This is because a G adjacent to the reporter dye may quench reporter fluorescence even after cleavage.
3. Choose the strand with a probe containing *more Cs than Gs*. The choice of probes with no more than 3 contiguous Gs increases the reaction yield because it avoids relatively stable secondary structures when 4 or more contiguous Gs are found.
4. Primer Express software selects probe T_m of 65–67°C, which has to be 7°C greater than matched primer T_ms, as determined by the nearest neighbor algorithm implemented in Primer Express.
5. Design separate probes for each of the two alleles. *Match the T_m of the two probes as closely as possible, but no more than 1.0°C apart.* This eliminates any preferential hybridization and subsequent probe cleavage due to a low T_m. Primer Express will select a single reporter as above, but the polymorphism and subsequent allele 2 probe must be designed manually.

3.1.2. Criteria for Selecting Allelic Discrimination Primer Sequences

The primers are chosen after the probes.

1. Select the forward and reverse primers to be *as close as possible to the probe* without overlapping it. The aim is to obtain the shortest possible amplicon (minimum 50 bp, maximum 150 bp). Shorter amplicons will amplify more efficiently than longer amplicons and this ensures a robust assay that yields reproducible results.
2. Primer Express T_m of 58–60°C.
3. The five nucleotides at the 3' end should only have 1–2 G + Cs. This decreases the stability of the 3' ends in order to reduce nonspecific priming.

3.2. Thermocycling Conditions

The thermal cycling profile was the two-temperature PCR recommended by the manufacturer. This profile ensures that the probe is hybridized to the template during the extension phase of the PCR. The thermocycling parameters were as follows: 50°C for 2 min and 95°C for 10 min, followed by 40 cycles of 95°C for 15 s and 62°C for 1 min.

3.3. Performing the TaqMan Assay

1. Dilute the primer stocks to 100 mM. The probes are supplied at a standard concentration of 100 μM. The volumes of reagents needed to perform the assay are provided in **Table 1**. The volumes are provided for a single PCR reaction, for a plate of 96 samples, and for multiples of that. Because of pipeting loss, it is essential to add enough reagents for more than 96 samples per plate, hence the figures in **Table 1** (*see* **Note 2**).

2. Prepare the master PCR mix by adding the appropriate volumes of TaqMan® universal PCR master mix, probes and primers. Vortex the mix and cover the tube with aluminium foil while keeping on ice (the fluorescent dyes are light sensitive).

3. Transfer two equal aliquots (for nine PCR reactions each) of this master mix to separate tubes labelled "allele 1" and "allele 2" and add the appropriate control DNA. For a 96-well plate, eight wells will serve as "allele 1" controls and another eight wells as "allele 2" controls. Use 50 ng of control DNA per PCR reaction, which should be similar to the unknown DNA samples' concentrations.

4. Using a multi-channel pipet, aliquot 25 μL of the master mix into the first eight wells of the 96-well plate (vertical or horizontal). These eight wells contain no DNA and act as the "no template control" (NTC) for the assay (*see* **Note 3**).

5. Aliquot 25 μL of "allele 1" control DNA into the next eight wells and repeat for "allele 2" control DNA.

6. This leaves 72 wells with the unknown DNA samples. Assuming the unknown DNA has already been aliquoted onto the plate, simply add master mix to make up the final reaction volume of 25 μL. The use of an automated multi-channel pipet saves considerable time and effort. There is no need to reconstitute the DNA with DH$_2$O before adding the master mix (*see* **Note 4**).

7. Apply the optical caps securely. It is advisable to centrifuge the plates briefly to ensure that the contents are thoroughly mixed.

8. Place the plates in the thermocycler. If running on the 7700, use the real-time mode. Using the allelic discrimination software, define a template that is identical to the layout of the samples on the plate and start the process. At the end of thermocycling (approx 2 h), save the output and analyze the real-time data. The plate can also be endpoint read, which will provide the output with the four clusters described earlier. Obtain a hard copy of the results and also save an electronic version that could be e-mailed or saved into a database for subsequent analysis (*see* **Notes 5–7**).

9. If running on an ordinary thermocycler, the plate will need to be read on the 7700 using the endpoint function. Again, use a template that is identical to the layout

Table 1
Volume of Reagents Needed for the TaqMan Allelic Discrimination Assays[a]

	1 PCR	1 Plate (100 PCR's)[b]	6 Plates (600 PCR's)[b]
PCR Master Mix (2X)	12.5 mL	1250 mL	7500 mL
DH$_2$O[c]	12.05 mL	1205 mL	7230 mL
Primers	0.2 mL each	20 mL	120 mL
Probes	0.025 mL each	2.5 mL	15 mL
DNA[c]	variable		
Total PCR volume	25 μL		

[a]Having such a table displayed in the lab allows for more efficient use of time and reagents. Calculate the volumes for the most frequent number of plates prepared at one time.
[b]Add enough for 100 PCRs per plate to overcome the inevitable pipeting loss.
[c]Assuming DNA (50 ng) has been preapplied and dried onto the plate. If DNA is applied fresh, subtract its volume from that of the DH$_2$O.

of the samples on the plate. It is essential that the position of the controls is accurate, i.e. the machine must be told which samples correlate with NTC, AL1, and AL2. If the plate has some empty wells, these should be labeled as "not in use" and not as unknowns, as this will affect the accuracy of all the results. Save the data as described above (*see* **Notes 5–7**).

4. Notes

1. For a novel assay, the most important technical aspect is the quality of the allelic discrimination. By following the criteria for probe and primer design outlined in **Subheading 3.1.**, most assays will work well, even with the first set of probes and primers. Some minor adjustments of probe and primer concentrations may be required. During this initial optimization phase, the assay has to be run in real-time mode. In that mode, there is no absolute requirement for having defined allelic controls on the plate. Each sample is read separately and its dye fluorescence profile allows the genotype to be called manually. As such, one can genotype a panel of DNA samples and select the "best" homozygous control samples for both alleles. This obviates the need to define these controls by other time-consuming methods such as SSCP or PCR-RFLP. In our lab, we use a panel of 96 DNA samples (for which cell lines have been created ensuring continuous supply of DNA) to define controls for all our TaqMan assays. If the SNP is reasonably frequent, we invariably find 1,1 and 2,2 samples among this panel. We select the appropriate control samples (two or three of each homozygous genotype) and submit them for sequencing to confirm the genotypes. Once confirmed, these samples could be used as the controls for all subsequent assays. If one is lucky, an assay could be successfully set up and optimised in less than 48 h. The time wastage occurs waiting for delivery of the probes (7–10 d) and primers (1–3 d).

2. As with any assay involving large numbers of samples, care has to be taken when pipeting samples and reagents. One sample out of phase could destroy many a promising hypothesis! It is essential to have extra controls on each plate. One approach would be to include water samples (instead of DNA samples) at defined positions on the plate and to run duplicate samples from the same and different plates.

3. To maximize efficiency for each TaqMan assay, a large number of 96-well plates could be prepared by addition of the PCR mix, primers and probe and then frozen at −70°C. Depending on how many PCR machines are available in the lab, these plates could then be processed appropriately. This saves technician time (because there is only one preparation stage) and maximises the efficiency of the lab. We have tested many TaqMan assays in such manner and found no difference between preprepared frozen plates and freshly prepared ones. Because several thermal cyclers can be used in parallel and plates can be read on the PRISM 7700 using SDS software in endpoint mode, hundreds of samples can be processed daily by a single technician.

4. For high-throughput genotyping, the DNA samples should be aliquoted on 96-well plates. Dilute the stock DNA to 10 ng/µL and aliquot 5 µL per well, giving 50 ng of DNA per PCR reaction. The DNA plates should be left to dry and could then be stored for many months in a cold room. On the day of assay, addition of the PCR mix reconstitutes the DNA sample. We find this the most efficient way of running large numbers of samples.

5. When reading the plates on the 7700, one occasionally obtains samples, or clusters of samples, that are clearly mislabeled by the machine. For example, the entire 1,2 cluster may be colored red (falsely indicating that it is 1,1), but its position is clearly where one expects to see the 1,2 samples and they are distinct from the 1,1 cluster. By checking the dye and allele components, one could easily confirm that the software mislabelled these samples and corrections could be easily made. It is essential that the corrected version is saved and electronically transferred at the time of the corrections. Unfortunately, these changes are not saved if the plate is read on another occasion or if the data is blindly transferred without checking for these mistakes.

6. Occasionally, the 7700 is unable to call a particular sample, which is then labeled as No Amp. If the real-time data is available, one could manually call some of these samples. The true No Amps are most often from poor quality or degraded DNA. It is also interesting to note that most No Amps tend to be heterozygotes, leading to heterozygote deficiency and problems with Hardy-Weinberg disequilibrium.

7. Some samples appear as outliers and these pose a particular problem. The genotype could be accurately deduced from real-time data but if the assay was only endpoint read, this will not be possible. The most common cause of these outlying samples is DNA concentration. Not infrequently, these samples will be either too dilute or too concentrated, and one could overcome the problem by manipulating the DNA concentration. In the difficult cases, it may be necessary to use sequencing to deduce the genotype.

References

1. Fridman, W. H., and E. Tartour. (1997) Cytokines and cell regulation. *Mol. Aspects Med.* **18,** 3–90.
2. Dinarello, C. A. (1996) Biologic basis for interleukin-1 in disease. *Blood* **87,** 2095–2147.
3. Landegren, U., Nilsson, M., and Kwok, P. Y. (1998) Reading bits of genetic information: methods for single-nucleotide polymorphism analysis *Genome Res.* **8,** 769–776.
4. El-Omar, E. M., Carrington, M., Chow, W. H., McColl, K. E., Bream, J. H., Young, H. A., et al. (2000) Interleukin-1 polymorphisms associated with increased risk of gastric cancer. *Nature* **404,** 398–402.
5. Livak, K. J. (1999) Allelic discrimination using fluorogenic probes and the 5' nuclease assay. *Genet. Anal.* **14,** 143–149.
6. Livak, K. J., Flood, S. J., Marmaro, J., Giusti, W., and Deetz, K. (1995) Oligonucleotides with fluorescent dyes at opposite ends provide a quenched probe system useful for detecting PCR product and nucleic acid hybridization PCR. *Methods Appl.* **4,** 357–362.
7. Livak, K. J., Marmaro, J., and Todd, J. A. (1995) Towards fully automated genome-wide polymorphism screening. *Nat. Genet.* **9,** 341–342.
8. Yuan, C. C., Peterson, R. J., Wang, C. D., Goodsaid, F., and Waters, D. J. (2000) 5' nuclease assays for the Loci CCR5-+/{Delta}32, CCR2-V64I, and SDF1-G801A related to pathogenesis of AIDS. *Clin. Chem.* **46,** 24–30.
9. PE Applied Biosystems. (1998) *Multiplex PCR with TaqMan VIC Probes.* User Bulletin No. 5. Foster City, CA.

36

Measurement of Cytokine and Chemokine Gene Expression Patterns Using cDNA Array

Zheng-Ming Wang and Roman Dziarski

1. Introduction

The purpose of the gene array techniques is to simultaneously analyze the expression or characteristics of a large number of genes (1–3). These techniques can be used to compare gene expression in various cells or in the same cells following various treatments, to analyze function of multiple genes sequenced in the human and other genome projects, to discover new genes, to detect mutations or gene polymorphism, to identify genes responsible for disease processes, to diagnose diseases, to monitor therapy, or to develop new therapies (1–17). When the human genome project is completed and when the entire human cDNA library becomes available on an array, it will be possible to identify all the genes that are expressed in a given cell type.

1.1. Principle of the Assay

The principle of the assay is based on hybridization of complementary nucleic acid sequences (**Fig. 1**):

1. RNA is extracted from tissue.
2. cDNA probe complementary to RNA, labeled with fluorescent dyes, biotin, or ^{32}P or ^{33}P, is synthesized.
3. Different target DNA sequences are immobilized in a grid-like or a dot-like pattern on a solid support (commercially available glass chips or membrane arrays).
4. The labeled cDNA probe is hybridized to the chip or the membrane and washed.
5. Hybridization of complementary sequences is detected based on the fluorescent or radioactive signal at the site of hybridization.

From: *Methods in Molecular Medicine, vol. 60: Interleukin Protocols*
Edited by: L. A. J. O'Neill and A. Bowie © Humana Press Inc., Totowa, NJ

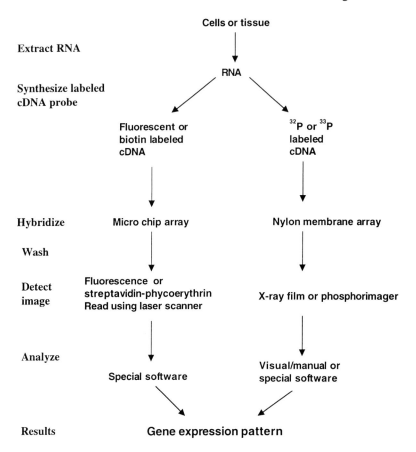

Fig. 1. Analysis of gene expression using micro-chip cDNA arrays *(left)* or membrane cDNA arrays *(right)*.

1.2. Types of DNA Arrays

The DNA array technology was basically developed from the nuclear run-on and dot or slot blot methods *(18)*, by combining standard nucleic acid hybridization with modern DNA chip technology *(1–3)*. DNA chip technology was initially developed for the genome sequencing project. Construction of DNA chips is based on the ability to attach nucleic acids to a solid matrix (usually a small glass or silicon chip) in a precise location in a form of a densely arranged array (containing as many as 100,000 different oligonucleotides), using a high-throughput robot. This arrangement of so many genes on a small chip allows simultaneous screening of a very large number of genes with a large number of probes in a very small volume *(1–3)*. The construction of these chips, however, is expensive, detection of DNA hybridization to these chips requires the use of specialized instruments (usually based on confocal laser scanning technology), and analysis of the data requires sophisticated computer programs (**Table 1**).

Several simpler versions of the DNA arrays have also been developed (**Table 1**), in which a few hundred to a few thousand DNA sequences are spotted on a nylon membrane, to which hybridization can be detected by simple autoradiography or phosphorimaging *(14,17)*. Currently, approx 20 different biotechnology companies offer a variety of DNA arrays designed for various applications (**Table 2**). These arrays can be classified into two groups (**Table 1**): chip arrays (microarrays), which typically contain thousands to tens of thousands of gene sequences and include both known and unknown (EST) sequences, and membrane-based arrays, which usually contain lower number of genes and are often targeted for a specific application (e.g., cytokine and chemokine array by R&D Systems, Minneapolis, MN). Some large membrane arrays or a series of small membranes, that contain large numbers of genes (similar to microchip arrays) are also available.

1.3. Overview of the Atlas cDNA Array for Detection of Cytokine Gene Expression in Monocytes

In this chapter, we will describe the use of a commercial 600 gene human Atlas cDNA array (Clontech, Palo Alto, CA) for detection of a gene expression pattern in human monocytes stimulated with bacteria or interferon-γ *(17)*. We have selected this array because it can provide information on the differential expression of a large number of known genes in cells exposed to various stimuli, yet it is relatively simple to use, inexpensive, and does not require special equipment for detection of hybridization and analysis of data (*see* **Note 1**).

The array consists of 588 inducible human cDNAs, 9 housekeeping control cDNAs, and 3 negative control DNA immobilized on a nylon membrane (**Fig. 2A**). In the first step (**Fig. 1**), RNA is extracted from control (unstimulated) monocytes, or monocytes that have been treated with various stimuli. In the second step, labeled cDNA probe is synthesized by reverse transcribing RNA in the presence of [α-^{32}P]dATP, using the cDNA Primer Mix, that contains a mixture of primers specific for the genes contained in this array. This primer mix ensures that cDNAs are only synthesized for the genes that are included in this array. The third step is hybridization of the labeled probe to the array membrane, followed by high-stringency wash. The fourth step is detection of hybridization by autoradiography or phosphorimaging. The last step is quantification of results and analysis of data.

Table 1
Comparison of Gene Array Techniques

Array type	Features/company	Advantages	Disadvantages
Microchip arrays	5000 to 30,000 genes on small glass or silicon slide chips	Can analyze a large number of both known and unknown (EST) genes in one assay with a small amount of probe. The companies offer custom service for reading and analyzing the arrays.	Fluorescent labeling efficiency is lower tha▮ radioactive labeling. The arrays are expensive produce and read. They have to be read usi▮ an expensive laser confo▮ scanning instrument, a▮ the data have to be analy▮ by special software. Usually the chip can be hybridized only once.
	Usually use fluorescent labeling		
	Affymetrix Hyseq Molecular Dynamics		
Membrane arrays	Single membranes or multiple sets of membranes. Small (5 × 7 cm) to large (22 × 22 cm) contain 100–30,000 genes. Series of several membranes can contain up to 100,000 genes. Contain either known genes (general or tissue-, cell-, or function -specific) or both known and unknown genes (EST).	Radioactive labeling efficiency is much higher than the fluorescent labeling. Arrays that contain fewer genes, do not require special equipment, and are less expensive. Can be done in any laboratory and developed using X-ray film or phosphorimager. Data can be analyzed visually or with standard image analysis software. Arrays that contain large numbers of genes require special software to analyze results. Membrane can be rehybridized at least 5 times. Special software also available, e.g., AtlasImage (Clontech), or Array Vision (Imaging Research).	Analyzing large numbers of genes without special equipment and softwar▮ is very laborious. Using special equipmen▮ and software significan▮ adds to the cost.
	Usually use radioactive labeling.		
	Research Genetics Clontech R&D Systems Genome Systems		

2. Materials

2.1. Atlas Human cDNA Expression Array Kit (Clontech)

This kit contains two sheets of the array membrane, which consist of 588 human cDNAs, 9 housekeeping control cDNAs, and three negative control plasmid and bacteriophage DNA immobilized on a 8 × 12 cm nylon membrane in duplicate dots (**Fig. 2A**). Each cDNA fragment is a 200–600 bp unique sequence of various

Table 2
Commercially Available Gene Arrays[a]

Company	Array format	Labeling/readout	Applications
Affymetrix Santa Clara, CA www.affymetrix.com	On-chip photolithographic synthesis of oligos onto silicon wafers	Fluorescence	Expression profiles, disease management, gene polymorphism
Brax Cambridge, UK	Short oligos synthesized off-chip	Mass spectrometry	Diagnostics, expression profiles, novel gene identification
Clontech Palo Alto, CA www.clontech.com	cDNA immobilized onto nylon membranes	Radioisotope	Differential gene expression for cellular pathways and targeted research
Genetic MicroSystems Woburn, MA (Affymetrix) www.geneticmicro.com	Surface tension spotting onto slides with ping-and-ring technology	Fluorescence	Highly parallel genomic research and drug discovery
Genome Systems St. Louis, MO (Icyte) www.geneomesystems.com	cDNA spotted onto nylon membranes	Radioisotope	Differential gene expression
German Cancer Institute Heidelberg, Germany www.dkfz-heidelberg.de	Protein-nucleic acid macro-chip with on-chip synthesis of probes	Fluorescence Mass spectrometry	Expression profiles and diagnostics
Hyseq Sunnyvale, CA www.hyseq.com	DNA sample printed onto 0.6 cm^2 or 18 cm^2 membranes, or 1.15 cm^2 glass HyChip	Radioisotope Fluorescence	Universal sequencing chip, expression profiles, novel gene identification, gene polymorphism
Incyte Pharmaceuticals Palo Alto, CA www.incyte.com	Piezoelectric printing for spotting PCR fragments and on-chip synthesis of oligos	Fluorescence Radioisotope	Expression profiles, gene polymorphism, diagnostics

Table 2 (cont.)
Commercially Available Gene Arrays[a]

Company	Array format	Labeling/readout	Applications
Luminex Austin, TX www.luminexcorp.com	Oligos coupled to fluorescent microspheres	Fluorescence	DNA and protein diagnostics, haplotype determination
Lynx Therapeutics Hayward, CA www.lynxgen.com	Beads loaded into a flow cell anchored in a clone array	Fluorescence	Massively parallel solid phase cloning
Molecular Dynamics, Inc. Sunnyvale, CA www.mdyn.com	500–5000 nt cDNAs printed by pen onto 10 cm^2 glass slide	Fluorescence	Expression profiling and novel gene identification
Nanogen San Diego, CA www.nanogen.com	Oligos captured onto electroactive spots on silicon	Fluorescence	Diagnostics and short tandem repeat identification
Protogene Laboratories Palo Alto, CA www.protogene.com	On-chip synthesis of oligos printed onto glass chip	Fluorescence	Expression profiles, gene polymorphism
Radius Biosciences Medfield, MA www.ultranet.com/ ~radius/	Custom spotted probes (DNA, RNA, peptides, proteins antibodies) onto any surface	Fluorescence Radioisotope	Gene expression, protein expression

Company	Method/format	Detection	Application
R & D Systems Minneapolis, MN www.rndsystems.com	cDNA immobilized onto nylon membrane	Radioisotope	Differential gene expression, cellular pathways, cytokines
Research Genetics Huntsville, AL www.resgn.com	cDNA immobilized onto nylon membrane	Radioisotope	Expression profiles
Sequenom San Diego, CA (Axys Pharmaceuticals) www.sequenom.com	Off-set printing of array, around 20–25-mer oligos	Mass spectrometry	Novel gene identification, candidate gene validation, diagnostics, and mapping
Synteni Fremont, CA www.synteni.com	500–5,000 cDNA printed by tip onto 4 cm^2 glass chip	Fluorescence	Expression profiles, identification of novel genes
TeleChem International Sunnyvale, CA www.hooket.net/~telechem	Oligos microspotted onto silylated slide	Fluorescence	Genomics for drug discovery and diagnostics

[a]Modified from **ref. 22**.

A

DNA pattern on Human Atlas cDNA Array

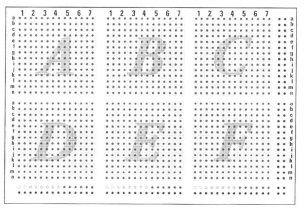

A: oncogenes, tumor suppressors, cell-cycle regulators
B: stress response, ion channels, signal transduction modulators and effectors
C: apoptosis, DNA synthesis, repair, and recombination
D: transcription factors, DNA-binding proteins
E: receptors, cell-surface antigens, cell adhesion molecules
F: growth factors, cytokines, chemokines, hormones

B

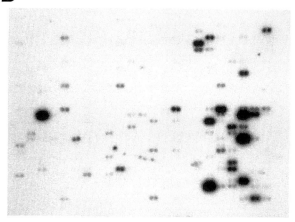

Fig. 2. **A**, Gene arrangement on the Atlas cDNA array and **B**, close-up of a gene expression pattern in human monocytes stimulated with bacterial peptidoglycan determined by the Atlas array.

inducible genes that has been amplified from a region of mRNA that lacks the poly-A tail, repetitive elements, or other highly homologous sequences. The genes include oncogenes, tumor suppressors, cell-cycle regulators, ion channels and transport, intracellular signal transduction modulators and effectors, stress response, apoptosis, DNA synthesis, repair and recombination, transcription factors and other

DNA-binding proteins, receptors, cell-surface antigens, cell adhesins, and cell-cell communication proteins (including cytokines). The list of genes, their position on the membrane, and their GeneBank accession numbers (and similar information on other types of Clontech arrays) can be obtained at http://atlasinfo.clontech.com.

Almost all reagents needed for the experiment, except few buffers, are provided in the kit.

2.2. Reagents that Need to be Purchased or Prepared

1. RNase-free DNase I. We use MessageClean kit (Gene Hunter, Nashville, TN).
2. 1X Cell lysis buffer: 4 *M* Guanidine thiocyanate, 0.5% sarcosyl, 25 m*M* sodium citrate, with freshly added 0.1 *M* 2-mercaptoethanol.
3. 10X Termination mix: 0.1 *M* EDTA, pH 8.0, 1.0 mg/mL glycogen.
4. Phenol:chloroform:isoamyl alcohol (25:24:1).
5. [α^{32}P] dATP(10 mCi/mL; 3000 Ci/mmol) (Perkin Elmer NEN).
6. Salmon testes DNA.
7. 10X DNA denaturing solution: 1*M* NaOH, 10 m*M* EDTA.
8. 2X Neutralizing solution: 1 *M* NaH$_2$PO$_4$, pH 7.0.
9. 20X SSC.
10. 20% (w/v) SDS.

2.3. Equipment

1. X-ray film and enhancing screens or phosphorimager.
2. Hybridization incubator.
3. Heat sealer to seal plastic bags.

2.4. Cells

Human monocytes, prepared as described below (*see* **Subheading 3.1.**).

2.5. Stimulants

1. Soluble peptidoglycan (PGN) is purified by vancomycin affinity chromatography from *Staphylococcus aureus (19)*. *S. aureus* cells are killed with gentamicin (800 μg/mL, 37°C, 2 h) *(17)*.
2. Lipopolysaccharide (LPS) from *Salmonella minnesota* Re 595 is from Sigma (St. Louis, MO).
3. Human recombinant interferon-γ (IFN-γ), produced in baculovirus-infected *Trichoplusia ni* cells (specific activity, 0.8–4 × 10^7 U/mL, endotoxin content <0.15 ng/μg) is from Pharmingen (San Diego, CA).

3. Methods
3.1. Monocyte Isolation and Stimulation

The use of endotoxin-free glassware, media, and reagents is crucial, because monocytes can be activated by even trace (picogram per mL) contamination with endotoxin.

1. Collect peripheral blood (400 mL) from healthy donors into syringes containing 1/20 vol of 200 U/mL heparin (to yield final concentration of 10 U of heparin/mL) and mix.
2. Distribute blood into 50 mL polypropylene centrifuge tubes (20 mL/tube), mix with 20 mL of RPMI 1640, and underlayer (using 23 cm Pasteur pipets) with 15 mL of Histopaque (density 1.077 g/mL, Sigma).
3. Centrifuge at 1900 rpm (600g) at room temperature for 20 min (in a slow accelerating centrifuge, to avoid mixing of the Histopaque with blood).
4. The red blood cells and polymorphonuclear leukocytes sediment to the bottom of the tube. Mononuclear cells form a layer at the interface of Histopaque and RPMI-diluted plasma. Aspirate mononuclear cells into 50 mL polypropylene centrifuge tubes and wash with RPMI (1400 rpm, 300g). When collecting the cells, avoid aspirating Histopaque, because it will increase the density of the medium and will prevent cells from sedimenting during centrifugation.
5. Suspend cells in RPMI 1640 with 20% autologous serum (commercial donor human AB serum or endotoxin-low fetal calf serum will also work, but may result in higher background stimulation of the cells), 10 mM HEPES, and 5×10^{-5} M 2-mercaptoethanol. Count cells and dilute to 10×10^6 cells/mL in the same medium with 20% serum. The yield is approx 2×10^6 mononuclear cells/ml of blood.
6. Distribute 6 mL of cells per 10-cm tissue culture plate (Falcon 3003, Beckton-Dickinson) and incubate for 1 h at 37°C, 5% CO_2 to let monocytes adhere to the plate.
7. Remove unattached cells after resuspending the cells by gently rocking the plates. Wash the adherent monocytes on the plates four times with warm (37°C) RPMI 1640 with 10 mM HEPES, by gently rocking the plates. Add 4 mL per plate of warm (37°C) RPMI 1640 with 10% autologous serum and 10 mM HEPES.
8. Incubate monocytes for 1–2 h at 37°C, 5% CO_2 (this step reduces the background activation of genes). Add appropriate stimulants (e.g., peptidoglycan at 10 µg/mL, *S. aureus* bacteria at 4×10^8 cells/mL, LPS at 10 ng/mL, or IFN-γ at 100 ng/mL, or vehicle alone to unstimulated control groups). Incubate monocytes with the stimulants at 37°C, 5% CO_2 for the desired lengths of time (e.g., 40 min, 2 h, 6 h). After the stimulation, isolate RNA.

3.2. RNA Preparation

The quality of RNA is crucial for the best results (*see* **Note 2**). Several methods can be used for RNA isolation. We usually use the single-step phenol-chloroform method *(20)*, described below.

1. Aspirate medium from the plates. Add 1 mL of 1X cell lysis buffer per plate to lyse the adherent monocytes (at room temperature).
2. Scrape the cells with a plastic scraper and release RNA from the cells by aspirating the cell lysates at least 10 times in and out of a syringe through a 20 G needle (*see* **Note 3**). Collect the cell lysates into 15 mL polypropylene tubes. We usually combine cell lysates from at least 2 plates/group, but the volumes indicated in this procedure are per 1 mL of lysate (1 plate).

3. Add 1.2 mL of phenol:chloroform:isoamyl alcohol and 0.1 mL of 2 *M* sodium acetate, pH 4, and vortex thoroughly.
4. Centrifuge at 5000 rpm (5,000*g*) at 4°C for 20 min, and carefully collect the top aqueous layer containing RNA into a new tube.
5. Reextract RNA two more times by repeating **steps 3** and **4**.
6. Transfer the supernatant into Beckman polyallomer 13×51 mm centrifuge tubes, and precipitate RNA by adding an equal volume of isopropanol and placing the tube at –20°C for 30 min.
7. Centrifuge at 15,000 rpm (27,000*g*) in a Sorvall SS-34 rotor at 4°C for 20 min. Discard the supernatant, add 5 mL of 70% ethanol, centrifuge as above, discard the supernatant, and air-dry the RNA pellet. Dissolve in 25 µL DEPC-dH$_2$O and transfer into a 1.5 mL tube (*see* **Note 4**).
8. Remove DNA from the RNA by digestion for 1 h at 37°C with 1 µL of RNase-free DNase I, using the MessageClean kit (Gene Hunter, Nashville, TN) (*see* **Note 5**).
9. To remove the DNase, add 50 µL of phenol/chloroform, mix, put on ice for 10 min, spin in a microcentrifuge at 14,000 rpm (16,000*g*) for 5 min at 4°C, collect the top layer into a new 1.5 mL tube, add 5 µL 3 *N* sodium acetate, and precipitate RNA by adding 200 µL of ethanol and placing the tube at –70°C for 1 h.
10. Centrifuge at 14,000 rpm (16,000*g*) for 5 min at 4°C, discard the supernatant, add 250 µL 70% ethanol, and centrifuge again for 10 min at 4°C. Discard the supernatant and dissolve the RNA precipitate in 20 µL DEPC-dH$_2$O. This is total RNA that can be used for the synthesis of cDNA probe (*see* **Subheading 3.3.**) or obtaining poly(A)$^+$ RNA (*see* **Subheading 3.2., step 12**).
11. Check the quality of RNA by running 5–10 µg of RNA on a denaturing formaldehyde/agarose/ ethidium bromide gel. The total RNA should appear as two bright 28S and 18S ribosomal RNA bands at approx 4.5 and 1.9 kb with minimal streaking (**Fig. 3**). The ratio of intensities of these bands should be 1.5–2.5 to 1. Excessive streaking with lower abundance of the 28S and 18S RNA bands indicates partially degraded RNA.
12. To increase the sensitivity of the array, poly(A)$^+$ RNA can be extracted from this total RNA, by oligo (dT)-cellulose chromatography using the QIAGEN Oligotex mRNA Mini kit (follow the instructions for the kit). The integrity of poly(A)$^+$ RNA should be checked by agarose electrophoresis. Mammalian poly(A)$^+$ RNA usually produces smears from 0.5 to 12 kb with weak ribosomal RNA bands.
13. Store RNA at –70°C.

3.3. cDNA Synthesis and Labeling

The reaction described below synthesizes ^{32}P-labeled first-strand cDNA from poly(A)$^+$ RNA or total RNA. The Atlas array comes with a control poly(A)$^+$ RNA, which can be labeled in parallel to check if the labeling reaction works.

1. To 1 µg of poly(A)$^+$ RNA or 2–5 µg of total RNA (2 µL) add 1 µL of 10X CDS primer mix (provided with the Atlas array) and incubate in a preheated thermal cycler at 70°C for 2 min and then at 50°C for 2 min (*see* **Notes 6** and **7**).

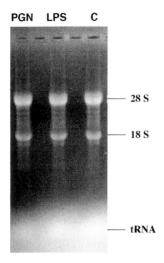

Fig. 3. Total monocyte RNA. RNA was extracted from untreated (C) or peptidoglycan (PGN) or LPS-activated human monocytes by the single-step phenol-chloroform method. 5 µg of each RNA was run on a 0.8% denaturing formaldehyde/agarose/ethidium bromide gel, and the 28S RNA, 18S RNA, and tRNA bands were visualized with UV light.

2. Add 2 µL of 5X reaction buffer, 1 µL of 10X dNTP, 3.5 µL of [α^{32}P] dATP (10 mCi/mL), 0.5 µL of 100 mM DTT, and 1 µL (50 U) of Moloney murine leukemia virus (MMLV) reverse transcriptase (Clontech), and incubate at 50°C for 25 min (total volume, 10 µL) (*see* **Notes 8** and **9**).
3. Stop the reaction by adding 1 µL of 10X termination mix.
4. Let the Chroma Spin-200 column (provided with the kit) warm up at room temperature for 1 h. Place the column in a 1.5 mL microcentrifuge tube and drain the column. Load the probe reaction mix onto the column and wash the column first with 40 µL of dH$_2$O and then with 250 µL of dH$_2$O.
5. Elute the labeled cDNA from the column with 6 × 100 µL of dH$_2$O. Collect 6 × 100 µL fractions and measure the amount of radioactivity in each fraction in a scintillation counter. Combine 2–3 fractions of the first peak of radioactive counts. The second peak with higher counts (fractions 5–6), containing the unincorporated radioactive nucleotides, should be discarded. The labeled probe should have a total of about 2–50 × 10^6 cpm. Pooled fractions containing the labeled probe are stored at –70°C and used for hybridization as soon as possible.

3.4. cDNA Array Hybridization

1. Heat-denature sheared salmon testes DNA (10 mg/mL in H$_2$0) by heating at 95–100°C for 5 min in a glass tube and then quickly chill on ice.
2. Prewarm the provided ExpressHyb (15 mL/membrane) at 68°C. Add 1.5 mg (0.3 mL) of heat-denatured sheared salmon testes DNA to 15 mL of prewarmed ExpressHyb and keep at 68°C until use (we keep the buffer in the hybridization incubator).

3. Cut two sheets of hybridization mesh (Amersham, Arlington Heights, IL) to a little larger size than the array membrane, put the array membrane between two hybridization mesh sheets, wet the sheets and the array with deionized water, roll up the two sheets with the array in between the sheets, and remove the air from between the array membrane and the sheets. Shake off any excess of water and put the mesh/array/mesh roll into the hybridization bottle. The sample side of the array membrane should face the inside of the hybridization bottle (*see* **Note 10**). Do not allow the membrane to dry.

4. Add 10 mL of prewarmed (68°C) hybridization solution and prehybridize at 68°C for 30 min to 1 h. Make sure that the solution is evenly distributed over the membrane. Keep the rest 5 mL of the buffer at 68°C for hybridization. Rotate the bottles at 3–5 rpm/min (*see* **Note 11**).

5. Prepare the probe mixture: Mix the column purified labeled cDNA (about 200 µL, $1–5 \times 10^7$ cpm) with 1/10th of the total volume (about 22 µL) of 10X DNA denaturing solution, and incubate at 68°C for 20 min (*see* **Notes 12** and **13**). Then add 5 µL Cot-1 DNA and 225 µL of the 2X neutralizing solution, and incubate at 68°C for 10 min.

6. Add the probe mixture to the remaining 5 mL of the hybridization buffer and mix.

7. Pour out the prehybridization buffer, add the 5 mL of probe-buffer mixture to the hybridization bottle, and hybridize overnight at 68°C, rotating at 3–5 rpm/min. Make sure that all regions of the membrane are evenly in contact with the hybridization mix.

8. Carefully remove the radioactive hybridization buffer and replace it with 125 mL of prewarmed (68°C) wash solution 1 (2X SSC, 1% SDS). Wash the array six times for 30 min in the hybridization incubator at 68°C, rotating at 3–5 rpm/min.

9. Perform three additional 30-min washes in 125 mL of prewarmed wash solution 2 (0.1X SSC, 0.5% SDS), rotating at 3–5 rpm/min.

10. Using smooth forceps, remove the array from the roller bottle and drain off any excess of the wash solution. Do not blot-dry or allow the membrane to dry. If the membrane even partially dries, later it will be difficult to remove (strip) the probe for rehybridization.

11. When no more solution is dripping off the membrane, immediately put the wet membrane in a plastic bag, press out all air bubbles, and seal the bag with a heat-sealer.

12. Expose the plastic-sealed array to an X-ray film at –70°C in a cassette with an intensifying screen. Usually an overnight exposure gives good results (**Figs. 2B** and **4**), but several exposure times (from few hours to few days) may need to be tried. Alternatively, a phosphorimager can be used.

3.5. Stripping cDNA from the Array for Reprobing and Preserving the Membranes

1. Cut the bag, remove the array, and immediately put it into 150–250 mL of boiling 0.5% SDS solution.

2. Continue to boil for 5–10 min.

3. Remove the solution from heat and allow to cool for 10 min with shaking (3–5 rpm/min).

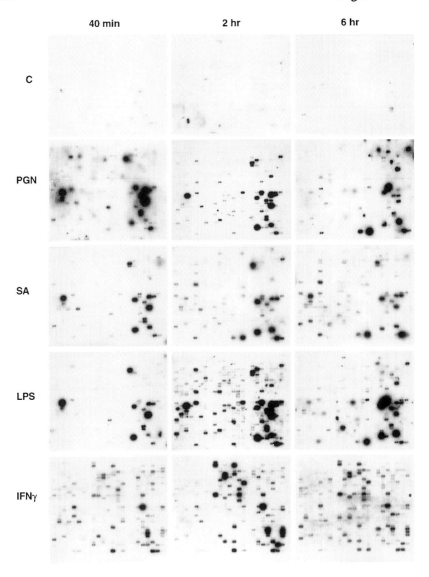

Fig. 4. Gene expression patterns in human monocytes unstimulated (C), or stimulated with bacterial peptidoglycan (PGN), *S. aureus* (SA), LPS, or IFN-γ determined by Atlas cDNA array (reproduced with permission from the *Journal of Biological Chemistry*, **ref. *17***).

4. Take out the array from the solution and rinse it in 2X SSC solution. Check the efficiency of stripping with a Geiger counter or by exposure to a phosphorimager or an X-ray film. One round of boiling is usually sufficient, but if radioactivity can still be detected, reboil the array again.

5. Rehybridize the array, or seal in a plastic bag and keep at –20°C or –70°C until needed (*see* **Note 14**).

3.6. Analysis of Results

1. The results can be compared visually (**Figs. 2** and **4**) and the spots can be identified by carefully aligning the film with the grid provided with the array. Because the membrane can sometimes stretch, care must be taken to avoid misalignment and resultant misidentification of the spots. In general, Phosphorimager gives smaller and sharper spots that are easier to identify and quantify.
2. The intensity of each spot can be quantified using either Phosphorimager or Kodak Digital Science Image Station 440CF and the Image Analysis Software 3.0. The results can be normalized based on hybridization to house-keeping genes, whose expression does not significantly change upon stimulation. This procedure allows direct comparison of the results from different membranes and donors. The results can be expressed as bar graphs **(Fig. 5)** or in a table format with the fold induction for each gene *(10,11,14)*. The standard analysis software provided with the phosphorimager or Kodak Image Station are sufficient for analysis, but laborious. A special array analysis software can also be purchased from Clontech.
3. Application of the Atlas cDNA array to the analysis of genes activated by bacterial and nonbacterial stimulants in human monocytes revealed that bacterial activators induce activation of over 120 genes, out of 600 genes tested (**Figs. 2** and **4**) *(17)*. Quantification of the amount of RNA induced revealed that 12–15 genes were very strongly induced (10–50-fold increase over the control), 20–25 genes showed intermediate induction (5–10-fold increase), and the remaining 80–90 genes showed lower induction (2–5-fold increase) **(Fig. 5)**. Chemokine genes were the highest induced genes, and cytokine genes were the second highest induced genes by all three bacterial stimulants **(Fig. 5)**. The gene expression patterns induced by the three bacterial stimulants were very similar, but not identical. By contrast, a nonbacterial monocyte activator, IFN-γ, induced more than 200 genes in human monocytes, but the gene expression pattern induced by IFN-γ was completely different from the gene expression pattern induced by the bacterial stimulants. These results were confirmed by the RNase protection assay *(17)*. These results demonstrate that cDNA arrays are very useful for the analysis of gene expression (*see* **Notes 15–17**).

   In summary, the advantages of using membrane-based cDNA arrays include simplicity, relatively low cost, and the ability to generate a large amount of information on the expression of hundreds of genes. However, if the array contains all known genes, this method will not reveal the expression of new unknown genes, although it can demonstrate the expression of genes that were previously not known to be expressed in a given cell type.

4. Notes

1. Careful selection of the array is crucial. For example, if an expression pattern of inducible mRNAs is to be determined, an array that includes inducible genes

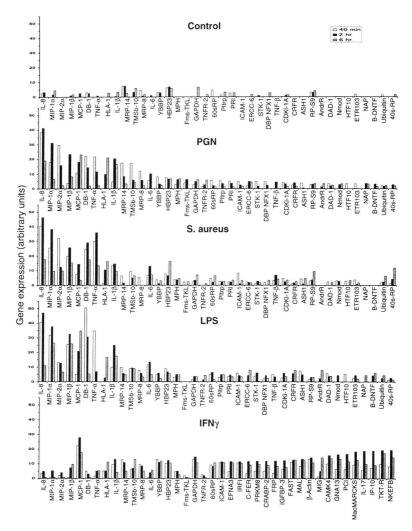

Fig. 5. Quantification of gene expression. Expression of the top 40 genes on Atlas cDNA array in human monocytes stimulated as in **Fig. 4**. For IFN-γ, 20 of the same genes shown for the bacterial stimulants are followed by the top 20 genes that were induced by IFN-γ. The results are means from 3 different donors and 3 different lots of membranes (reproduced with permission from the *Journal of Biological Chemistry*, **ref. 17**).

should be selected. Arrays that are based on cDNA from unstimulated cells may not contain cDNAs for many inducible genes.

2. Good quality of the RNA preparation **(Fig. 3)** is the most important guarantee for obtaining reliable results. Wear gloves to perform the experiments. Use separate pipets and RNase-free tubes, tips, glassware, and reagents, including water (use

DEPC-treated water, *see* **Note 4**). Keep RNA on ice all the time, and store at –70°C to prevent degradation. We find that RNA prepared by various methods (phenol-chloroform extraction, cesium chloride gradient centrifugation, or QIAGEN RNeasy kit) can be used, as long as it is of high quality. After preparing RNA, run the gel to check your RNA quality (**Fig. 3**) before you start to prepare gene array experiment. When comparisons between different treatments, diseases, etc., are made, the same method of RNA isolation should be used and the quality of RNA in the samples that are being compared should be similar.

3. Alternative methods to release RNA from the cell are using a homogenizer (which, however, is impractical when small numbers of cells are handled), or using a shredder column (from QIAGEN, Valencia, CA).

4. For RNase-free water, add 0.1% diethylpyrocarbonte (DEPC) to double-distilled, deionized water, stir well and incubate at 37–42°C for 8–24 h, and autoclave for at least 45 min. RNase-free water is also commercially available (e.g., from Ambion, Austin, TX).

5. If enough RNA is available, perform DNase digestion only on a portion of RNA, in case the RNA sample is not RNase free (which can result in a significant degradation of RNA).

6. We find that using 1 µg of mRNA for probe preparation will enhance the signal for the weakly expressed genes, but may also yield much more variable results (perhaps because of the difficulty to accurately measure the amounts of mRNA, that is obtained in very small amounts). Using 2–5 µg of total RNA yields less variation and still very good results, especially if quantification of the results is intended. Also, there may be a significant loss of RNA during mRNA preparation. By eliminating this sample loss, fewer cells can be used for isolating total RNA. The use of total RNA was also found suitable for chip-based microarrays *(21)*.

7. If the hybridization signal is weak, use 2 µL of the CDS primer mix.

8. Using ^{33}P instead of ^{32}P for labeling the probe will yield sharper spots, but will result in lower sensitivity. Also, for very strong spots, images from Phosphorimager are sharper than from an exposure of an X-ray film.

9. Always keep the MMLV reverse transcriptase on ice and return it to the freezer as soon as possible after use.

10. Using hybridization mesh improves the results. Better results are obtained when the sample side of the array membrane faces the inside of the bottle. However, if by mistake the sample side faces the wall of the bottle, using the mesh will still yield good hybridization, which would not be the case without the mesh.

11. Rotate the bottles at 3–5 rpm/min during prehybridization, hybridization, and washing. The use of higher speed for washing (recommended in the manual) yields fuzzy, "blossoming," or "bleeding" spots, especially for spots with high or medium signal. If a hybridization incubator in not available, plastic bags can be used, but the results will be poorer.

12. For hybridization, we use $1–5 \times 10^7$ cpm of the probe, rather than $2–10 \times 10^6$ cpm recommended by Clontech (because our probe labels to a higher specific activity than indicated in Clontech's manual).

13. If high nonspecific background is obtained, test hybridization of each labeled probe to a blank nylon membrane (provided with Atlas array) to test for the level of nonspecific background. Use a small piece of the membrane, so a small amount of the probe is used up. However, in our assays, we have not seen high background. If there is not enough RNA for this background test hybridization, a test for genomic DNA contamination of RNA using a PCR reaction may be done. Select primers that will amplify an abundant housekeeping gene. RNA should contain less than 0.001% genomic DNA or produce no visible PCR product after 35 cycles. Higher DNA contamination will result in a high background hybridization, and high hybridization signals on the genomic DNA lanes of the array will be obtained.

14. Sealing the membrane (instead of simply wrapping it) will prevent it from drying (this is especially important when using phosphorimager at room temperature) and will allow excellent preservation upon freezing. Even if the array is kept for more than a year at $-70°C$, the membrane can be reprobed and will still give good re-hybridization results. The membrane can be rehybridized at least 5 times, and the first three hybridizations do not result in much loss of the signal.

15. This method (with only minor modifications in the procedure for obtaining and treating the cells) can be used for the analysis and comparison of gene expression in various primary cells, cells from patients with different diseases, or in vitro cultured cell lines exposed to various treatments. We have obtained very similar results using the same human Atlas cDNA array for the analysis of gene expression in human THP-1 monocytic cell line, and we have shown that bacterial stimulants induce activation of mostly the same genes in this monocytic cell line and in primary human monocytes (*17*).

16. This cDNA array method is convenient to use and does not require any special equipment, so it can be performed in any laboratory equipped to perform basic molecular biology experiments. The method is also highly sensitive, because the mixture of gene-specific primers used for synthesizing the probe yields probes that are significantly less complex than probes generated using oligo(dT) or random primers. Reducing probe complexity increases the sensitivity approx 10 times. The method also has a good liner correlation between each hybridization signal and the abundance of each RNA, and, therefore, the array can be used for evaluation of RNA abundance. With the same array and the same RNA, the detection is linear for a given RNA present at levels of 0.002% to 3% of total RNA. However, equal concentrations of RNA for different genes in the probe may give different signals, which makes the results only semi-quantitative. We found that the same membrane lot and RNA obtained from cells from the same donor even in separate independent experiments still yields very consistent results. However, different donors show some variation in the expression of the same genes. Moreover, we have also noticed that there is some variation in the strength of hybridization of the same genes when different lots of the membrane are used. Therefore, to increase the reliability of the data, we recommend averaging the results from at least three donors tested with three different membrane lots.

17. This procedure can also be used with other membrane-based cDNA arrays produced by Clontech and by other manufacturers. By following exactly the same

Chemokines + Receptors   Cytokines + Receptors   Interleukins + Receptors   TNF + Receptors

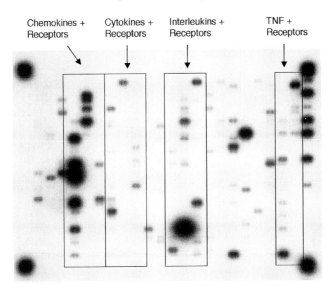

Fig. 6. Expression of chemokine and cytokine genes in human monocytes stimulated with LPS, determined by the 375 gene chemokine and cytokine cDNA array from R&D Systems. Both chemokine mRNA (left side of the membrane) and cytokine mRNA (right side of the membrane) were highly induced.

procedure, we have also obtained very good hybridization results with a 375 gene cytokine/chemokine array manufactured by R&D Systems (**Fig. 6**). The results obtained by the Clontech and R&D Systems arrays (i.e., genes induced by the same stimulants in human monocytes) were very similar.

References

1. Ramsay, G. (1998) DNA chips: state of the art. *Nature Biotech.* **16,** 40–44.
2. Marshall, A. and Hodgson, J. (1998) DNA chips: an array of possibilities. *Nature Biotech.* **16,** 27–31.
3. Young, R. A. (2000) Biomedical discovery with DNA arrays. *Cell* **102,** 9–15.
4. Schena, M., Shalon, D., Davis, R. W., and Brown, P. O. (1995) Quantitative monitoring of gene expression patterns with a complementary DNA microarray. *Science* **270,** 467–470.
5. Schena, M., Shalon, D., Heller, R., Chai, A., Brown, P. O., and Davis, R. W. (1996) Parallel human genome analysis: microarray-based expression monitoring of 1000 genes. *Proc. Natl. Acad. Sci. USA* **93,** 10,614–10,619.
6. DeRisi, J., Peneland, L., Brown, P. O., Bittner, M. L., Meltzer, P. S., Ray, M., et al. (1996) Use of a cDNA microarray to analyse gene expression patterns in human cancer. *Nature Genet.* **14,** 457–460.
7. Zhang, L., Zhou, W., Velculescu, V. E., Kern, S. E., Hruban, R. H., Hamilton, S. R., et al. (1997) Gene expression profiles in normal and cancer cells. *Science* **276,** 1268–1272.

8. Heller, R. A., Schena, M., Chai, A., Shalon, D., Bedilion, T., Gilmore, J., et al. (1997) Discovery and analysis of inflammatory disease-related genes using cDNA microarrays. *Proc. Natl. Acad. Sci. USA* **94,** 2150–2155.

9. Lashkari, D. A., DeRisi, J. L., McCusker, J. H., Namath, A. F., Gentile, C., Hwang, S. Y., et al. (1997) Yeast microarrays for genome wide parallel genetic and gene expression analysis. *Proc. Natl. Acad. Sci. USA* **94,** 13,057–13,062.

10. Zhu, H., Cong, J.-P., Mamtora, G., Gingeras, T., and Shenk, T. (1998) Cellular gene expression altered by human cytomegalovirus: global monitoring with oligonucleotide arrays. *Proc. Natl. Acad. Sci. USA* **95,** 14,470–14,475.

11. Der, S. D., Zhou, A., Williams, B. R. G., and Silverman, R. H. (1998) Identification of genes differentially regulated by interferon α, β, or γ using oligonucleotide arrays. *Proc. Natl. Acad. Sci. USA* **95,** 15,623–15,628.

12. Alon, U., Barkai, N., Notterman, D. A., Gish, K., Ybarra, S., Mack, D., and Levine, A. J. (1999) Broad patterns of gene expression revealed by clustering analysis of tumor and normal colon tissues probed by oligonucleotide arrays. *Proc. Natl. Acad. Sci. USA* **96,** 6745–6750.

13. Kaminski, N., Allard, J. D., Pittet, J. F., Zuo, F., Griffiths, M. J. D., Morris, D., et al. (2000) Global analysis of gene expression in pulmonary fibrosis reveals distinct programs regulating lung inflammation and fibrosis. *Proc. Natl. Acad. Sci. USA* **97,** 1778–1783.

14. Cohen, P., Bouaboula, M., Bellis, M., Baron, V., Jbilo, O., Poinot-Chazel, C., et al. (2000) Monitoring cellular responses to *Listeria monocytogenes* with oligonucleotide arrays. *J. Biol. Chem.* **275,** 11,181–11,190.

15. Wilson, S. B., Kent, S. C., Horton, H. F., Hill, A. A., Bollyky, P. L., Hafler, D. A., et al. (2000) Multiple differences in gene expression in regulatory Vα24JαQ T cells from identical twins discordant for type I diabetes. *Proc. Natl. Acad. Sci. USA* **97,** 7411–7416.

16. Hughes, T. R., Marton, M. J., Jones, A. R., Roberts, C. J., Stoughton, R., Armour, C. D., et al. (2000) Functional discovery via a compendium of expression profiles. *Cell* **102,** 109–126.

17. Wang, Z.-M., Liu, C., and Dziarski, R. (2000) Chemokines are the main pro-inflammatory mediators in human monocytes activated by *Staphylococcus aureus,* peptidoglycan, and endotoxin. *J. Biol. Chem.* **275,** 20,260–20,267.

18. Wang, Z.-M., Yasui, M., and Celsi, G. (1994) Glucocorticoids regulate the transcription of Na^+-K^+-ATPase genes in the infant rat kidney. *Am. J. Physiol.* **267,** C450–C455.

19. Rosenthal, R. S. and Dziarski, R. (1994) Isolation of peptidoglycan and soluble peptidoglycan fragments. *Meth. Enzymol.* **235,** 253–285.

20. Chomczynski, P. and Sacchi, N. (1987) Single-step method of RNA isolation by acid guanidinium thiocyanate-phenol-chloroform extraction. *Anal. Biochem.* **162,** 156–159.

21. Mahadevappa, M. and Warrington, J. A. (1999) A high-density probe array sample preparation method using 10- to 100-fold fewer cells. *Nature Biotech.* **17,** 1134–1136.

22. Slabiak, T. (2000) Hybridization array technologies: DNA chip technology. Bio Online (http://bio.com/articles/dnachip/dnachip.html), 1–4.

Index